OXFORD MEDICAL PUBLICATIONS

Paediatric
Rheumatology

T0369591

Oxford Specialist Handbooks

Oxford Specialist Handbooks in Paediatrics
Paediatric Rheumatology

Second Edition

Edited by

Helen Foster

MBBS(Hons), MD, Cert Med Ed, DCH, FRCP, FRCPCH

Professor Paediatric Rheumatology, Newcastle University
Honorary Consultant in Paediatric Rheumatology,
Great North Children's Hospital, Newcastle Hospitals
NHS Foundation Trust,
Newcastle upon Tyne, UK

Paul A. Brogan

BSC(Hon), MBChB(Hon), MSC, PhD, MRCPCH, FRCPCH

Professor of Paediatric Vasculitis, and
Honorary Consultant in Paediatric Rheumatology,
UCL Institute of Child Health, and Great Ormond
St Hospital for Children NHS Trust,
London, UK

OXFORD
UNIVERSITY PRESS

Preface

The purpose of this book

Paediatric Rheumatology, Second Edition is an indispensable resource for the recognition and management of rheumatological diseases of the young. As well as covering common and rare rheumatological problems, it includes chapters on rheumatological emergencies, designed for quick reference, and essential core clinical skills of relevance to the full spectrum of paediatric rheumatological disease. This Second Edition is fully updated with state-of-the-art descriptions of new autoinflammatory diseases, advances in genetics, and up-to-date guidance on treatments. Highlights include alignment of management approaches for paediatric rheumatological diseases with recent evidence-based/consensus European guidelines, a description of North American treatment approaches to juvenile idiopathic arthritis (JIA), updated chapters on more specialist interventions (including immunization in the immunosuppressed, haematopoietic stem cell transplantation) and approaches to management of rheumatological diseases in low-resource/income countries. Bone diseases are also described in detail including Chronic Recurrent Multifocal Osteomyelitis, skeletal dysplasias and metabolic bone diseases. There are many colour plates depicting rashes observed in paediatric rheumatological conditions.

This book is fully endorsed by the British Society for Paediatric and Adolescent Rheumatology (BSPAR) and we acknowledge the commitment and contributions from many members of BSPAR in this revision. We have successfully engaged with the breadth of the BSPAR community, with representation from the majority of centres across the UK and have contributions from all current UK trainees in paediatric rheumatology working in partnership with consultant supervisors. We have also for this Second Edition engaged with our paediatric rheumatology colleagues from around the world to bring a different perspective that is increasingly relevant with population movement across the globe.

This Second Edition thus provides fully updated clinical guidelines and the supporting information needed to successfully manage children and young people with rheumatological diseases. This Second Edition maintains the 'pocket-sized' format with bullet points to allow easy reference to up-to-date evidence based (where possible) and consensus-derived opinion. The handbook is divided into sections to cover essential elements of the clinical assessment, the approach to investigations and management along with important key facts of knowledge and practical advice. It includes advice on the care of acute emergencies, chronic disorders, the spectrum of common conditions presenting to clinicians (primary care, general paediatricians, adult rheumatologists, allied health) through to those managed predominantly within specialized centres. The principles of collaborative multidisciplinary working within clinical networks and shared care are endorsed. Many of the chapters will be applicable to the day-to-day care of patients on a general paediatric ward or in the outpatient clinic. Acute emergencies that can occur in multisystem disease and issues arising from the use of potent immunosuppressive treatments are dealt with in detail. The importance of transitional care and collaboration with adult rheumatology teams is emphasized.

This handbook will provide guidance for trainees, general paediatricians, general practitioners, adult rheumatologists and the multidisciplinary team specialists (doctors, nurses, physiotherapists, occupational therapists, podiatrists, and psychologists) who care for children with rheumatological conditions. Building on the success of the first edition, we bring together updated practical guidance for the use of outcome measures, clinical scores of disease activity, and drug prescribing relevant to paediatric rheumatology. 'State-of-the-art treatment' of paediatric rheumatology conditions includes an ever increasing number of biologic and novel therapies—we provide practical guidance for the use of such treatments with guidelines, an update on regulatory approvals for these drugs, treatment algorithms, and emphasis of the role of the multidisciplinary team to deliver optimal clinical care.

We are very proud of our extensive authorship, including doctors and allied health professionals, many of whom are international leaders in their field. We also have input from parents of children with rheumatic disease to emphasize their role in working together with healthcare professionals—much of what we do in clinical practice lacks a robust evidence base and we emphasize the importance of input from consumers on how to involve and fully engage children and their families with clinical decision-making and research opportunities to facilitate growth of evidence to inform best practice.

This Second Edition of our highly successful book is a measure of the growing collaboration of paediatric rheumatology both within the UK and with our colleagues further afield to develop and share knowledge, promote highest quality clinical care, education, and training to facilitate access to optimal care for all children and young people with rheumatic disease.

As was the case for the First Edition, all profits from the sales of this Second Edition of the handbook will be donated to BSPAR.

Helen Foster

Paul A. Brogan

Foreword: UK Paediatric Rheumatology Clinical Studies Group

The importance of supporting the very best clinical research to improve the care of children with rheumatic and musculoskeletal health has been exemplified by the establishment by the National Institute of Health Research (NIHR) Clinical Research Network (CRN): Children[1,2] and Arthritis Research UK Paediatric Rheumatology Clinical Studies Group (CSG).[3] This partnership of expertise has supported a major opportunity and development in recent years of delivering a comprehensive and long lasting, national clinical research programme for paediatric rheumatology and musculoskeletal disease.

Following a detailed, widespread consultation and consensus process, involving all relevant stakeholders including consumers (see Foreword for comment on consumer input), the CSG's primary task was to define the key strategic priorities in paediatric rheumatology with respect to:

'What are the key clinical research priorities that will change clinical practice in paediatric rheumatology?'

To achieve this, the CSG:
- Looks to address the gaps in the evidence base in the management of children and young people with rheumatic or musculoskeletal conditions.
- Works with all interested parties towards developing a comprehensive portfolio of key research clinical trials and related studies covering the entire spectrum of major disease areas in paediatric rheumatology in the UK.
- Has a strong multidisciplinary membership including: four consumer representatives, clinicians, clinical academics, basic scientists, allied health professionals, and a pharmacist expert in paediatric formulations.

The CSG's 'goal' has been that:
- 'All children and young people in the UK with a rheumatological condition may be given the opportunity to be enrolled in a clinical trial or well-conducted clinical study from point of diagnosis onwards, and in so doing improve the care and outcome of them and patients with similar conditions in the future;
- That all children have the option of contributing towards a related, fully informed and consented Biobank (e.g. DNA and serum) for subsequent investigation into the cause of their condition.'

To facilitate this process, the CSG has developed (to date) 10 'topic specific groups' (TSGs) to foster collaboration and support multidisciplinary efforts to address the key priority areas within paediatric rheumatology, as well as organizing *ad hoc* meetings to focus on specific projects.

- Each TSG has members of the CSG as 'link-persons' to support communication and integration of the activities of the TSGs within the wider CSG research agenda and support structures.
- The 10 TSGs are: Auto-inflammatory diseases; Bone Health; Consumer-led Research; Formulations and Pharmacy; Juvenile Dermatomyositis; Juvenile Idiopathic Arthritis and Associated Uveitis; Juvenile-onset Systemic Lupus Erythematosus; Childhood Scleroderma; Non-inflammatory Musculoskeletal Disorders; Childhood Vasculitides.

In addition, the CSG supports investigators in the following way:

- Welcoming and publicizing expressions of interest in working towards these priority studies, calling for submission of protocols and proposals to address these priorities.
- Working with stakeholders and funding bodies and to identify barriers to research participation and identifying strategies to facilitate engagement and collaboration in clinical research.
- Supporting protocols where relevant can also include pilot and feasibility studies to provide proof of concept for definitive studies in terms of recruitment, data acquisition.
- Encouraging consideration of research 'add-ons' to bring value-added benefit to the children participating in these studies, e.g. pharmacogenetic and qualitative studies.
- Being advisory to investigators, the NIHR CRN: Children and to the Arthritis Research UK and assist with their development.
- Working in close collaboration with other NIHR CRN: Children's Theme and Arthritis Research UK CSGs, as well as other topic-specific research networks in all areas of mutual interest.

Professor Michael Beresford
Institute of Translational Medicine,
University of Liverpool and Alder Hey
Children's NHS Foundation Trust,
Liverpool, UK

References

http://www.crn.nihr.ac.uk/children/

Rose AC, Van't Hoff W, Beresford MW, Tansey SP. NIHR Medicines for Children Research Network: improving children's health through clinical research. *Expert Rev Clin Pharmacol.* 2013;6(5):581–7

http://www.arthritisresearchuk.org/research/research-funding-and-policy/our-clinical-study-groups/paediatric-rheumatology.aspx

Foreword: Parent and young person involvement in research—a consumer perspective

The social and psychological aspects of living with any chronic condition can create a different type of expertise to that of clinicians and researchers. Consumer involvement is concerned with creating a forum where the experience, knowledge, and expertise of both healthcare professionals and the public can come together in an equal partnership to benefit healthcare research. High-quality research, optimal accrual to research projects, and improved patient outcomes are dependent on listening to the voices of patients (children and young people), their families, carers and patient organizations (hereafter referred to as patient and public involvement or PPI). It is also important to take account of their experiences, priorities, and perspectives. Engaged effectively, and early in the research process, patients and the public can contribute to all aspects of clinical research and health service development, including:

- Identifying and prioritizing research questions that are relevant to clinical practice.
- Commissioning research to highlight areas of concern for patients.
- Designing research studies and associated documentation to enhance the feasibility of the project by identifying potential barriers to study participation.
- The management of studies (e.g. as members of a steering group).
- Analysis or interpretation of research results to address key issues relevant to patients.
- Dissemination of research results throughout the lay community.

Providing opportunities for patients and the public to become involved in research is likely to contribute to superior disease self-management skills, which are particularly important for young people transitioning from paediatric to adult care services. Involvement in different aspects of research and health service development may also lead to improved shared-decision making between patients, their families and healthcare professionals.

Key principles for productive and effective PPI partnerships in research and health service development include:

- All members of the research group should understand the benefits of PPI and the value of their unique perspective.
- Participation of new PPI members will be facilitated if they are formally introduced and effort is made to find out about their background and experiences.

- In advance of meetings, it is important to consider the PPI angle on all agenda items and identify which may be of particular interest to PPI members so they may prepare for discussions.
- Documents to be discussed at an upcoming meeting should be circulated to PPI members in advance of the meeting, to facilitate their understanding
- Include introductions at the start of a meeting and clarify the meeting purpose, using plain English where possible, and minimal jargon.
- During the meetings, encourage questions and invite the PPI members to comment on all issues.
- PPI contributions are often based on personal experiences of a condition. Wherever possible, opinions should be representative of the broader community.
- After a meeting, it is important to minute contributions made by PPI members with a follow-up process for feedback

PPI is increasingly reported in clinical, health and social care research, with a growing commitment from professionals to embed PPI as an integral part of research. The launch of the journal *Research Involvement and Engagement* has supported the wider dissemination of best practice PPI amongst the research community. It is one of the first journals co-produced by patients and researchers as equal partners. However, barriers for effective PPI still remain in current practice. In a recent NIHR publication, individuals expressed difficulties in the delivery of PPI in their research. INVOLVE have a large repository of guidance and information available, which is a good resource for researchers and clinicians.

Ms Sharon Douglas and Mr Simon Stones
Clinical Study Group, Longniddry,
Scotland, UK

Further reading

INVOLVE. 2015. http://www.invo.org.uk

Research Involvement and Engagement. 2015. http://www.researchinvolvement.com

TwoCan Associates for the UKCRC and NCRI. Patient and public involvement in research groups – Guidance for Chairs. TwoCan Associates, 2010. http://www.twocanassociates.co.uk/pubs.php.

Foreword: British Society for Paediatric and Adolescent Rheumatology

I am delighted as the current President of The British Society for Paediatric and Adolescent Rheumatology (BSPAR) to provide a Foreword for this edition of the Oxford Handbook of Paediatric Rheumatology.

BSPAR is a multidisciplinary group committed to advancing the care of paediatric rheumatology patients through encouraging training, research and collaboration between all members of the multidisciplinary team, including parents and patients. BSPAR has recently integrated with the British Society of Rheumatology (BSR) in order to help influence the care of rheumatology patients from early life to old age.

This handbook has been produced by a dedicated editorial team and with contributions from a large and truly multidisciplinary authorship. This highlights the fundamental principle that underpins the ethos of BSPAR—namely the sense of teamwork that helps individual teams deliver day-to-day healthcare to children and young people with rheumatologic disorders and also drives us towards our goal of high-quality research continually improving the delivery of clinical care.

Throughout our activities it is our patients and their families who directly benefit from the improved training and dissemination of information that BSPAR provides to the medical and allied health carers with whom they come into direct contact. Through education and training, all healthcare professionals improve the service which they provide to their patients. The first handbook was an invaluable tool for many working in this field. This updated version will include the new advances that have been made in this rapidly evolving specialty.

Dr Clarissa Pilkington
Consultant in Adolescent and Paediatric Rheumatology
Great Ormond Street Hospital for Children
NHS Foundation Trust, London, UK

Foreword: British Society for Paediatric and Adolescent Rheumatology

Foreword: British Society for Paediatric and Adolescent Rheumatology

Dr Clarissa Pilkington

Consultant in Adolescent and Paediatric Rheumatology
Great Ormond Street Hospital for Children
BSPAR [...]

Foreword: Paediatric rheumatology training in the UK

In the UK, training in paediatric rheumatology follows completion of general paediatric training and is overseen by the Royal College of Paediatrics and Child Health (RCPCH) with a Competency Based Framework and a process of assessment. Training in paediatric rheumatology is through the national training programme for the training of specialists in paediatrics (called the 'Grid') with competitive entry organized by RCPCH. This programme of training is a minimum of 2 years, recommended to be in more than one accredited centre, and trainees complete a programme of formative and summative assessments that are competency based. Ultimately trainees acquire a Certificate of Completion of Training (CCT) to be eligible to be appointed to Consultant posts working in the National Health Service. Training for general paediatricians with an interest in rheumatology is also encouraged and such candidates are not appointed to the Grid but are recommended to have 1 year's training in a recognized paediatric rheumatology centre, completing a Special Interest (SPIN) Module in paediatric rheumatology, either before or after CCT. The Competency Frameworks for Speciality Paediatrics form the basis of the curriculum for training and there is a Framework for the Specialist in Paediatric Rheumatology and also for the general paediatrician with an interest in rheumatology. Academic training is encouraged within the specialty. Trainees can join an integrated clinical academic training programme early in their career (ST1–ST4) as an Academic Clinical Fellow (ACF), or after completing a PhD or research MD as an Academic Clinical Lecturer (ACL). Further details on the format of training and the Competency Frameworks are given on the British Society of Paediatric and Adolescent Rheumatology website (⅋ http://www.bspar.org.uk/pages/trainees_area_members.asp) and the RCPCH website (⅋ http://www.rcpch.ac.uk/Training/Competency-Framework). Work is on-going updating the European Training Syllabus, with UK representation, through the European Academy of Paediatrics.

Increasingly throughout the UK and elsewhere, there are networks of clinical services working together to deliver paediatric rheumatology care, often across large geographical areas and encompassing various models of care with specialist expertise linking with other, and often smaller units. The role of adult rheumatologists is still very important as part of these clinical networks, although in many areas the focus of the adult rheumatology team is increasingly towards transitional care. There is a great need to raise awareness of paediatric rheumatology and the importance of early and prompt access to appropriate specialist care. There is a shortage of specialist paediatric rheumatology multi-disciplinary teams in the UK and further afield. The role of shared care between specialist services with local general paediatric and adult rheumatology teams is increasingly important so that high-quality clinical care can be delivered and equitably. Such clinical networks require personnel with training and support, highlighting the need for training, training positions, and a mechanism for support and teaching resources. This content of this handbook is largely based on the content of the Competency Frameworks for Paediatric Rheumatology and aims to address learning needs of paediatric rheumatology trainees, general paediatricians with an interest in rheumatology, as well as other healthcare professionals working within the specialty and clinical networks. Through BSPAR, a competency framework for allied health professionals (AHPs) working in paediatric rheumatology has been developed and covers recommended competencies for therapists working at primary, secondary, and tertiary care levels. Core competencies have also been developed for Paediatric Rheumatology Clinical Nurse Specialists and Advanced Nurse Practitioners.

Dr Anne-Marie McMahon
Chair of the UK Royal College of Paediatrics and
Child Health Specialist Advisory Committee for
Paediatric Rheumatology, and
Sheffield Children's Hospital NHS Foundation Trust,
Sheffield, UK

Contents

Contents

Detailed contents

10 Rashes in paediatric rheumatology 525

Contributors

Dr Mario Abinun
Great North Children's Hospital,
Newcastle upon Tyne NHS
Hospitals Foundation Trust,
Newcastle upon Tyne, UK
Chapter 4, Chapter 6, Chapter 8

Mr Alwyn Abraham
Leicester Royal Infirmary,
Leicester, UK
Chapter 1, Chapter 2

Dr Wijh Abreswil
Great North Children's Hospital,
Newcastle upon Tyne NHS
Hospitals Foundation Trust,
Newcastle upon Tyne, UK
Chapter 6, Chapter 9

Dr Ali al-Hashimi
University of Liverpool,
Liverpool, UK
Chapter 8

Dr Beverley Almeida
Great Ormond Street
Hospital for Children NHS
Foundation Trust,
London, UK
Chapter 1

Dr Muthana Al-Obaidi
Great Ormond Street Hospital
for Children NHS Foundation
Trust, London, UK
Chapter 3

Dr Nicola Ambrose
University College London
Hospital, London, UK
Chapter 3

Dr Tania Amin
Leeds Children's Hospital,
Leeds, UK
Chapter 4, Chapter 7, Chapter 9

Dr Kate Armon
Consultant Paediatric
Rheumatologist,
Addenbrookes Hospital,
Cambridge University Hospitals
NHS Foundation Trust,
Cambridge, UK
Chapter 2

Dr Eileen Baildam
Alder Hey Children's Foundation
NHS Trust, Liverpool, UK
Chapter 4

Dr Kathy Bailey
Nuffield Orthopaedic Centre,
Oxford University Hospitals,
Oxford, UK
Chapter 4

Dr Peter Bale
Addenbrookes Hospital,
Cambridge University Hospital
NHS Trust, Cambridge, UK
Chapter 2

Ms Catrin Barker
Alder Hey Children's NHS
Foundation Trust,
Liverpool, UK
Chapter 8

Mr Tom Beckingsale
Newcastle upon Tyne NHS
Hospitals Foundation Trust,
Newcastle upon Tyne, UK
Chapter 2

Professor Michael Beresford
Department of Women's and
Children's Health, Institute of
Translational Medicine, University
of Liverpool; and Alder Hey
Children's NHS Foundation Trust,
Liverpool, UK
Chapter 4

Professor Nick Bishop
Sheffield Children's
Hospital, Sheffield, UK
Chapter 5

Dr Emily Boulter
Princess Margaret Hospital,
Perth, Australia
Chapter 4

Dr Mary Brennan
Royal Hospital for Sick Children,
Edinburgh, UK
Chapter 3, Chapter 4, Chapter 9

Professor Paul A. Brogan
UCL Institute of Child Health and
Great Ormond St Hospital for
Children NHS Foundation Trust,
London, UK
Chapter 1, Chapter 9

Dr Richard Brough
Shrewsbury and Telford NHS
Trust, Royal Shrewsbury
Hospital, Shrewsbury, UK
Chapter 2

Dr Jennifer Campbell
Consultant Clinical Geneticist,
Yorkshire Regional Genetics
Service, Department of Clinical
Genetics, Chapel Allerton
Hospital, Leeds, UK
Chapter 5

Dr Alice Chieng
Royal Manchester Children's
Hospital, Manchester, UK
Chapter 4

Dr Julia Clark
Lady Cilento Children's Hospital,
Brisbane, Australia
Chapter 6

Ms Liz Clayton
Great North Children's Hospital,
Newcastle upon Tyne NHS
Hospitals Foundation Trust, UK
Chapter 1, Chapter 2

Dr Gavin Cleary
Alder Hey Children's Hospital,
Liverpool, UK
Chapter 4, Chapter 10

Dr Jacqui Clinch
Bristol Royal Hospital for Children,
Bristol and Royal National Hospital
for Rheumatic Diseases, Bristol, UK
Chapter 2, Chapter 9

Dr Hannah Connell
Consultant Clinical Psychologist,
Bath Centre for Pain Service,
Royal United Hospitals NHS
Foundation Trust, Bath, UK
Chapter 2

Dr Elizabeth Coulson
Northumbria Healthcare NHS
Foundation Trust, Northumbria,
UK
Chapter 3

Dr Joyce Davidson
Royal Hospital for Sick Children,
Glasgow, UK
Chapter 3, Chapter 9

Dr Karen Davies
New Cross Hospital,
Wolverhampton, UK
Chapter 9

Dr Penny Davis
Birmingham Children's Hospital,
Birmingham, UK
Chapter 2

Dr Hans de Graaf
University Hospital Southampton
NHS Foundation Trust
Southampton, UK
Chapter 2

Dr Anita Dhanrajani
Hospital for Sick Children,
Toronto, Canada
Chapter 6

Dr Deborah Eastwood
Great Ormond Street Hospital
for Children NHS Foundation
Trust, London, UK
Chapter 5

Mr Clive Edelsten
Great Ormond Street Hospital
for Children NHS Foundation
Trust, London, UK
Chapter 4

Dr Despina Eleftheriou
Great Ormond Street Hospital
NHS Foundation Trust and UCL
Institute of Child Health,
London, UK
Chapter 4

Dr Jill Ferrari
Department of Nursing and
Health, University of East
London, UK
Chapter 7

Dr Daniel Fishman
Luton and Dunstable NHS
Foundation Trust, Luton, UK
Chapter 3

Dr Charlene Foley
National Children's Research
Centre, Dublin, Ireland
Chapter 4

Ms Catherine Forster
Great North Children's Hospital,
Newcastle upon Tyne NHS
Hospitals Foundation Trust,
Newcastle upon Tyne, UK
Chapter 7

Professor Helen Foster
Newcastle University and Great
North Children's Hospital,
Newcastle NHS Hospitals
Foundation Trust, Newcastle
upon Tyne, UK
*Chapter 1, Chapter 2, Chapter 3,
Chapter 9*

Dr Mark Friswell
Great North Children's Hospital,
Newcastle upon Tyne NHS
Hospitals Foundation Trust,
Newcastle upon Tyne, UK
Chapter 8, Chapter 9

Dr Janet Gardner-Medwin
University of Glasgow,
Scotland, UK
Chapter 3, Chapter 4

Mr Craig Gerrand
Newcastle upon Tyne NHS
Hospitals Foundation Trust,
Newcastle Upon Tyne, UK
Chapter 2

Dr Claire Gowdy
Freeman Hospital,
Newcastle-Upon-Tyne, UK
Chapter 1

Ms Rachel Guyll
Great North Children's Hospital,
Newcastle upon Tyne NHS
Hospitals Foundation Trust,
Newcastle upon Tyne, UK
Chapter 7

Professor Sophie Hambleton
Newcastle University and the
Great North Children's Hospital,
Newcastle upon Tyne NHS
Hospitals Foundation Trust,
Newcastle upon Tyne, UK
Chapter 6

Dr Kirsty Haslam
Bradford Teaching Hospitals
NHS Foundation Trust,
Bradford, UK
Chapter 2

Dr Nathan Hasson
The Portland Hospital, London, UK
Chapter 5

Dr Daniel Hawley
Sheffield Children's NHS
Foundation Trust, Sheffield, UK
Chapter 4, Chapter 9

Dr Anne Hinks
Arthritis Research UK Centre for
Genetics and Genomics,
Centre for Musculoskeletal
Research, University of
Manchester, UK
Chapter 3

Mr Michael Hughes
Great North Children's Hospital,
Newcastle upon Tyne NHS
Hospitals Foundation Trust,
Newcastle upon Tyne, UK
Chapter 7

Dr Richard Hull
Queen Alexandra Hospital,
Portsmouth, UK
Chapter 3

Professor Kimme Hyrich
Centre for Musculoskeletal
Research, the University of
Manchester, UK
Chapter 1

Dr Talal Ibrahim
Sidra Medical and Research
Center, and Weill Cornell
Medicine-Qatar, Doha, Qatar
Chapter 1, Chapter 2

Dr Yiannis Ioannou
University College London,
London, UK
Chapter 3

Dr Sharmila Jandial
Great North Children's Hospital,
Newcastle NHS Hospitals
Foundation Trust, Newcastle
upon Tyne, UK
Chapter 1

Dr Simon Jones
Consultant in Paediatric
Inborn Errors of Metabolism,
Manchester Centre for
Genomic Medicine; Honorary
Senior Lecturer, University of
Manchester; St Marys Hospital,
Manchester University Hospitals
NHS Foundation Trust, UK
Chapter 4

Dr Akhila Kavirayani
Oxford University Hospitals NHS
Foundation Trust, Oxford, UK
Chapter 2, Chapter 9

Dr Alison Kelly
Bristol Royal Hospital for Children,
Bristol, UK
Chapter 4

Ms Jane Kelly
Alder Hey Children's Foundation
Trust, Liverpool, UK
Chapter 8

Dr Khulood Khawaja
Mafraq Hospital, Abu Dhabi, UAE
Chapter 4

Dr Raju Khubchandani
Jaslok Hospital, Mumbai, India
Chapter 6

Dr Orla Killeen
Our Lady's Children's Hospital,
Crumlin, Dublin, Ireland
Chapter 2, Chapter 4

Professor Yuki Kimura
Joseph M Sanzari Children's
Hospital, Hackensack Meridian
Health, New Jersey, USA
Chapter 9

Dr Helen Lachmann
UK National Amyloidosis Centre,
University College London
Medical School, London, UK
Chapter 4

Dr Alice Leahy
Southampton Children's Hospital,
Southampton, UK
Chapter 6, Chapter 8

Dr Martin Lee
Newcastle Hospitals NHS
Foundation Trust, Newcastle, UK
Chapter 7

Dr Valentina Leone
The Leeds Teaching Hospitals NHS
Trust, Leeds, UK
Chapter 6

Dr Clodagh Lowry
The Children's University
Hospital, Dublin, Ireland
Chapter 4

Ms Sue Maillard
Great Ormond Street Hospital
for Children NHS Foundation
Trust, London, UK
Chapter 4, Chapter 7

Dr Cynthia K Manos
Children's Hospital of Philadelphia,
Philadelphia, USA
Chapter 9

Dr Stephen Marks
Great Ormond Street Hospital
for Children NHS Foundation
Trust, London, UK
Chapter 4

Dr Kate Martin
Gloucestershire Hospitals NHS
Trust, Cheltenham General
Hospital, Cheltenham, UK
Chapter 2

Dr Neil Martin
Royal Hospital for Children,
Glasgow, UK
Chapter 4, Chapter 5, Chapter 9

Dr Joanne May
Oxford University Hospitals NHS
Foundation Trust, Oxford, UK
Chapter 2, Chapter 9

Dr Liza McCann
Alder Hey Children's NHS
Foundation Trust, Liverpool, UK
Chapter 8, Chapter 9

Dr Janet McDonagh
Centre for Musculoskeletal
Research and NIHR Manchester
Musculoskeletal Biomedical
Research Unit, University of
Manchester; Central Manchester
University Hospitals NHS
Foundation Trust, Manchester
Academic Health Science Centre,
Manchester, UK
Chapter 7

Dr Flora McErlane
Great North Children's Hospital,
Newcastle upon Tyne NHS
Hospitals Foundation Trust,
Newcastle upon Tyne, UK
*Chapter 1, Chapter 3, Chapter 4,
Chapter 9*

Dr Anne-Marie McMahon
Sheffield Children's Hospital,
Sheffield, UK
Chapter 2

Professor Kirsten Minden
German Rheumatism Research
Center, Berlin and Charité
University Medicine Berlin,
Germany
Chapter 9

Dr Andrea Myers
Northumbria Healthcare NHS
Trust, The School of Medical
Education, Newcastle University,
Tyne and Wear, UK
Chapter 2

Dr Kiran Nistala
Great Ormond St Hospital NHS
Foundation Trust, London, UK
Chapter 3

Dr Susan O'Connell
Lyme Borreliosis Unit, Health Protection Agency Laboratory, Southampton, UK
Chapter 6

Dr Clare Pain
Alder Hey Children's NHS Foundation Trust, Liverpool, UK
Chapter 4, Chapter 8

Dr Jason Palman
Luton and Dunstable NHS Foundation Trust, Luton, UK
Chapter 3

Dr Sanjay Patel
Southampton Children's Hospital, Southampton, UK
Chapter 2, Chapter 4

Dr Clarissa Pilkington
Great Ormond Street Hospital for Children NHS Foundation Trust, London, UK
Chapter 4

Professor Athimalaipet Ramanan
Professor of Paediatric Rheumatology, University of Bristol; Bristol Royal Hospital for Children and Royal National Hospital for Rheumatic Diseases, Bath, UK
Chapter 4, Chapter 9

Dr Valerie Rogers
Bristol Royal Hospital for Children, Bristol and Royal National Hospital for Rheumatic Diseases, Bath, UK
Chapter 4

Dr Ricardo Russo
Hospital de Pediatria Juan P. Garrahan, Buenos Aires, Argentina
Chapter 2, Chapter 4

Dr Sunil Sampath
Centre for Musculoskeletal Research, University of Manchester, UK
Chapter 1

Dr Satyapal Rangaraj
Nottingham Children's Hospital, Nottingham University Hospitals NHS Trust, Nottingham, UK
Chapter 6, Chapter 9

Professor Chris Scott
Red Cross War Memorial Children's Hospital, University of Cape Town, Cape Town South Africa
Chapter 6

Dr Debajit Sen
University College London Hospital, London, UK
Chapter 4

Dr Ethan Sen
Bristol Royal Hospital for Children, Bristol, UK
Chapter 9

Dr Eve Smith
Alder Hey NHS Hospital, Liverpool, UK
Chapter 2

Dr Glenda Sobey
The Children's Hospital, Sheffield, UK
Chapter 5

Professor Taunton Southwood
School of Infection and Immunity, College of Medical and Dental Sciences, University of Birmingham, UK
Chapter 1

Ms Liz Stretton
Nottingham Children's Hospital,
Nottingham University Hospitals
NHS Trust, Nottingham, UK
Chapter 8

Ms Helen Strike
Paediatric and Adolescent
Rheumatology, Bristol Royal
Hospital for Children,
Bristol, UK
Chapter 9

Dr Alexandra Tabor
University Hospital of North
Staffordshire, Stoke-on-Trent,
Staffordshire, UK
Chapter 1, Chapter 4

Dr Rachel Tattersall
Sheffield Children's Hospital
NHS Foundation Trust and
Sheffield Teaching Hospitals
NHS Foundation Trust,
Sheffield, UK
Chapter 3

Professor Wendy Thomson
Arthritis Research UK Centre for
Genetics, and Genomics
Centre for Musculoskeletal
Research, University of
Manchester, UK
Chapter 3

Dr John D. Tuckett
Freeman Hospital,
Newcastle-Upon-Tyne, UK
Chapter 1

Dr Bas Vastert
University Medical Center,
Utrecht, The Netherlands
Chapter 9

Dr Josephine Vila
Newcastle upon Tyne NHS
Hospitals Foundation Trust,
Newcastle upon Tyne, UK
Chapter 7

Dr Joanna Walsh
NHS Greater Glasgow and
Clyde, UK
Chapter 3, Chapter 7, Chapter 9

Dr Kate Webb
University College London,
London, UK
Chapter 4

**Professor Lucy
Wedderburn**
UCL Institute of Child Health,
London, UK
Chapter 3

Dr Pamela Weiss
Children's Hospital of
Philadelphia, Perelman School
of Medicine, University of
Pennsylvania, USA
Chapter 9

Ms Pamela Whitworth
Birmingham Children's Hospital,
Birmingham, UK
Chapter 9

Dr Nick Wilkinson
Evelina Children's Hospital,
London, UK
Chapter 1

Dr Charlotte Wing
University College London,
London, UK
Chapter 3

Dr Mark Wood
Leed's Children's Hospital ,
Leeds, UK
Chapter 2

Dr Michael Wright
Northern Genetics Service,
Newcastle upon Tyne Hospitals
NHS Foundation Trust,
Newcastle upon Tyne, UK
Chapter 5

Professor Nico Wulffraat
University Medical Center,
Utrecht, the Netherlands
Chapter 9

Mrs Ruth Wyllie
Great North Children's Hospital,
Newcastle upon Tyne NHS
Hospitals Foundation Trust,
Newcastle upon Tyne, UK
Chapter 7

Symbols and abbreviations

⊃	cross-reference
↑	increase/d
↓	decrease/d
♂	male
♀	female
~	approximately
±	plus/minus
2D	two-dimensional
3D	three-dimensional
AAV	ANCA-associated vasculitides
ACE	angiotensin-converting enzyme
ACL	anticardiolipin
ACR	American College of Rheumatology
ALL	acute lymphoblastic leukaemia
ALP	alkaline phosphatase
ALPS	autoimmune lymphoproliferative syndrome
ANA	antinuclear antibody
ANCA	anti-neutrophil cytoplasmic antibody
anti-CCP	anti-cyclic citrullinated protein
AP	anteroposterior
aPL	antiphospholipid [antibody]
APS	antiphospholipid syndrome
APTT	activated partial thromboplastin time
ARF	acute rheumatic fever
AS	ankylosing spondylitis
ASIC	anterior superior iliac crest
ASOT	anti-streptolysin O titre
AYA	adolescents and young adults
AZA	azathioprine
BAFF	B-cell activating factor
BASDAI	Bath Ankylosing Spondylitis Disease Activity index
BASFI	Bath Ankylosing Spondylitis Functional Index
BD	Behçet's disease
BJHS	benign joint hypermobility syndrome
BNFC	British National Formulary for Children

BP	blood pressure
BPRG	British Paediatric Rheumatology Group
BSA	body surface area
BSPAR	British Society of Paediatric and Adolescent Rheumatology
CAA	coronary artery aneurysm
cANCA	cytoplasmic anti-neutrophil cytoplasmic antibody
CANDLE	chronic atypical neutrophilic dermatosis with lipodystrophy and elevated temperature .
CAPS	catastrophic antiphospholid syndrome or cryopyrin associated periodic syndrome
CARRA	Childhood Arthritis and Rheumatology Research Alliance
CAU	chronic anterior uveitis
CCP	cyclic citrullinated protein
CD	Crohn's disease
CF	cystic fibrosis
CHAQ	Child Health Assessment Questionnaire
CINCA	chronic infantile, neurological, cutaneous and articular syndrome
CMV	cytomegalovirus
CNS	central nervous system or clinical nurse specialist
cPACNS	primary angiitis of the central nervous system in children
cPAN	cutaneous polyarteritis nodosa
CRMO	chronic recurrent multifocal osteomyelitis
CRP	C-reactive protein
CRPS	complex regional pain syndrome
CSF	cerebrospinal fluid
CSS	Churg–Strauss syndrome
CT	computed tomography
CTA	computed tomography angiography
CTD	connective tissue disease
CTP	consensus treatment plan
CVD	cardiovascular disease
CXR	chest x-ray
CYC	cyclophosphamide
DADA2	Deficiency of adenosine deaminase 2
DAS	Disease Activity Score
DD	Degos disease
DDH	developmental dysplasia of the hip
DIRA	deficiency of IL-1 receptor antagonist

DITRA	deficiency of IL-36 receptor antagonist
dL	decilitre
DMARD	disease-modifying antirheumatic drug
DMSA	dimercaptosuccinic acid
dRVVT	dilute Russell viper venom test .
DXA	dual-emission X-ray absorptiometry
EBV	Epstein–Barr virus
ECG	electrocardiogram
EEG	electroencephalogram
EGPA	eosinophilic granulomatosis with polyangiitis [formerly known as Churg–Strauss syndrome]
ELISA	enzyme-linked immunosorbent assay
EMA	European Medicines Agency
EMG	electromyography
ENA	extractable nuclear antigen
EOS	early-onset sarcoidosis
ERA	enthesitis-related arthritis
ERT	enzyme replacement therapy
ESR	erythrocyte sedimentation rate
ESRF	end-stage renal failure
EULAR	European League Against Rheumatism
FBC	full blood count
FCAS	familial cold autoinflammatory syndrome
FII	factitious or induced illness
FMD	fibromuscular dysplasia
FMF	familial Mediterranean fever
G6PD	glucose-6-phosphate dehydrogenase
GAG	glycosaminoglycan
GBM	glomerular basement membrane
GFR	glomerular fi ltration rate
GI	gastrointestinal
GN	glomerulonephritis
GP	general practitioner
GPA	granulomatosis with polyangiitis
GvHD	graft-versus-host disease
GWAS	genome-wide association study
HA	healthy adults
HC	healthy children
HEEADSSSS	Home, Exercise, Education, Activities, Drugs, Sexual health, Suicide, Sleep, Safety
HIV	human immunodeficiency virus

HLA	human leucocyte association
HLH	haemophagocytic lymphohistiocytosis
HSCT	haematopoietic stem cell transplantation
HSN	Henoch–Schönlein nephritis
HSP	Henoch–Schönlein purpura
HUVS	hypocomplementaemic urticarial vasculitic syndrome
IA	intra-articular
IAC	intra-articular corticosteroid
IBD	inflammatory bowel disease
IC	indeterminate colitis
IDSA	Infectious Diseases Society of America
Ig	immunoglobulin
IGRA	interferon gamma releasing assays
ILAR	International League of Associations for Rheumatology
IM	intramuscular
INR	international normalized ratio
IV	intravenous
IVIG	intravenous immunoglobulin
IVMP	intravenous methylprednisolone
JAMAR	Juvenile Arthritis Multidimensional Assessment Report
JAPAI	Juvenile Arthritis Parent Assessment Index
JDM	juvenile dermatomyositis
JIA	juvenile idiopathic arthritis
JSLE	juvenile-onset systemic lupus erythematosus
jSSc	juvenile systemic sclerosis
KD	Kawasaki disease
kg	kilogramme/s
L	litre/s
LAC	lupus anticoagulant
LDH	lactate dehydrogenase
LFT	liver function test
LMWH	low-molecular-weight heparin
LN	lupus nephritis
LS	localized scleroderma
LTBI	latent tuberculosis infection
LV	livedoid vasculopathy
MAS	macrophage activation syndrome

MC&S	microscopy, culture and sensitivity
MCPJ	metacarpophalangeal joint
MCTD	mixed connective tissue disease
MDHAQ	Multi-Dimensional Health Assessment Questionnaire
MDT	multidisciplinary team
MED	multiple epiphyseal dysplasia
MESNA	sodium 2-mercapto-ethanesulphonate
mg	milligramme/s
MHC	major histocompatibility complex
min	minute/s
MKD	mevalonate kinase deficiency
mL	millilitre/s
ML	mucolipidoses
mm	millimetre/s
MMF	mycophenolate mofetil
MPA	microscopic polyangiitis
MPO	myeloperoxidase
MPS	mucopolysaccharidoses
MRA	magnetic resonance angiography
MRI	magnetic resonance imaging
MSK	musculoskeletal
MSUS	musculoskeletal ultrasound
MTPJ	metatarsophalangeal joint
MTX	methotrexate
MVK	mevalonate kinase
MWS	Muckle–Wells syndrome
NAI	non-accidental injury
NAPS	NALP12 associated periodic syndrome
NBO	non-bacterial osteitis
NBT	nitroblue tetrazolium
NFC	nailfold capillary
NICE	National Institute for Health and Clinical Excellence
NOMID	neonatal onset multisystem inflammatory disease
NTI	narrow therapeutic index
OCD	osteochondritis dissecans
OI	osteogenesis imperfecta
OT	occupational therapist
PA	posterior–anterior
PACNS	primary angiitis of the central nervous system

PAH	pulmonary arterial hypertension
PAN	polyarteritis nodosa
pANCA	perinuclear anti-neutrophil cytoplasmic antibody
PAPA	pyogenic sterile arthritis, pyoderma gangrenosum, and acne [syndrome]
PCR	polymerase chain reaction
PET	positron emission tomography
PFAPA	periodic fever, aphthous stomatitis, pharyngitis, and cervical adenitis
pGALS	paediatric Gait Arms Legs Spine
PGAS	Physician Global Assessment Score
PIPJ	proximal interphalangeal joint
PK	pharmacokinetic
PO	per os (orally)
PR3	proteinase 3
pREMS	paediatric Regional Examination of the Musculoskeletal System
PROMs	patient or parent reported outcome measures
PRT	paediatric rheumatology team
PTH	parathyroid hormone
PUO	pyrexia of unknown origin
PVL	Panton–Valentine leukocidin
PXE	pseudoxanthoma elasticum
QoL	quality of life
RA	rheumatoid arthritis
RCPCH	Royal College of Paediatrics and Child Health
RCT	randomized control trial
RD	Raynaud's disease
RF	rheumatoid factor
RICE	Rest, ice, compress, elevate
RP	Raynaud's phenomenon
SAPHO	synovitis acne pustulosis hyperostosis osteitis
SAVI	STING-associated vasculopathy with onset in infancy
sec	second/s
SEDC	spondyloepiphyseal dysplasia congenita
SIADH	syndrome of inappropriate anti-diuretic hormone secretion
sJIA	systemic juvenile idiopathic arthritis
SLE	systemic lupus erythematosus
SmPC	summary of product characteristics
SNP	single nucleotide polymorphism

SPECT	single-photon emission computerized tomograph
SSc	systemic sclerosis
SSZ	sulphasalazine
TA	Takayasu arteritis
TA	triamcinolone acetonide
TB	tuberculosis
TGF	transforming growth factor-beta
TH	triamcinolone hexacetonide
TMJ	temporomandibular joint
TNF	tumour necrosis factor
TPMT	thiopurine methyltransferase
TRAPS	TNF alpha receptor associated periodic fever syndrome
TRM	transplant-related mortality
TST	tuberculin skin test
U&E	urea and electrolytes
UA:UC	spot urine albumin:creatinine ratio
UC	ulcerative colitis
US	ultrasound
VAS	visual analogue score
VZIG	varicella-zoster immunoglobulin
VZV	varicella zoster virus
WCC	white cell count
yr	year/s

Clinical skills and assessment

Epidemiology of paediatric musculoskeletal conditions

Musculoskeletal symptoms are common in the paediatric population; however, inflammatory musculoskeletal diseases are not. This chapter briefly presents the estimated incidence and prevalence of some of the more common conditions seen in the paediatric rheumatology clinic.

Inflammatory musculoskeletal conditions

Juvenile idiopathic arthritis (JIA), the most common chronic inflammatory rheumatic disease of childhood, is a clinically heterogeneous group of disorders characterized by chronic inflammatory arthritis. Determining the incidence and prevalence, both within the UK and internationally, has been complicated by changing classification criteria (American College of Rheumatology [ACR] versus European League Against Rheumatism [EULAR] versus League of Associations for Rheumatology [ILAR]) as well as differences in case ascertainment.

The earliest epidemiological studies of JIA performed in populations from Western Europe and North America showed an incidence varying from 1.6 (France, 1982) to 13.9 (North-America, 1970) and prevalence between 8.6 (France, 1982) and 96 (North-America, 1970) per 100,000 persons. Recent studies report a higher JIA incidence, from 3.2 (France, 2001) to 23 (Finland, 2000) and prevalence between 15.7 (France, 2006) and 83.7 (Estonia, 2000) per 100,000 persons.

Ethnicity has been found to play a role in both JIA susceptibility and outcomes. Children of European ancestry have been found to be at the highest risk of developing all types of JIA compared to other ethnic groups, except rheumatoid factor (RF)+ve polyarticular JIA. Also, native North American children are at a higher risk than children of European descent of developing a polyarticular course of disease, such as extended oligoarticular JIA, RF−ve polyarticular JIA, and RF+ve polyarticular JIA. Prevalence of the enthesitis-related arthritis in studies from China, India, and Turkey were much higher than reported from many western countries. African-American children with poly-articular JIA had higher odds of having joint damage, and children of Asian origin reported less JIA related pain and disability. Incidence of JIA-related uveitis was found to be low in India and Kuwait, while a large study in a multiethnic JIA cohort found no association between uveitis and ethnicity.

Juvenile-onset systemic lupus erythematosus

Childhood-onset juvenile systemic lupus erythematosus (SLE) was found to account for <1% of patients in paediatric rheumatology clinics in a UK registry, compared to 1.5–3% in Canada and 4.5% in the USA. A recent review reported a worldwide incidence of JSLE as 0.4–2.5 and prevalence as 1.9–25.7 per 100,000 persons, the higher prevalence was reported from the Hawaiian Islands. Caucasian children with JSLE reported lower health-related quality of life compared to non-Caucasians.

Juvenile dermatomyositis

The incidence of juvenile dermatomyositis in the UK and Ireland is reported at a rate of 0.19 per 100,000 children. This compares with rates of 0.25–0.41 per 100,000 for children in a US registry.

Juvenile scleroderma

Scleroderma in childhood remains very rare. A recent UK study has estimated the annual incidence to be 3.4 per million children for localized scleroderma; and 0.27 per million for the systemic disease.

Non-inflammatory musculoskeletal conditions

Hypermobility

The prevalence of hypermobility in children as a phenomenon, as opposed to benign joint hypermobility syndrome (BJHS), is common and decreases with age. This has been measured in a number of studies previously and, depending on the age or ethnicity of the study population or the inclusion criteria, has been reported to range from 2.3% to as high as 64%. There is wide divergence in the joint laxity observed amongst different ethnic groups. The Europeans are most stiff; the Bantu tribes of intermediate joint laxity; and those originally from the Indian subcontinent of most marked joint laxity.

However, the presence of hypermobility in children does not equate to having BJHS. The latter is defined as the presence of a degree of joint hypermobility measured by a prearranged and validated scoring system, associated with musculoskeletal symptoms and signs, and other connective tissue problems likely to be attributable to it.

Considerable overlap between benign hypermobility and mild variants of Ehlers–Danlos syndrome, Marfan syndrome, and osteogenesis imperfecta has been reported.

Complex regional pain syndrome

The common alternative name in the literature for complex regional pain syndrome (CRPS) is reflex sympathetic dystrophy. The incidence of CRPS in children is unknown. A Canadian study which reviewed children with idiopathic musculoskeletal pain of the upper limb attributed 52% of cases to CRPS. In a population study in the USA, the overall risk of CRPS was 5.4 per 100,000 person years. However, this mainly reflected adult CRPS, as the median age at diagnosis was 46 years. In two large paediatric series of CRPS, most cases occurred in girls (~85%) and the mean age at diagnosis was ~13 years (range 5–17 years).

Further readings

Bowyer S, Roettcher P, and the members of the Pediatric Rheumatology Database Research Group. Pediatric rheumatology clinic populations in the United States: results of a 3 year survey. *J Rheumatol* 1996;23:1968–74.

Malleson PN, Fung MY, Rosenberg AM. The incidence of pediatric rheumatic diseases: results from the Canadian Pediatric Rheumatology Association Disease Registry. *J Rheumatol* 1996;23:1981–7.

Symmons DP, Jones M, Osborne J, et al. Pediatric rheumatology in the United Kingdom: data from the British Pediatric Rheumatology Group National Diagnostic Register. *J Rheumatol* 1996;23:1975–80.

History taking, physical examination, and approaches to investigation

- The differential diagnosis of musculoskeletal pain in children is broad (Box 1.1). Taking a history and performing a physical examination (general and musculoskeletal) are integral to making an accurate diagnosis.
- In history taking it is worth asking open questions (Table 1.1), probing for features that may suggest mechanical or inflammatory pathology (Table 1.2), seeking any suggestion of systemic disease and 'red flags' (Box 1.2) to warrant urgent concern or clues in the history to suggest inflammatory musculoskeletal disease (Box 1.3).
- Appropriate clinical assessment requires knowledge of normal development, normal variants (see ➜ Normal variants of lower limb development, pp. 9–10), normal and abnormal gait patterns (see ➜ The gait cycle and abnormal gait patterns, p. 11), clinical presentations at different ages (e.g. the hip, see ➜ Hip pain and hip problems in children and adolescents, pp. 111–18), and an approach to initial investigations. Further details are given in chapters relating to individual diseases.

Key points to note in the clinical assessment

- A common pitfall in making a diagnosis is to inappropriately attribute a child's problem to trauma (which is a common event in the life of all ambulant children).
- The history (often given by the parent or carer), may be based on observations and interpretation of events made by others (such as teachers or friends), and may be rather vague and ill-defined with non-specific complaints such as 'my child is limping' or 'my child is not walking quite right'.
  - Consider the age and development of the child and modify the questioning and consultation style accordingly.
  - The young child may deny having pain when asked directly, and this should not be taken to mean that the child does not have any pain.
- Physical examination needs to be comprehensive:
  - Assessment of pain is important (see ➜ Pain syndromes and the assessment of pain, pp. 84–8).
  - A musculoskeletal assessment (e.g. pGALS—see ➜ pGALS, pp. 18–22) will identify areas of significant joint abnormality which may not be apparent from the history alone. Some aspects of pGALS, such as gait observation, may be modified or need to be postponed in the acutely unwell child.
  - A more detailed regional musculoskeletal examination (see ➜ pREMS, pp. 23–7) is an adjunct to pGALS and always required where abnormalities in pGALS are observed. Remember the possibility of referred pain (particularly hip pathology with a presentation of knee pain).
  - Indolent presentations of chronic musculoskeletal disease can impact on growth (either localized or generalized). It is important to assess height and weight, review growth charts in the Parent Held Record where available, and look for evidence of disproportionate growth (e.g. asymmetrical leg length) or muscle wasting.

- Additional clinical skills are required pending the clinical scenario and include capillaroscopy (see ➲ Nailfold capillaroscopy in rheumatic disease, pp. 39–42) and muscle testing (see ➲ Juvenile dermatomyositis, pp. 280–7).
- Musculoskeletal ultrasound is increasingly being used as an adjunct to clinical examination in order to detect synovitis (see ➲ Musculoskeletal ultrasound in juvenile idiopathic arthritis, pp. 28–32).

Box 1.1 The differential diagnosis of musculoskeletal pain in children and adolescents

Life-threatening conditions
- Malignancy (leukaemia, lymphoma, bone tumour)
- Sepsis (septic arthritis, osteomyelitis)
- Non-accidental injury (NAI).

Joint pain with minimal or no swelling
- Hypermobility syndromes
- Orthopaedic syndromes (e.g. Osgood–Schlatter disease, Perthes disease)
- Idiopathic pain syndromes (reflex sympathetic dystrophy, fibromyalgia)
- Metabolic (e.g. hypothyroidism, lysosomal storage diseases)
- Tumour (benign and malignant).

Joint pain with swelling
- Trauma (haemarthrosis)
- Infection
- Septic arthritis and osteomyelitis (viral, bacterial, mycobacterial):
  - Reactive arthritis (post-enteric, sexually acquired)
  - Infection related (rheumatic fever, post-vaccination)
- JIA
- Arthritis related to inflammatory bowel disease
- Connective tissue diseases (SLE, scleroderma, dermatomyositis, vasculitis)
- Metabolic (e.g. osteomalacia/rickets, cystic fibrosis)
- Haematological (e.g. haemophilia, haemoglobinopathy)
- Tumour (benign and malignant)
- Chromosomal (e.g. Down's related arthritis)
- Auto-inflammatory syndromes (e.g. periodic syndromes, chronic recurrent multifocal osteomyelitis)
- Sarcoidosis
- Developmental/congenital (e.g. achondroplasia).

Table 1.1 Key questions to ask when taking a musculoskeletal history

Questions to parent/carer (and the child as appropriate)	Points to check for	Comments
What have you or anyone else noticed?	Behaviour, mood, joint swelling, limping, bruising	Limping, whether intermittent or persistent, *always* warrants further assessment. Deterioration in school performance (e.g. sport, handwriting) is always significant. Joint swelling is always significant but can be subtle and easily overlooked by the parent (and even healthcare professionals!), especially if the changes are symmetrical
		Rather than describing stiffness, the parents may notice the child is reluctant to weight-bear or limps in the mornings or 'gels' after periods of immobility (e.g. after long car rides or sitting in a classroom).
What is the child like in him/herself?	Irritability, grumpy, 'clingy', reluctant to play, systemic features (e.g. fever, anorexia, weight loss)	Young children may not verbalize pain but may present with behavioural changes or avoidance of activities previously enjoyed
		Systemic features including 'red flags' to suggest malignancy or infection.
Where is the pain? (Ask the child to point) and what is it like?	Take a pain history and focus on locality, exacerbating/relieving factors, timescale pattern.	Asymmetrical persistent site of pain is invariably a cause for concern. Referred pain from the hip may present with non-specific pain in the thigh or knee.
How is he/she in the mornings and during the day?	Diurnal variation and daytime symptoms (e.g. limping, difficulty walking, dressing, toileting, stairs?)	Pain on waking or daytime symptoms suggestive of stiffness or gelling (after periods of inactivity), are indicative of inflammatory joint (or muscle) disease.
What is he/she like with walking and running? Has there been any *change* in his/her activities?	Motor milestones and suggestion of delay or regression of achieved milestones, including speech and language. Avoidance of activities that previously enjoyed (e.g. sport, play) are noteworthy.	Regression of achieved motor milestones, functional impairment or avoidance of activity (including play, sport, or writing), are more suggestive of acquired joint or muscle disease (and especially inflammatory causes). An assessment of global neurodevelopment is indicated with delay or regression in speech, language, feeding or motor skills. 'Clumsiness' is a non-specific term but may mask significant musculoskeletal or neuromuscular disease
		Delay in walking and especially if accompanied by problems with speech, feeding frequent falls may indicate muscle disease such as muscular dystrophies.

Table 1.1 Contd.

Questions to parent/carer (and the child as appropriate)	Points to check for	Comments
How is he/she at school/nursery?	School attendance (any suggestion of school avoidance, bullying)	Behavioural problems in the young child may manifest as non-specific pains (headaches, tummy aches, or leg pains). Sensitive questioning may reveal stressful events at home or school.
Does he/she wake at night with pain?	Pattern of night waking	Night waking is a common feature of growing pains (and usually intermittent, and often predictable). Conversely persistent night waking, especially if there are other concerns (such as unilaterality, limping, unusual location, or systemic features) are of concern and invariably necessitate further investigation.
Can you predict when the pains may occur?	Relationship to physical activity (including during or after sporting activities)	Mechanical pains (e.g. related to hypermobility) tend to be worse later in the day, evenings and often after activities or busy days.
What do you do when he/she is in pain?	Response to analgesics, anti-inflammatory medication, massages, heat or ice packs and reaction of parent	Lack of response to simple analgesia is a concern. Vicious circle of reinforced behaviour can occur.
What is your main concern?	Sleep disturbance, cosmetic appearance anxiety about serious disease (arthritis, cancer, family history), pain control.	A family history of muscle disease, arthritis or autoimmune disease may indicate a predisposition to muscle or joint disease. Observed 'abnormalities' (such as flat feet, curly toes) may be part of normal development. The parent or carer will undoubtedly have anxieties and concerns about their child, may fear severe illness and with possible expectation of investigations (e.g. blood tests or imaging).

Table 1.2 Distinguishing mechanical from inflammatory musculoskeletal presentations

Mechanical		Inflammatory
Pain	Worse on weight bearing and after activity such as walking	Often eased by movement and may be seemingly absent in young children and manifest as behavioural change or avoidance of activity
Joint swelling	Usually mild and maybe transient	Tends to be persistent
Morning stiffness or gelling after rest	Usually absent	Often marked
Instability (giving way)	May be present	Usually absent
Locking	May be present	Usually absent
Loss of full movement	May be present	Often present

Box 1.2 RED FLAGS (to raise concern about infection or malignancy or non-accidental malignancy)
- Fever, systemic upset
- Bone/joint pain with fever
- Weight loss, sweats, persistent night waking
- Incongruence between history and clinical presentation pattern of physical findings.

Box 1.3 Important points when considering inflammatory joint or muscle disease
- The lack of reported pain does not exclude arthritis.
- There is need to probe for symptoms such as:
  - Gelling (e.g. stiffness after long car rides)
  - Altered function (e.g. play, handwriting skills, writing, regression of milestones)
  - Deterioration in behaviour (irritability, poor sleeping).
- There is need to examine all joints as often joint involvement may be 'asymptomatic' or illocalized.
- There is need to assess muscle strength (e.g. proximal muscle weakness such as Gowers test).

Normal variants of lower limb development

See Table 1.3.

Table 1.3 Normal variants of lower limb development

	Indications for concern and referral to physiotherapy or paediatric orthopaedics unless specified	Comments (see ➔ Foot and ankle problems, pp. 123–5, ➔ The role of the podiatrist, pp. 427–9, and ➔ Joint hypermobility, pp. 126–30)
Tip-toe walking Common in healthy young children	• Toe walking is persistent or asymmetrical • Associated developmental delay • Child unable to squat or stand with their heels on the floor (tightness of calf muscles) • Child >3yr old, and unable to stand from floor sitting without using hands	• Can associate with clubfoot or neurological disease (e.g. muscular dystrophy, cerebral palsy, poliomyelitis). Careful neuromuscular assessment required. Check for gastrocnemius contracture and shoes for sole wear. Physiotherapy may help mild cases but surgery may be required.
Flat feet Common and normal for babies and toddlers, resolves with development of longitudinal arch usually by 4–6yr of age	• Signs of pressure on the foot, e.g. blistering • The longitudinal arch does not form normally when the child stands on tip toe • The foot is stiff (i.e. the normal arch does not form when the child stands on tip toe or the big toe is passively extended)	• Persistence often familial, more common in hypermobility • Insoles may help but shouldn't be worn all the time—walking in bare in feet helps promote foot development • A non-flexible flat foot may indicate tarsal coalition (often teens) • In newborn exclude vertical talus
Pes Cavus Not common— the opposite of flat feet and is when the arch is extremely pronounced	• Often associated with toe clawing, calluses, heel varus, and pain with difficult to fit footwear • May be physiological (familial— so check parents' feet!), residual from clubfoot abnormality, or associated with neurological abnormalities. Paediatric neurology/orthopaedics referral usually needed	• Careful neuromuscular/ musculoskeletal assessment required. Neurological conditions to consider include—spina bifida, spinal dysraphism, poliomyelitis, Charcot–Marie–Tooth, Friedrich's ataxia • Insoles may help and surgery may be required

Table 1.3 Contd.

Curly toes Most resolve by 4yr	• Surgery rarely needed	• Check shoes are well fitting
Knock knees Usually resolve by the age of 6yr	• Associated with pain or asymmetrical • Extreme (>6cm intermalleolar distance at ankles) or persistent (>6yr)	• A gap of 6–7cm between the ankles is normal (between 2–4yr) • Late feature of arthritis of knee (e.g. JIA)
Bow legs Common and normally seen in children until the age of 2yr	• Associated with pain or asymmetrical or the child is short in stature or has other medical problems • Extreme (>6cm intercondylar distance at knees) or persistent (>6yr)	• Conditions to exclude include rickets, skeletal dysplasias, syndromes associated with dwarfism (e.g. achondroplasia, Blount's disease • Late feature of arthritis of knee (e.g. JIA)
Out-toeing Feet point outwards and usually resolves by 4yr	• Recent onset in a teenager—check hips for a slipped upper femoral epiphysis.	

JIA, juvenile idiopathic arthritis.

Further reading

Staheli, L.T. *Fundamentals of Pediatric Orthopedics—Foot and lower limb.* Philadelphia, PA: Lippincott-Raven, 2008.

The gait cycle and abnormal gait patterns

A child with an abnormal gait is a common presentation and can be due to many different causes (Tables 1.4 and 1.5). Clearly there is considerable overlap with neurological problems and careful clinical assessment, recognition of different gait patterns, and knowledge of potential differential diagnoses is very helpful (Table 1.6).

General effects of neuromuscular disease on joint action

- Muscle weakness reduces stability.
- Muscle weakness and spasticity reduces range of motion.
- Muscle weakness and spasticity reduces efficiency.
- Muscle weakness and spasticity encourages compensatory movements.
- Longstanding weakness and spasticity may cause joint contracture.
- Longstanding contracture and compensatory movements may causebone deformities (lever arm dysfunction).

Indications for neuromuscular assessment

- To study abnormal inefficient gait or gait that is deteriorating
- To identify specific targets for surgical correction, e.g. osteotomies, muscle lengthening
- Allows detailed assessment of gait by multidisciplinary team
- Assess outcomes of intervention, i.e. orthoses, physiotherapy, or surgery.

Limitations of gait analysis

- Expense, training, and operator experience dependent
- Variation between observers, of assessments, and of recommendations.

Table 1.4 The normal gait cycle and abnormal patterns observed in neuromuscular disease

Gait cycle phase	Normal characteristics	Abnormal characteristics in neuromuscular disease	Examples of abnormality in musculoskeletal disease
Loading response	• Dorsiflexed ankle for weight acceptance • Heel strike (for shock absorption)	• Lack of dorsiflexion range due to weakness, contracture or calf muscle spasticity • High stepping gait (no heel strike), e.g. poliomyelitis and other paralytic disorders	• Tip-toe walking with short gastrocnemius muscles or painful hindfoot (e.g. Sever's disease)

Table 1.4 Contd.

Gait cycle phase	Normal characteristics	Abnormal characteristics in neuromuscular disease	Examples of abnormality in musculoskeletal disease
Mid stance	• Stable ankle • Dorsiflexors contract, plantar flexors relax • Knee extends • Hip extends	• Peroneal weakness may reduce ankle stability, e.g. common peroneal nerve palsy • Hamstring contracture or spasticity may reduce knee extension	• Painful ankle (e.g. JIA)
Terminal stance	• Full hip extension • Full knee extension • Allows contralateral limb clearance	• Pelvic lurch due to abductor weakness affects hip stability (Trendelenburg gait) • Psoas spasticity and contracture prevents hip extension, e.g. spastic diplegia	• Leg-length discrepancy (longer leg scuffs the ground or circumducts)
Pre/early swing	• Ankle plantar flexion • Power generation for propulsion	• Weak calf muscle generates less power, e.g. poliomyelitis	• Restricted ankle (e.g. JIA)
Mid swing	• Hip max flexion • Knee max flexion • Ankle dorsiflexion for clearance	• Poor clearance due to tibialis anterior and peronei weakness, e.g. Charcot–Marie–Tooth and other peripheral neuropathies	• Loss of full extension due to inflammatory joint (knee) or muscle (quadriceps) disease
Terminal stance	• Knee extends (allows adequate step length) • Ankle dorsiflexes for heel strike (foot pre-positioning)	• Lack of full extension due to quads weakness, e.g. spastic diplegia • Lack of dorsiflexion range due to weakness, contracture or calf muscle spasticity, e.g. spastic hemiplegia	• Pain inhibition of hip abductors in Legg–Calve–Perthes disease

Table 1.5 Neuromuscular assessment

Component	Risk factors	Examples
History	Prenatal infection or bleeding	Varicella zoster, abruption
	Postnatal special care	Postnatal respiratory distress
	Family history of neuromuscular disorder	Charcot–Marie–Tooth disease
	Deteriorating mobility	Deteriorating gait, fatigue
	Milestones not achieved	Poor head control, not sitting unsupported by age 12 months
Examination	Muscle weakness	
	↑ muscle tone	Spasticity
	Joint contracture	Tip toeing, hamstring tightness
	Bone deformity	Femoral neck anteversion, cavovarus or plano valgus feet
Gait analysis	Abnormal gait	High stepping or crouch gait
	Slow motion playback	Lack of heel strike (calf muscle spasticity)
	Force plate studies	Loss of knee extension (hamstring spasticity)
	Joint motion sensors	Loss of hip extension
	Electromyography	Abnormal muscle contraction

Table 1.6 Abnormal gait patterns seen in musculoskeletal disease

	Description	Potential causes
Antalgic gait	Due to pain on the affected side, where the stance phase (the length of time spent bearing weight) on the affected side is shorter. May present with limp or non-weight-bearing	• Multiple causes and sites, including trauma, sepsis, JIA, Legge–Calve–Perthes disease
Trendelenburg gait	Results from hip abductor muscle weakness and whilst weight-bearing on ipsilateral side, the pelvis drops on contralateral side, rather than rising as is normal With bilateral hip disease—a waddling 'rolling sailor' gait with hips, knees and feet externally rotated. This gait is also observed secondary to painful hip conditions due to pain inhibition of normal muscle activity	• Hip joint disease (e.g. Legge–Calve–Perthes disease, slipped capital femoral epiphysis, developmental dysplasia of the hip, JIA involving the hip) • Muscle disease (juvenile dermatomyositis or inherited myopathies) • Neurologic conditions (spina bifida, cerebral palsy, and spinal cord injury)
Circumduction gait ('peg leg')	A circular movement of the leg with excessive hip abduction as the leg swings forward	• A lack of full knee extension (JIA, trauma)—in JIA may be due to leg-length discrepancy • Unilateral spasticity as in hemiplegic cerebral palsy
Waddling gait	A wide-based gait suggests proximal muscle weakness	• Inflammatory myopathies
Spastic gait	Refers to stiff walking with foot-dragging and the foot inverted	• Upper motor neuron neurologic disease (e.g. diplegic or quadriplegic cerebral palsy, stroke)
Ataxic gait	Due to instability with an alternating narrow to wide base of gait	• Neurological disease (e.g. ataxic cerebral palsy affecting the cerebellum, cerebellar ataxia, and Friedreich's ataxia)
Toe-walking gait ('equinus')	Absent heel contact	• Habitual toe walking (common and associated with normal foot examination and normal walking on request) • Persistent toe walking (spastic upper motor neuron neurologic disease (e.g. diplegic cerebral palsy), JIA, and mild lysosomal storage disorders

Normal gait and musculoskeletal development

- It is important to be aware of normal motor milestones (Table 1.7) and normal variants in gait and leg alignment (see ➲ Normal variants of lower limb development, pp. 9–10).
- Patterns of abnormal gait are important to recognize and are based on understanding of the gait cycle (see ➲ The gait cycle and abnormal gait patterns, p. 11).
- There is considerable variation in the way normal gait patterns develop—such variation may be familial (e.g. 'bottom-shufflers' often walk later) and subject to racial variation (e.g. African black children tend to walk sooner and Asian children later than average).
- The normal toddler has a broad-base gait for support, and appears to be high stepped and flat footed with arms outstretched for balance.
- The legs are externally rotated with a degree of bowing. Heel strike develops around 15–18 months with reciprocal arm swing.
- Running and change of direction occur after the age of 2yr, although this is often accompanied by frequent falls until the child acquires balance and coordination.
- In the school-age child, the step length increases and step frequency slows. Adult gait and posture occur around the age of 8yr.

The approach to investigation

- The approach to investigation is based on the differential diagnosis derived from the clinical setting; details of investigations required and their interpretation are given in this handbook for the various diseases.
- With regard to suspected inflammatory joint disease, it must be remembered that JIA is a diagnosis of exclusion, there is no diagnostic test and pending the clinical scenario the child may undergo multiple tests to confirm the diagnosis (Table 1.8).
- It is important that the child is referred for a paediatric rheumatology assessment as soon as a diagnosis of JIA is suspected and certainly before invasive tests such as arthroscopy or procedures requiring general anaesthetic (e.g. magnetic resonance imaging [MRI] in the young child) are contemplated.
- Delay in making a diagnosis of JIA is well reported and often exacerbated through waiting for procedures that may be unnecessary.

Table 1.7 Normal musculoskeletal development

Sits without support	6–8 months
Creep on hands and knees	9–11 months
Cruise/or bottom shuffle	11–12 months
Walk independently	12–14 months
Climb up stairs on hands and knees	~15 months
Run stiffly	~16 months
Walk down steps (non-reciprocal)	20–24 months
Walk up steps, alternate feet	3yr
Hop on one foot, broad jump	4yr
Skipping	5yr
Balance on one foot for 20sec	6–/yr
Adult gait and posture	8yr

Table 1.8 Investigations in the child with suspected JIA—cautionary notes

FBC and blood film	May be normal in JIA, especially oligo-articular subtype
	Anaemia of chronic disease may be present in polyarticular JIA and systemic onset JIA
	Raised white cell count and raised platelets a feature of systemic onset JIA
	A blood film is helpful to exclude leukaemia but suspicion of this requires a bone marrow examination
Acute phase reactants ESR, CRP	May be raised, and often very high in systemic JIA
Ferritin	May be raised and often extremely high in systemic JIA or macrophage activation syndrome
Antinuclear factor	May be absent in 50% of JIA and may be found in viral illnesses, non-rheumatic disease, and many healthy children as well as connective tissue disease (such as SLE)
	In the presence of JIA, ANA indicates high risk of chronic anterior uveitis, which affects 30% of children with JIA and is potentially blinding if undetected and untreated
Rheumatoid factor	Rarely found in children with JIA (<10% of cases) but associates with poor prognosis
Slit lamp examination	*All children with suspected JIA require prompt referral to ophthalmology for eye screening for uveitis which is invariably asymptomatic in the early stages and if undetected and untreated, can lead to blindness*

Table 1.8 Contd.

Synovial fluid examination	Not required to make a diagnosis of JIA but is mandatory to exclude sepsis in the child with a single hot swollen joint (and any suspicion of tuberculosis)
Arthroscopy and synovial biopsy	Not required to make a diagnosis of JIA. Seldom indicated and not recommended before child has been assessed by a paediatric rheumatologist
Radiographs	May be normal in early JIA—loss of joint space and joint damage occur in severe or untreated disease. Useful to exclude other pathology (and tumour)
Ultrasound	Ultrasonography is sensitive to early changes, is well tolerated by young children, and is increasingly more available
MRI	MRI is sensitive to early changes of inflammatory arthritis but may not be available and in young children invariably requires sedation. Referral to paediatric rheumatology should not be delayed whilst awaiting MRI scanning. Gadolinium contrast should be remembered—often not given to children who have MRI prior to paediatric rheumatology assessment, resulting in need for repeat scans

ANA, antinuclear antibody; CRP, C-reactive protein; ESR, erythrocyte sedimentation rate; FBC, full blood count; MRI, magnetic resonance imaging.

pGALS: paediatric Gait, Arms, Legs, Spine musculoskeletal assessment

- The pGALS musculoskeletal assessment (Box 1.4) is a simple evidence-based approach to examination based on the adult GALS (Gait, Arms, legs, Spine) screen and has been shown to have high sensitivity to detect significant joint abnormalities.
- Key to distinguishing normal from abnormal is knowledge of ranges of movement in different age groups and ethnicity, looking for asymmetry, and careful examination for subtle changes.
- When performing pGALS it is important to understand which joints are being assessed with each movement; many manoeuvres assess several joints at a time and the examiner needs to be aware of identifying the area of abnormality.
- pGALS is primarily aimed at the school-aged child, but younger children will often perform pGALS, especially if they copy the examiner and see this as a game.
- pGALS incorporates a series of simple manoeuvres, takes an average of 2 min to perform, and we provide simple practical tips facilitate the examination (Box 1.5 and Tables 1.9 and 1.10).
- The pGALS assessment includes three questions relating to pain and function although a negative response does *not* exclude significant musculoskeletal disease and at a minimum the examination should be done in all clinical scenarios where musculoskeletal disease is a concern (Box 1.6). The questions may be modified if the child does not get dressed or undressed or walk up and down stairs/steps e.g any problems with squatting or walking?
- It is essential to perform all parts of pGALS as joint involvement may be apparently 'asymptomatic'—symptoms may not be localized, and it is important to check for verbal and non-verbal clues of joint discomfort such as facial expression or withdrawal of limb.
- The information needs to be interpreted in the context of the physical examination elsewhere (e.g. chest, abdomen, neurological examinations in the case of the limping child) or in the presence of any 'red flags' in the unwell child.
- Documentation of findings in the case notes is simple, using a grid (Fig. 1.1).

Box 1.4 The pGALS assessment

Opening questions
- 'Do you (or does your child) have any pain or stiffness in your joints, muscles, or your back?'
- 'Do you have any difficulty getting yourself dressed without any help?'
- 'Do you have any difficulty going up and down stairs?'

Gait
- Observe the child walking.
- 'Walk on your tip-toes/walk on your heels.'

Arms (see Table 1.9)
- 'Put your hands out in front of you.'
- 'Turn your hands over and make a fist.'
- 'Pinch your index finger and thumb together.'
- 'Touch the tips of your fingers with your thumb.'
- Squeeze the metacarpophalangeal joints.
- 'Put your hands together/put your hands back to back.'
- 'Reach up and touch the sky.'
- 'Look at the ceiling.' (*assesses neck*)
- 'Put your hands behind your neck.'

Legs (see Table 1.10)
- Feel for effusion at the knee.
- 'Bend and then straighten your knee' (active movement of knees and examiner feels for crepitus).
- Passive flexion (90°) with internal rotation of hip.

Spine (see Table 1.10)
- 'Open your mouth and put 3 of your [*child's own*] fingers in your mouth.'
- Lateral flexion of cervical spine—'Try and touch your shoulder with your ear.'
- 'Look at the ceiling.'
- Observe the spine from behind.
- 'Can you bend and touch your toes?' Observe curve of the spine from side and behind.

Reproduced with permission from Foster HE, Kay LJ, Friswell M, Coady D, Myers A. pGALS – a paediatric musculoskeletal screening examination for school aged children based on the adult GALS screen. *Arthritis Care & Research*, Volume 55, Issue 5, pp. 709–16, Copyright © 2006 John Wiley and Sons Ltd.

Box 1.5 Practical tips: while performing pGALS
- Get the child to copy you doing the manoeuvres.
- Look for verbal and non-verbal clues of discomfort (e.g. facial expression, withdrawal).
- Do the full pGALS assessment as extent of joint involvement may not be obvious from the history.
- Look for asymmetry (e.g. muscle bulk, joint swelling, range of joint movement).
- Consider clinical patterns (e.g. non-benign hypermobility and Marfanoid habitus or skin elasticity, and association of leg-length discrepancy and scoliosis).

Table 1.9 pGALS incorporates a series of simple manoeuvres

Figure	Manoeuvres	What is being assessed?
	'Touch the tips of your fingers'	• Manual dexterity • Coordination of small joints of fingers and thumbs
	Squeeze the metacarpophalangeal joints for tenderness	• Metacarpophalangeal joints
	'Put your hands together palm to palm' and 'put your hands together back to back'	• Extension of small joints of fingers • Wrist extension • Elbow flexion
	'Reach up, 'touch the sky'' and 'Look at the ceiling'	• Elbow extension • Wrist extension • Shoulder abduction • Neck extension
	'Put your hands behind your neck'	• Shoulder abduction • External rotation of shoulders • Elbow flexion

Table adapted and used with permission by Arthritis Research UK. Figures reproduced with permission from Foster HE, Kay LJ, Friswell M, Coady D, Myers A. pGALS – a paediatric musculoskeletal screening examination for school aged children based on the adult GALS screen. *Arthritis Care & Research*, Volume 55, Issue 5, pp. 709–16; Copyright © 2006 John Wiley and Sons Ltd.

(Continued)

Table 1.9 Contd.

Figure	Manoeuvres	What is being assessed?
	'Try and touch your shoulder with your ear'	• Cervical spine lateral flexion
	'Open wide and put three (*child's own*) fingers in your mouth'	• Temporomandibular joints (and check for deviation of jaw movement)
	Feel for effusion at the knee (patella tap, or crossfluctuation)	• Knee effusion (small effusion may be missed by patella tap alone)
	Active movement of knees (flexion and extension) and feel for crepitus	• Knee flexion • Knee extension
	Passive movement of hip (knee flexed to 90°, and internal rotation of hip)	• Hip flexion and internal rotation
	'Bend forwards and touch your toes'	• Forward flexion of thoraco-lumbar spine (and check for scoliosis)

Table adapted and used with permission by Arthritis Research UK. Figures reproduced with permission from Foster HE, Kay LJ, Friswell M, Coady D, Myers A. pGALS – a paediatric musculoskeletal screening examination for school aged children based on the adult GALS screen. *Arthritis Care & Research*, Volume 55, Issue 5, pp. 709–16, Copyright © 2006 John Wiley and Sons Ltd.

Box 1.6 Practical tips: when to perform pGALS

- Child with muscle, joint, or bone pain.
- Unwell child with pyrexia
- Child with limp
- Delay or regression of motor milestones
- The 'clumsy' child in the absence of neurological disease
- Child with chronic disease and known association with musculoskeletal presentations

Documentation of the pGALS examination

Documentation of the pGALS screening assessment is important and a simple pro forma is proposed with the following example–a child with a swollen left knee with limited flexion of the knee and antalgic gait.

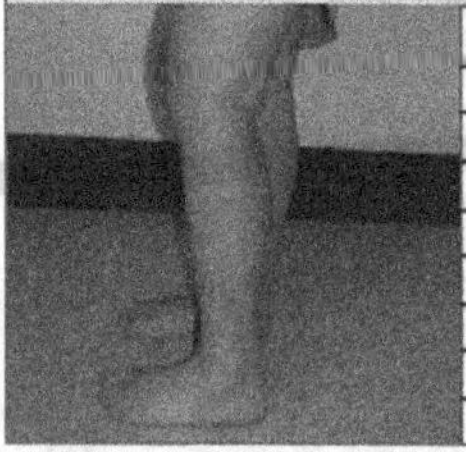

pGALS screening questions		
Any pain?	Left knee	
Problems with dressing?	No difficulty	
Problems with walking?	Some difficulty on walking	
	Appearance	Movement
Gait		✗
Arms	✓	✓
Legs	✗	✗
Spine	✓	✓

Fig. 1.1 Documentation of pGALS findings.

Reproduced with permission from Arthritis Research UK. *pGALS – a screening examination of the musculoskeletal system in school-aged children*, ℞ http://www.arthritisresearchuk.org/shop/products/publications/information-for-medical-professionals/hands-on/series-5/ho15-series-5.aspx, accessed 01 Dec. 2016, Copyright © 2008 Arthritis Research UK.

Further reading and resources

Free educational resources to demonstrate pGALS and the manoeuvres are available:

Paediatric musculoskeletal matters – a free online paediatric musculoskeletal resource approved by BSPAR and produced by Newcastle University, UK; ℞ www.pmmonline.org

Foster HE, Jandial S. pGALS – paediatric Gait, Arms, Legs, Spine. A simple examination of the musculoskeletal system. *Pediatr Rheumatol Online* 2013;11:44

A pGALS app is available and can be downloaded from app stores.

pREMS: paediatric Regional Examination of the Musculoskeletal System

- Detailed musculoskeletal assessment is indicated where the history focusses on a particular area, or if an abnormality is seen on performing pGALS.
- The approach to detailed assessment is based on the 'look, feel, move,' principle described in the adult regional examination of the musculoskeletal system (called REMS), with active movements performed first and then passively by the examiner.
- A paediatric version of REMS (called pREMS) has been developed from observation of clinicians in clinical practice and is the first consensus-based regional musculoskeletal examination for school-aged children.
- pREMS is similar to adult REMS using the same general principles (Box 1.7) although it differs by anatomical region reflecting different pathologies from those observed in adults (Box 1.8).
- Video demonstrations of pREMS for each joint are available on 'paediatric musculoskeletal matters', a free online resource for paediatric musculoskeletal medicine, approved by BSPAR and produced by Newcastle University, UK; www.pmmonline.org

Box 1.7 General principles of pREMS

Introduction
- Introduce yourself to child and parent/carer.
- Explain what you want to examine, gain verbal consent to examine.
- Be aware of normal variants in leg alignment, joint range, gait, developmental milestones.

Look for:
- Swellings, rashes (e.g. psoriasis/vasculitis), muscle wasting, scars, leg-length discrepancy.
- Deformity/dysmorphism/'disproportions'/discomfort (check for non-verbal signs), i.e. non-verbal signals.

Feel for:
- Temperature, swelling, tenderness (along bones and joint line).

Movement
- Full range of movement—active and passive (note any asymmetry).
- Restriction—mild, moderate, or severe.

Function and measure
- Functional assessment of joint/anatomical region to include power of muscles and stability.
- Measurement of height/leg length.

Box 1.8 Examination schedules by anatomical region

The options refer to additional manoeuvres suggested pending common clinical scenarios. Details on the examination techniques used are available (see ➋ 'Further reading', p. 27).

Examination of the hand and wrist

- Inspect hands (palms and backs) for muscle wasting, skin, and nail changes.
- Feel for radial pulse, tendon thickening, and bulk of thenar and hypothenar eminences.
- Feel for skin temperature.
- Squeeze metacarpophalangeal joints (MCPJs).
- Bimanually palpate swollen or painful joints, including wrists.
- Look and feel along ulnar border.
- Assess full finger extension and full finger tuck.
- Assess wrist flexion and extension, abduction and adduction—active and passive.
- Assess function: grip and pinch, picking up small object, writing/drawing.
- Options—assess for hypermobility syndromes, muscle power, capillaroscopy, peripheral neuropathy.

Examination of the elbow

- Look for carrying angle, scars, swellings or rashes, deformity.
- Feel for skin temperature.
- Palpate over head of radius, joint line, medial and lateral epicondyles.
- Assess full flexion and extension, pronation and supination—actively and passively.
- Assess function—e.g. hand to nose or mouth, hands behind head.
- Options—assess for hypermobility syndromes, muscle power, instability tests, entheses.

Examination of the shoulder

With the patient standing or sitting:

- Inspect shoulders, clavicles, and sternoclavicular joints from the front, side, and behind, and assess shoulder height.
- Inspect skin in axillae and palpate for lymphadenopathy.
- Assess skin temperature.
- Palpate bony landmarks and surrounding muscles.
- Assess movement and function: hands behind head, hands behind back.
- Assess (actively and passively) external rotation, flexion, extension, and abduction.
- Observe scapular movement.
- Options—assess for hypermobility syndromes, muscle power, instability.

Box 1.8 *Contd.*
Examination of the hip

With the patient supine lying on couch:
- Look for flexion deformity and leg-length discrepancy.
- Check for scars, rashes.
- Feel the greater trochanter for tenderness.
- Assess full hip flexion, internal and external rotation, abduction and adduction.
- Perform Thomas' test.
- Hip abduction (lying on side).

Patient lying prone on couch:
- Sacroiliac joint palpation.
- Hip internal (and external) rotation.
- Hip extension.

With the patient standing:
- Assess posture and leg alignment.
- Look for gluteal muscle bulk.
- Perform the Trendelenburg test.
- Assess function (gait with turning and running, ancillary movements).
- Options—assess for hypermobility, muscle power, enthesitis, thigh–foot angle (child with in-toeing).

Examination of the knee

With the patient standing:
- Look for varus/valgus deformity, hyperextension, and popliteal swellings.
- Inspect skin for pattern of bruising and rashes.
- Assess gait (see Examination of the hip, this Box).

With the patient lying on couch:
- Look from the end of the couch for varus/valgus deformity, muscle wasting, scars, and swellings.
- Look from the side for fixed flexion deformity.
- Check for passive hyperextension and leg-length discrepancy.
- Feel skin temperature.
- With the knee slightly flexed palpate the joint line and the borders of the patella.
- Feel the popliteal fossa.
- Perform a patellar tap and cross fluctuation (bulge sign).
- Assess full flexion and extension (actively and passively).
- Option: assess stability of knee ligaments—medial and lateral collateral—and perform anterior draw test.
- Option: tests for anterior knee pain/patellar maltracking/apprehension/patella glide.
- Option—assess for hypermobility, enthesitis, hamstring tightness, iliotibial band tightness/thigh–foot angle.

Box 1.8 *Contd.*
Examination of the foot and ankle

With the patient lying supine on couch:
- Look at dorsal and plantar surfaces of the foot.
- Feel the skin temperature.
- Palpate for peripheral pulses.
- Squeeze the MTPJs.
- Palpate the midfoot, ankle joint line, and subtalar joint.
- Assess movement (actively and passively) at the subtalar joint (inversion and eversion), the big toe (dorsi- and plantar flexion), the ankle joint (dorsi- and plantar flexion), and mid-tarsal joints (passive rotation).
- Look at the patient's footwear.
- Option: assess for hypermobility, thigh–foot angle, enthesitis, muscle power, capillaroscopy

With the patient standing:
- Look at the forefoot, midfoot (foot arch), and the hindfoot.
- Assess gait cycle (heel strike, stance, toe off), running and turning, ancillary movement.
- Assess muscle bulk (calves).

Examination of the spine

With the patient standing:
- Inspect from the side and from behind.
- Inspect skin and natal cleft.
- Inspect limb/trunk proportions.
- Inspect facial and jaw profile.
- Palpate the spinal processes and paraspinal muscles and temporomandibular joints (TMJs).
- Assess movement: lumbar flexion and extension and lateral flexion; cervical flexion, extension, rotation and lateral flexion, thoracic rotation.
- Assess TMJ opening.
- Options: Schober's test, 'stork test'.*

With the patient sitting on couch (standing in younger child):
- Assess thoracic rotation.

With the patient lying on couch:
- Perform straight leg raising and dorsi-flexion of the big toe.
- Assess limb reflexes.
- Options: assess for leg-length discrepancy, hypermobility, sacroiliac joint irritation on palpation.

* 'Stork test'—standing on one leg and extension of spine causes pain (suggestive of spondylolysis)—see ➜ Back pain in children and adolescents, pp. 105–7.

Further reading

Paediatric Musculoskeletal Matters—🔗 www.pmmonline.org—a free educational resource about paediatric musculoskeletal medicine produced by Newcastle University, UK

Coady, D, Walker D, Kay L. Regional Examination of the Musculoskeletal System (REMS): a core set of clinical skills for medical students. *Rheumatology* 2004;**43**(5):633–9.

Foster HE, Kay L, May CR, *et al*. pREMS—a consensus approach to pediatric regional musculoskeletal examination. *Arthritis Care Res* 2011; **63**(11):1503–10.

Clinical skills in the evaluation of arthritis Szer IS. Malleson PN. *Arthritis in Children and Adolescents* Eds Szer, Kimura, Malleson and Southwood. Oxford University Press 2006; 3–18.

Houghton KM. Review for the generalist: evaluation of anterior knee. *Pediatr Rheumatol* 2007;**5**:8. 🔗 http://www.ped-rheum.com/content/pdf/1546-0096-5-8.pdf.

Houghton KM. Review for the generalist: evaluation of pediatric foot and ankle pain. *Pediatr Rheumatol* 2008;**6**:6. 🔗 http://www.ped-rheum.com/content/pdf/1546-0096-6-6.pdf.

Houghton KM. Review for the generalist: evaluation of pediatric hip pain. *Pediatr Rheumatol* 2009;**7**:10. 🔗 http://www.ped-rheum.com/content/pdf/1546-0096-7-10.pdf.

Houghton KM. Review for the generalist: evaluation of low back pain in children and adolescents. *Pediatr Rheumatol* 2010;**8**:28. 🔗 http://www.ped-rheum.com/content/pdf/1546-0096-8-28.pdf.

Staheli, L.T. *Fundamentals of Pediatric Orthopedics—Foot and lower limb*. Philadelphia, PA: Lippincott-Raven, 2008.

Imaging in juvenile idiopathic arthritis

Imaging is commonly used in the diagnosis and follow-up of children with rheumatological problems, to assess disease activity, monitor progression and identify treatment response. Imaging is a valuable adjunct to clinical examination and plays a key role in guiding management. Ultrasound (US) and magnetic resonance imaging (MRI) are the modalities of choice to identify early inflammation, having different strengths and weaknesses (Table 1.10).

Plain film radiographs

- Radiographs demonstrate late, potentially irreversible, destructive changes (Fig. 1.2).
- Radiographs also show complications unique to the paediatric skeleton, such as epiphyseal overgrowth and premature physeal fusion.

Table 1.10 Strengths and weaknesses of different imaging modalities in the assessment of paediatric rheumatological conditions

	Strengths	Weaknesses
Plain film radiographs	Cheap and readily available Images are easily comparable to chart progression	Demonstrates late manifestations Relatively insensitive in the early stages Exposure to ionizing radiation
US	Readily available Short well-tolerated examinations Non invasive Excellent assessment of soft tissue inflammation, synovitis, tenosynovitis, tendonopathy, bursitis, joint effusion Guided injections or aspiration of fluid Dynamic assessment whilst moving the joint	Operator dependent and thus comparison with previous studies may also be difficult Unable to assess bone oedema Poor assessment of deeper structures
MRI	Excellent assessment of soft tissue inflammation, synovitis, tenosynovitis, tendonopathy, bursitis, joint effusion Able to detect bone marrow oedema Less operator dependent	Expensive Limited availability Long examinations May require general anaesthetic/sedation Invasive, often requiring intravenous cannulation

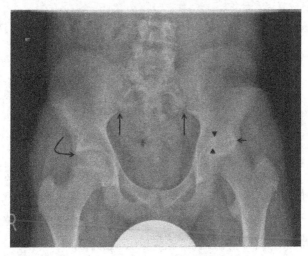

Fig. 1.2 Plain film radiograph of an adolescent patient with previous inflammatory arthropathy of the left hip, demonstrating erosions and secondary degenerative changes, characterized by joint space narrowing (short straight arrow) and subchondral sclerosis (arrowheads). Note the normal joint space of the right hip (curved arrow) and the normal sacroiliac joints (long straight arrows).

Ultrasound

- Ultrasound machines are user friendly and with some practice one can develop a systematic approach to produce easily recognizable images. Familiarity with the individual ultrasound machine is essential and attendance at an ultrasound course is required to enable accurate interpretation of the images acquired.
- The ultrasound probe both transmits and receives high frequency sound. The amount of sound reflected back by a structure is represented by the brightness of the image. 'Grey scale' refers to the processed image displayed. Hypoechoic (black) areas of the image represent cartilage and fluid. Pressure with the ultrasound probe allows discrimination of compressible fluid from non-compressible cartilage. Hyperechoic (bright) areas are seen typically at the edges of bone or other foci of calcification. Intermediate (grey) areas of the image represent soft tissue such as muscle, tendon, and synovial tissue (Fig. 1.3).
- Power Doppler signal represents blood flow. Abnormal synovial blood flow represents synovitis. However, power Doppler signal is prone to artefact, for example excess pressure on the ultrasound probe will eliminate abnormal blood flow from the synovium. Normal nutrient arteries may mimic synovitis, and comparison with the contralateral side is often helpful.

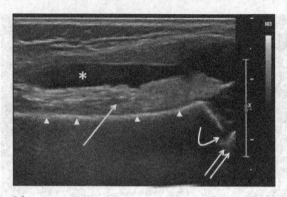

Fig. 1.3 Ultrasound of the knee in a 3-year-old girl with active inflammatory arthritis. Hypoechoic fluid distension of the suprapatellar pouch of the knee (asterix). Thickened synovium (arrow) is seen between the joint fluid and the anterior cortex of the femur, the hyper-reflective linear at the deepest aspect of the image (arrow heads). Note the normal appearances of the physeal cleft (curved arrow) between the metaphysis of the femur and the distal epiphysis (double arrow).

- Scans are usually performed assessing structures along both their longitudinal and transverse axes.
- Low frequency probes (5–10Hz) are used for large or deep areas such as the hip; however, spatial resolution is poor. High frequency probes (10–15Hz) should be used for small joints and superficial structures as they offer better spatial resolution; however, penetration is limited. Machines with a 'hockey-stick' probe are particularly useful for assessing the small joints of children.

Magnetic resonance imaging

- MRI is extremely sensitive for the detection of early inflammatory change involving the synovium, bone marrow, and cartilage.
- A typical study utilizes T1-weighted sequences to identify bone marrow oedema and the presence of erosions, both of which are low signal. Fluid-weighted sequences, in which fluid and oedema are bright, include T2, STIR, and proton density weighted sequences. Fluid-weighted sequences are used to identify joint effusions, synovial inflammation, tenosynovitis, cartilage lesions and bone marrow oedema (Fig. 1.4).
- Gadolinium-based contrast agents are employed with T1-weighted sequences, usually incorporating fat saturation. Areas with high blood flow are high signal on such sequences. The use of a contrast agent demonstrates synovial enhancement in synovitis, allowing differentiation of synovitis from a joint effusion, both of which give similar high signal on unenhanced imaging.

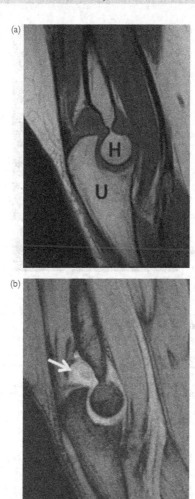

Fig. 1.4 (a) T1w sequence. (b) STIR sequence. (c) T1FS + contrast

MRI of the elbow in a teenager with inflammatory arthropathy. The T1 weighted sequence shows distension of the joint capsule with low signal material. The alignment between the trochlea of the distal humerus (H) and the proximal ulna (U) is maintained and there is no erosive change. The STIR sequence shows that the joint is distended with material of high water content (white arrow), but this imaging is unable to discriminate synovitis from joint effusion. No bone marrow oedema. The use of contrast material in Fig 3c demonstrates enhancing thickened synovitis (arrowhead) with central non-enhancing fluid (black arrow) of a joint effusion.

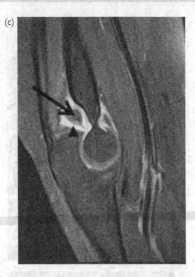

Fig. **1.4** *Contd.*

Further reading

British Society for Rheumatology ultrasound courses: ℘ http://www.rheumatology.org.uk/education.

EULAR musculoskeletal imaging and courses: ℘ http://www.eular.org.

Colebatch-Bourn *et al.* EULAR-PReS Points to consider for the use of imaging in the diagnosis and management if JIA in clinical practice *Ann Rheum Dis* 2015;**74**:1946–1957.

McNally EG. *Practical Musculoskeletal Ultrasound.* Philadelphia, PA: Elsevier, 2005.

Muller LO, Humphries P, Rosendahl, K. The joints in juvenile idiopathic arthritis. *Insights Imaging* 2015; **6**:275–284.

Wakefield RJ, D'Agostino MA. *Essential Applications of Musculoskeletal Ultrasound in Rheumatology.* Philadelphia, PA: Saunders, 2010.

Autoantibodies

Antibodies are immunoglobulins produced in response to an antigen and form an important part of the adaptive immune system and our humoral response to infection. Autoantibodies are formed in response to self-antigens. The presence of autoantibodies does not imply or inevitably result in autoimmune diseases, although in some autoimmune diseases the associated antibodies are directly involved in the pathogenesis, e.g. anti-glomerular basement membrane (GBM) disease, myasthenia gravis, and anti-neutrophil cytoplasmic antibody (ANCA)-associated vasculitides. This section describes some of the important and/or frequently observed autoantibodies in paediatric rheumatology.

Anti-neutrophil cytoplasmic antibodies

(see ➔ The ANCA-associated vasculitides, pp. 196–200)

- Antibodies against lysosomal enzymes in neutrophils and (to a lesser extent) monocytes.
- The main enzymes targeted are myeloperoxidase (MPO) and proteinase 3 (PR3); however, other antigens may also be targeted.
- There are 2 main patterns of staining detectable by indirect immunofluorescence: perinuclear (pANCA) and cytoplasmic (cANCA).
- About 90% of cANCA is directed against PR3 (PR3-ANCA) and 70% of pANCA is against MPO (MPO-ANCA).
- PR3-ANCA is commonly seen in Granulomatosis with Polyangiitis (GPA); although it can be detected in some cases of microscopic polyangiitis (MPA).
- MPO-ANCA is typically associated with:
  - Microscopic polyangiitis
  - Eosinophilic granulomatosis with polyangiitis (EGPA; formerly known as Churg–Strauss syndrome) (occasional)
  - Idiopathic renal limited pauci-immune glomerulonephritis.
- ANCAs are not 100% specific for the ANCA-associated vasculitides: they can also be positive in chronic infections or malignancy including tuberculosis, HIV, and Hodgkin's lymphoma. Atypical ANCA (BPI-ANCA) are sometimes observed in cystic fibrosis, and are not necessarily associated with vasculitis in that scenario.
- Atypical pANCA are detected in some forms of inflammatory bowel disease and may be associated with sclerosing cholangitis, and can also be drug induced.

Antinuclear antibodies (ANAs)

- ANAs are directed against the cell's nuclear contents. Titres vary between laboratories but are usually reported to be 'positive' at 1:40–1:80. In clinical practice titres may be significant at 1:320 or higher.
- A positive ANA titre alone is not diagnostic of a specific condition, nor is ANA necessarily a useful screening test for autoimmune disease. A positive ANA can be found in up to 15% of normal children.
- A positive ANA can be associated with a variety of conditions including:
  - SLE
  - Drug-induced lupus

- Undifferentiated connective tissue disease
- Sjögren's syndrome
- Juvenile dermatomyositis
- Scleroderma and systemic sclerosis
- Morphoea
- JIA, particularly those who have (or may develop) uveitis.
- Positive ANA is rare in systemic juvenile idiopathic arthritis (sJIA).
- ANA can also occur in immunoglobulin A (IgA) deficiency, viral infections, and neoplasias, and may also be drug-induced.

Anti ds-DNA antibodies

These autoantibodies are highly specific for SLE and are seen in the majority of children with lupus nephritis. Titres can be useful in monitoring disease activity; however, they do not always correlate with disease activity in all patients.

Rheumatoid factor and anti-cyclic citrullinated protein (anti-CCP) antibodies

- Classic RF is IgM directed against IgG. RFs of other immunoglobulin isotypes have been reported but their significance is uncertain.
- <10% of children with JIA are RF+ve. Those who are positive are usually older girls with a polyarticular disease course.
- RF can also be positive in SLE and in a minority of patients with systemic sclerosis.
- RF may also be elevated as an acute phase reactant, e.g. in bacterial endocarditis, and so a positive result should be confirmed by repeating.
- Anti-CCP antibodies are also found in children with RF+ve polyarthritis.
  - Anti-CCP antibodies are less prevalent in JIA than adult RA but are detectable in a significant proportion of RF+ve patients with polyarticular-onset JIA.
  - There may be a significant relation between anti-CCP positivity and erosive joint disease in polyarticular RF+ve JIA.

Antiphospholipid antibodies

(see ➔ Antiphospholipid syndrome (APS), pp. 293–6)
- These are a heterogeneous group of antibodies which bind to phospholipids in the cell membrane and include IgG and IgM anticardiolipin (ACL) Ab, and beta 2-glycoprotein 1 antibodies. The lupus anticoagulant (LAC) is typically measured using the dilute Russell viper venom assay (see ➔ Antiphospholipid syndrome (APS), pp. 293–6).
- May be positive in 1° antiphospholipid syndrome, SLE, some vasculitides, viral infections (often associated with transient ACL positivity), drug induced, and up to 8% of the normal population.
- Not all ACL are pathogenic, nor is the mechanism of ACL pathogenicity fully understood. This is an area of ongoing research.

Anti-C1q antibodies

- Cause low C1q and are seen in almost all patients with hypocomplementaemic urticarial vasculitic syndrome (HUVS), but also in a variety of other autoimmune conditions such as SLE.

Extractable nuclear antigens (ENAs)
- A number of ENAs have been identified. In fact not all ENAs are truly nuclear; some can be directed against cytoplasmic components. The following may be present in paediatric rheumatology patients (Table 1.11).

Other autoantibodies
- There are many other organ-specific and non-organ-specific autoantibodies associated with paediatric autoimmune disease beyond the scope of this chapter.
- These include antibodies against components of the nephron and lung (notably anti-GBM antibodies); renal tubules; striated muscle (see ➔ JDM Chapter 4 pp. 280–7); endocrine and reproductive organs; components of the brain (associated with the emerging and increasingly described autoimmune encephalopathies; see Table 1.12); peripheral nervous system (including myasthenia gravis); the gastrointestinal tract; skin; and many others.
- Not all of these fulfil Koch's postulates as the defined cause of the disease, although some are directly involved in the pathogenesis of the associated disease.
- Increasingly, paediatric rheumatologists are asked to provide advice in relation to suspected or proven autoimmune brain disease. Table 1.12 provides a brief (non-exhaustive) description of more commonly described brain autoantibodies and their commonly associated symptoms.

Table 1.11 Common ENAs in paediatric rheumatology

Antibody	Common disease association
Anti-RNP	Mixed connective tissue disease (MCTD), SLE, scleroderma
Anti-histone	Drug-induced lupus
Anti-Smith	SLE—possible association with central nervous system (CNS) disease when present along with anti RNP
SS-A/anti-Ro SSB/anti-La	SLE, Sjögren's syndrome Anti-Ro and anti-La are associated with recurrent spontaneous abortions, heart block in neonatal lupus, and may be detectable in ANA−ve lupus.
Anti-SCL-70	Diffuse systemic sclerosis.
Anti-centromere	Systemic sclerosis and related disorders; may be associated with an increased risk of developing calcinosis and telangiectasia. May be a risk factor for developing pulmonary hypertension, gastrointestinal involvement, and Raynaud's phenomenon.
Anti-LKM	Some forms of autoimmune hepatitis
Smooth muscle antibodies	Post-viral infection; some forms of autoimmune hepatitis

Table 1.12 Brain autoantibodies and their disease/symptom association

Brain autoantibody/syndrome	Common symptoms
Anti N methyl-D-aspartate receptor (NMDAR) encephalitis	Cortico-subcortial encephalopathy with psychiatric features, dyskinesias, mutism, reduced conscious level and occasionally limbic encephalitis
Voltage gated potassium channel (VGKC)-complex: mainly LGI1-Abs	Limbic encephalitis with amnesia, seizures, psychiatric disturbance, facio-brachial dystonic seizures
Voltage gated potassium channel (VGKC)-complex: mainly CASPR2-Abs	Morvan's phenotype with confusion, amnesia, insomnia, autonomic dysfunction, neuromyotonia, and pain
AMPAR-Ab limbic encephalitis	Limbic encephalitis (amnesiac, seizures); psychosis
GABA-R-Ab limbic encephalitis	Limbic encephalitis with prominent seizures
GlyR-Ab associated disorders	Combinations of startle (hyperekplexia), stiffness, rigidity, brainstem disturbance, occasionally seizures
Glutamic acid decarboxylase (GAD)- Ab limbic encephalitis	Temporal lobe epilepsy with mild cognitive involvement
Anti- myelin oligodendrocyte glycoprotein (MOG)-Abs	Monophasic or relapsing demyelinating disease
Anti-aquaporin-4 (AQP4)-Ab	Neuromyelitis optica (NMO): single or recurrent attacks of optic neuritis, myelitis, or brain/brainstem disease.

LGI1: leucine rich glioma inactivated 1; AMPAR: AMPA receptor; GABA-R: GABA receptor; GlyR: glycine receptor; CASPR2 contactin associated protein 2.

Further reading

Hacohen Y et al. Paediatric autoimmune encephalopathies: clinical features, laboratory investigations and outcomes in patients with or without antibodies to known central nervous system autoantigens. J Neurol Neurosurg Psychiatry 2013;84:748–755.

Thermography in rheumatic disease

Introduction

Thermography is a non-invasive technique able to detect infrared radiation and provide an image of the temperature distribution across the body surface. The skin temperature is influenced by the skin vasculature or by the conduction of heat generated in structures deeper to the skin surface and this can be detected by thermography.

Indications

- Assessment of inflamed joints.
- Response to cold challenge of the hands in Raynaud's phenomenon.
- Detection of disease activity and monitoring of treatment in scleroderma.

Preparation

- The environmental temperature should be 22–24°C.
- Patients should remove their clothing from the area to be examined for at least 15 min prior to examination to balance the body temperature with the environment.
- The infrared camera should be allowed to acclimatize with the room temperature and be calibrated.

Techniques

- The infrared camera should be focused and the distance from the camera to patient should be recorded.
- A thermograph (static, single image) of the relevant lesion is taken.
- For comparison, images of the matching opposite site or surrounding skin are also taken.

Images and interpretation

- Images are analysed for skin asymmetries with corresponding opposite sites or surrounding skin. Lesions are considered active (or positive) on thermography and appear red when the affected area is more than 0.5°C warmer than the matching opposite limb or body site. Alternatively this can be 0.5°C warmer than the surrounding skin if bilateral sites are involved.
- In Fig. 1.5 the lesion on the right leg as indicated by the 3 arrowheads was clinically causing limb-length discrepancy. The corresponding thermal image prior to treatment shows ↑ temperature on the affected area representing an active lesion.
- Thermography can also be used after the onset of treatment, in which you would expect to see cooling of the initial 'hot', active lesion.

Limitations

- Changes in heat conduction through the skin from deep tissues in lesions associated with extensive subcutaneous atrophy can lead to 'false-positive' thermograms so older scleroderma lesions can often appear 'active' despite their clinical inactivity.
- Thermography is only a substitute measure of blood flow, laser Doppler techniques provides a direct measure of blood flow.

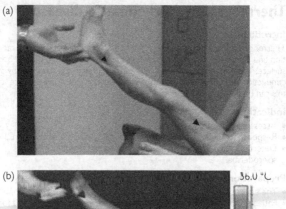

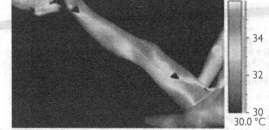

Fig. 1.5 (a) Clinical and (b) thermographic images of a patient with linear morphoea.

Nailfold capillaroscopy in rheumatic disease

Introduction

- Nailfold capillaroscopy is a useful, non-invasive investigation.
- Morphological changes of the finger nailfold capillaries (NFCs) can be directly visualized with magnification and appear to reflect microvascular abnormalities in many rheumatological conditions.
- Nailfold capillaroscopy can be employed when clinical features suggest an underlying connective tissue disease (CTD) or vasculopathy (Table 1.13).

Preparation

- The environmental temperature should be 20–24°C.
- Both hands must be uncovered at least 30 min before the examination to balance the body temperature with the environment.
- Place a drop of water, immersion oil, or aqua gel over the edge of the nailfold and look through this to reduce the reflections of the keratin layer.

Techniques

- Hand-held ophthalmoscope:
  - Set the magnification (dioptres) to at least +20 or preferably +40.
  - Use the 'non-ophthalmoscope' hand to hold the patient's fingertip and bring the ophthalmoscope to within about 0.5cm of the nailfold with the drop of fluid (typically KY-jelly) on it.

Table 1.13 When to consider nailfold capillaroscopy

Underlying cause	Clinical features
Non-specific/constitutional	Fever, anorexia, nausea, lethargy, easy fatiguability, non-specific pain, weakness
Raynaud's phenomenon (RP)	Primary Raynaud's disease: if RP occur in the absence of a definable underlying disease
	Secondary Raynaud's syndrome: if RP is associated with a connective tissue disease/vasculopathy
Juvenile dermatomyositis (JDM)	Muscle weakness, heliotrope rash, Gottron's papules
Progressive systemic sclerosis/scleroderma	Raynaud's syndrome, peripheral skin tightening and ulceration, respiratory symptoms, abdominal pain, malabsorption
Other vasculopathy/vasculitis	(Although many do not appear to have prominent nailfold capillaroscopy abnormalities)
SLE and undifferentiated CTD	Fever, malaise, joint pain, myalgia, fatigue, malar rash

- Small adjustments in the distance between the ophthalmoscope head and the nailfold will bring the capillaries into sharp focus.
- Hand-held dermatoscope:
  - Easier to use than a hand-held ophthalmoscope and can be attached to a digital camera, but does not give as much magnification (×10)
  - 2 types: either an oil immersion (technique as for ophthalmoscope) or cross-polarized dermatoscope which can be placed directly on the nailfold.
- Direct capillaroscopy using a dissecting stereomicroscope (such as an Olympus SZ-40).

Images and interpretation

Six parameters aid more precise definition:

- Capillary density, capillary width, capillary tortuosity, visible avascular areas, capillary disarrangement, number of abnormal vessels (Fig. 1.6a–e).

Healthy children (HC) have a lower density of capillaries than healthy adults (HA) (Fig. 1.7). JDM and scleroderma (grouped as CTD) demonstrate significantly reduced capillary density compared with HC and other childhood rheumatological diseases (JIA, SLE, primary Raynaud's disease (RD), and vasculitis).

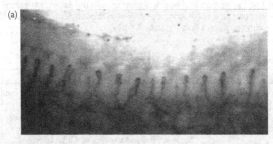

Fig. 1.6 (a) Nailfold capillaries. Normal pattern of NFCs (original magnification ×66). Regular pattern of thin 'hairpin' loops. There is an uncommon normal anatomical variation where the capillaries loop more vertically up towards the surface of the skin, so the horizontal 'hairpin' appearance may not always be seen. (b) Naked eye view. Note the tiny red dots on the nailfolds. (c) Hand-held ophthalmoscope at +40 dioptres. Note irregular size and pattern of capillaries. (d) Abnormal NFCs (original magnification ×66). Dilated capillaries with reduced number in the field of view. (e) Abnormal NFCs (original magnification ×66). Abnormal 'bushy' shapes and bare areas suggesting capillary drop out.

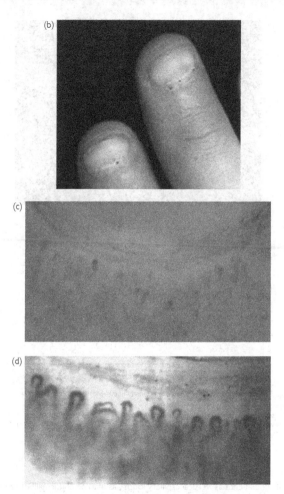

Fig. 1.6 *Contd.*

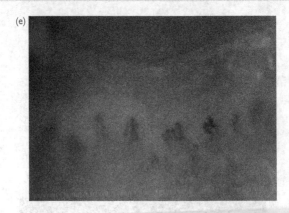

Fig. 1.6 Contd.

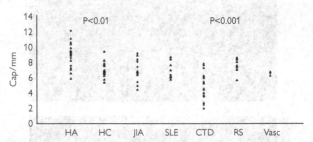

Fig. 1.7 Differences in nailfold capillary density in childhood rheumatic diseases.

Reproduced with permission from Dolezalova P, Young SP, Bacon PA, et al. Nailfold capillary microscopy in healthy children and in childhood rheumatic diseases: a prospective single blind observational study. *Annals of Rheumatic Disease*, Volume 62, Issue 5, pp. 444–9, Copyright © 2003 BMJ Publishing Ltd.

Limitations
- If the patient has 'vertical capillary loops', as marked abnormalities can only be visualized if present in the horizontal plane.
- Fingernail/cuticle biters may traumatize the nailfold and disrupt the capillary appearance.
- It is unclear whether nailfold capillaroscopy is useful for disease monitoring. Some patients with a previous CTD may continue to have abnormal NFCs for years after disease remission.

Outcome measures in paediatric rheumatology

The paediatric rheumatic disorders and their treatments can significantly compromise quality of life (QoL). The accurate assessment of disease outcomes is key to understanding the impact of the disease on the individual child, as well as standardizing clinical research and enabling outcomes-based commissioning of clinical services. However, the heterogeneous nature of rheumatic disorders and the normal developmental changes of childhood ensure that no single measure can reliably capture overall disease outcomes. Measures of disease activity and pain guide immediate intervention, but broader holistic assessments of mental, physical, family, and social functioning, life satisfaction, and well-being capture more information about the impact of the disease on the patient and family.

Composite disease activity scores incorporate multiple domains within a single measurement and are more precise than their individual components. With this in mind, there has been a concerted and important international effort to develop and validate outcome instruments specific to paediatric rheumatic disorders in recent years. Since there is a degree of subjectivity, each measure has to be reliable (repeatable on more than one occasion), valid (ask the right questions), and responsive (sensitive to true changes in patient's condition to guide effective care). A summary of the outcome measure often used in paediatric rheumatology is given in Table 1.14.

Core outcome variables

Core outcome variables (core sets of variables central to the assessment of disease activity) have been established for JIA, juvenile SLE, and juvenile dermatomyositis (Table 1.14). The core set variables have been used to develop response criteria for use in therapeutic trials, e.g. the definition of improvement in JIA (the so-called ACR paediatric 30, 50, and 70 response criteria). More recently, the core set variables have been used to develop composite disease activity scores, quantifying the absolute level of disease activity at a single point in time. For example, the juvenile arthritis disease activity score (JADAS) comprises the sum of active joint count (AJC), physician global, parent global, and ESR. Finally, a number of internationally agreed definitions of disease status (e.g. high disease activity, minimal disease activity, and inactive disease) aim to simplify the monitoring of disease activity over time and inform changes to the therapeutic regime.

Interpretation of outcome measures

Interpretation of outcome measures needs to consider a child's changing cognitive skills, needs, and expectations and a parent's physical and emotional well-being, relationships, and adjustment. Parents are used as proxy respondents and the level of parent/child agreement varies for disability, pain, and QoL measurements. Adolescents may be less positive than parents about health and well-being. Parent and physician reports tend to agree in 70% of cases with over-rating by parents in 20% (typically due to pain intensity) and over-rating by physician in 12% (typically rated to CRP and a number of active joints). Other problems include ceiling and floor effect,

Table 1.14 Outcome measures in paediatric rheumatology

Outcome measure	Definition	Comments
JIA (disease activity and damage assessments)		
ACR Core outcome variables (COV)	Active Joint Count (AJC) Limited Joint Count (LJC) Physician global (PhysGA) (10cm VAS) Parent global (PGA) ESR / CRP CHAQ	
Definition of improvement	ACR Pedi30: 3 of any 6 of the core set criteria improved by at least 30% with no more than 1 worsening by > 30%	Describes change in disease activity over time. More significant levels of improvement at the 30%, 70%, 90% level (ACR Pedi50, Pedi70, Pedi90), are also employed as outcome measures in interventional trials.
Definition of disease flare	Three of any 6 of the core set criteria worsening by at least 30% with no more than 1 improving by greater than 30%. Contingencies: If the AJC/LJC are included, there must be at least a 2 joint increase. If the physician or parent global scales are included, there must be at least a 2cm worsening (0–10cm scale). For systemic onset JIA: fever spikes >38°C for at least 2 of the preceding 7 days not due to infection.	Describes change in disease activity over time. Integral to the innovative design of randomized double blind controlled withdrawal trials, allowing all children access to the trial drug from point of entry to trial.
Juvenile arthritis disease activity score (JADAS)	Linear sum of 4 components: 1) AJC assessed in 1 of 3 ways: JADAS-10: any involved joint (max ten) JADAS-27: 27 joints including cervical spine, elbows, wrists, 1st–3rd metacarpophalangeals, proximal interphalangeals, hips, knees and ankles JADAS-71: 71 joint count 2) Physician global (10cm VAS) 3) Parent global (10cm VAS) 4) ESR/CRP* *ESR normalized on a 0–10 scale using the following formula to avoid excessive weight in the overall index: [ESR(mm/hr) – 20]/10	Describes disease activity at a single point in time. Allows comparison of current disease activity or responsiveness between 2 patients or 2 groups of patients. The 3 variable JADAS (JADAS3 or cJADAS) may be more feasible in the clinical setting.

Table 1.14 Contd.

Outcome measure	Definition	Comments
JADAS response criteria for JIA	Oligoarticular disease course: Inactive Disease (ID) Minimal Disease Activity (MDA) Polyarticular disease course: ID = 1, MDA = 3.8	May be used to monitor the disease course over time, enabling tighter disease control and treatment towards clinical targets. Similar response criteria have been developed for the 3 variable cJADAS
ACR criteria for clinical inactive disease (CID)	No joints with active arthritis No fever, rash, serositis, splenomegaly or generalized lymphadenopathy attributable to JIA No active uveitis as defined by the SUN working group ESR/CRP within normal limits or, if elevated, not attributable to JIA Physician Global (PhysGA) best possible on scale used Duration of morning stiffness ≤ 15min	All criteria must be met. Allows remission to be used as an end point in JIA clinical trials.
Criteria for inactive disease and clinical remission	On medication: criteria for inactive disease met for at least 6 consecutive months on medication. Off medication: criteria for inactive disease met for at least 12 consecutive months off medication.	
Minimal disease activity	Oligoarticular JIA: PhysGA ≤ 2.5cm and no swollen joints Polyarticular JIA: PGA ≤ 3.4cm, PGE ≤ 2.1cm, maximum of one swollen joint	
Juvenile arthritis damage index (JADI)	Assesses articular (36 joints) and extra-articular (5 organs including eyes) damage	Not employed routinely in clinical practice.

Table 1.14 Contd.

Outcome measure	Definition	Comments
JSLE (disease activity and damage assessments)		
British Isles Lupus Assessment Group index (BILAG)	Scoring based on the physicians intention to treat and used in association with biological data and global assessments.	An assessment of disease activity can be used serially in the clinical setting or clinical studies/clinical trials. BILAG has been adapted for paediatric use. An alternative is to use SLEDAI, SLAM or ECLAM (see ➔ British Isles Lupus Assessment Group (BILAG) 2004 Index, p. 262 and Table 4.11)
Systemic Lupus International Collaborative Clinics (SLICC)	See lupus section (➔ SLICC/ACR Damage Index (paediatric), p. 272)	Usually performed annually.
JDM (disease activity and damage assessments)		
Measurement of muscle strength (MMT8)	Tests strength of 8 muscle groups.	Measurement of muscle strength. (see ➔ JDM pp. 280–7)
Childhood myositis assessment scale (CMAS)	14-item quantitative assessment of muscle strength and endurance. Used in JDM along with global assessments of activity and CHAQ	Measurement of muscle function. Scored out of 53. Requires trained personnel. Manual myometry testing may be an alternative (see ➔ Juvenile dermatomyositis, pp. 280–7)
JDM PRINTO core dataset	1) Physician global assessment 2) Parent global assessment 3) Muscle strength (MMT, CMAS) 4) Function (CHAQ) 5) Global disease activity tool (DAS) 6) HR QOL score (CHQ)	Can be difficult to use in routine clinical practice. An alternative is the IMACS core dataset. A provisional JDM minimal dataset has been developed to provide a minimum standard of care and inform future research.
Paediatric vasculitis (disease activity and damage assessments)		
Paediatric vasculitis activity score (PVAS)	Scoring based on the physicians intention to treat	Adapted from the adult BVAS (Birmingham Vasculitis Activity Score) tool and validity is being assessed

Table 1.14 Contd.

Outcome measure	Definition	Comments
Paediatric vasculitis damage index (pVDI)	Cumulative index of items persisting for 3 months or more	Adapted from VDI and validity is being assessed
Physical function		
Childhood health assessment questionnaire (CHAQ)	Standard tool. Takes 10min to complete 8 domains, focusing on disability and discomfort. Easy to score and interpret	Translated in to many languages. Forms for child (8–19yr) & parent (patient 2–19yr). Insensitive to short term changes in children.
Juvenile arthritis functional assessment scale (JAFAS)	Comprehensive assessment of function in children >7yr using 10 timed tasks	Requires standardized equipment and trained health professionals. Responsiveness not known.
Juvenile arthritis functional assessment report (JAFAR)	23-item evaluation of both child (>7yr) and parent reports	
Juvenile arthritis functionality scale (JAFS)	Short 15-item questionnaire of function in lower limbs, hand/wrist and upper segment.	Responsive and discriminative.
Functional status measure FSII (R)	Health status (eating, play behaviour, sleep, and emotional health) of children 0–16yr.	
Child activity limitations interview (CALI)	Assesses impairment due to recurrent pain in school age children and adolescents.	
Health status and quality of life		
Child health questionnaire (CHQ)	Domains in health perception, function, behaviour, mental health, impact on parents, family cohesion, limitations in family activity, activities with friends, change in health, bodily pain, school, work, self-esteem. Age range 5–18 yrs	Adapted from the SF-36. Sensitive to clinical change in children with JIA. Time consuming to complete.
Paediatric Quality of Life Inventory (PedsQoL)	A quick (23-item) measure for healthy and sick children aged 2–18yr assessing physical, emotional, social and school functioning.	Versions for both parents and children. A PedsQL rheumatology module takes 10–15min.

Table 1.14 Contd.

Outcome measure	Definition	Comments
Juvenile arthritis quality of life questionnaire (JAQQ)	Disease specific measure of physical and psychosocial function.	Useful in adolescents.
KIDSCREEN	A cross-cultural multidimensional construct covering physical, emotional, mental, social, and behavioural components of well-being and function as perceived by patients and parents. Age range 8–18yrs.	A comprehensively validated QoL tool with recently developed shorter versions including one of 10 items that takes 5min to complete.
EQ-5D-Y	The youth version (ages 0 10yrs) of the preference-based EuroQoL includes 5 domains and a visual analogue scale for self related health.	A quick QoL tool with good overlap and correlation with the adult tool.
CHU-9D	A preference based PROM for patients aged 7–17yrs that allows weighting of 9 questions covering emotions, participation, sleep and pain	A quick QoL tool that allows economic evaluation.

e.g. a patient may continue to improve or deteriorate but the test does not capture this change.

Physicians, parents, and children frequently disagree in the assessment of disease activity, implying that there are aspects of the disease and its treatment that cannot be captured by clinicians or researchers. Patient-reported outcome measures (PROMs) provide a detailed insight from the patient and/or family of the impact of the disease and its treatment on the overall well-being and quality of life of the child. PROMs are important outcomes in clinical studies and clinical trials, with the potential to improve the evaluation of routine clinical care pathways.

A subgroup of these measures are preference-based PROMs, which can be used for quality-adjusted life years. These tools allow weighting of outcomes according to patient group preferences. For example, the impact on schooling may be more important than absolute AJC. These measures include EuroQoL 5D Youth and Child Health Utility 9D, and like other PROMs have not been adequately tested in the general population for responsiveness and generally show poor proxy-reliability.

Recent collaborative efforts have worked towards a consensus-based approach to datasets useful in clinical practice and to address service evaluation and to facilitate research opportunities. CAPTURE JIA has been developed in the UK (Thomson W et al., paper in progress) and testing in practice is in progress; CAPTURE (Consensus [derived], Accessible [information], Patient [focused], Team [Focused], Universally [collected (UK)], Relevant [to all], Essential [data items].

Further reading

Brunner HI, Ravelli A. Developing outcome measures for paediatric rheumatic diseases. *Best Pract Res Clin Rheumatol* 2009;23;609–624.

McErlane F, Beresford MW, Baildam EM *et al*. Recent developments in disease activity indices and outcome measures for juvenile idiopathic arthritis. *Rheumatology* 2013;52:1941–51.

Common and important clinical problems

Musculoskeletal presentations and child maltreatment

Child maltreatment is common, serious, and can be fatal. The true incidence of child abuse is difficult to ascertain (and it is probably under-diagnosed and under-reported) but a UK survey of more than 6000 parents, children and young people conducted in 2009 reports a prevalence of severe maltreatment of 5.9% in under 11s and 18.6% in 11–17 year olds. In England in 2013–14 over 650,000 children were referred to children's social care, either as a child in need or a child in need of protection. In the same year there were over 480,00 children subject to a child protection plan. Early detection and intervention may help to prevent further abuse and limit resulting damage to the child. It is therefore important that *all* medical staff who have contact with children are aware of the possibility of child maltreatment and consider this where there are features of concern and that professionals are familiar with the procedures to be followed if abuse or neglect is suspected or they believe that a child is suffering, or may be likely to suffer, significant harm.

Possible musculoskeletal presentations of non-accidental injury (NAI) include:

- A child with a limp or loss of function of a limb, which may result from a fracture or soft tissue injury with no history of trauma or an inadequate history.
- Joint swelling which may be due to haemarthrosis resulting from trauma (although JIA is a much more common cause of joint swelling in childhood).
- Direct impact injury to fingers may cause fusiform swelling which may mimic symmetrical small-joint arthritis.
- Cold injury may produce redness and swelling of hands and feet.

Conversely, NAI may occasionally be suspected in cases where the underlying cause is a rheumatological disease:

- Vasculitis or panniculitis presenting with bruising, purpura, or soft tissue swelling in the absence of a history of trauma.
- Henoch–Schönlein purpura should be identifiable by its characteristic evolution from urticarial lesions to purpura and by the associated abdominal pain and arthritis. The typical distribution is a symmetrical rash on the buttocks and lower limbs but the rash may occur elsewhere.
- Chilblains have been misdiagnosed as NAI.
- Infantile cortical hyperostosis or Caffey's disease may present with multiple areas of soft tissue swelling, bone lesions, and irritability in a young infant and has been mistaken for NAI.
- Degos disease is a rare occlusive vasculopathy that can present with subdural effusions and an ulcerative skin rash which may mimic cigarette burns.
- Remember children with rheumatological disease may also be subjected to abuse and considering safeguarding issues is an important role of the paediatric rheumatology MDT (see ➲ The multidisciplinary team, pp. 418–19).

Features in the presentation suggestive or supportive of a diagnosis of abuse or neglect

- Usually, one single feature is not diagnostic of abuse, but it is the overall pattern of presentation that is suspicious.
- Vague, unwitnessed, inconsistent, discrepant history.
- Inappropriate carer response, e.g. delayed presentation.
- Previous or ongoing social concerns.
- Repeated presentations to A&E departments with episodes of poorly explained trauma.
- *Bruises* in children should be assessed in the context of the child's medical and social history, developmental stage, and explanation given. Maltreatment may be suggested by bruises:
  - In children who are not independently mobile.
  - Away from bony prominences.
  - To particular sites, e.g. face, back.
  - That are multiple and in clusters (e.g. fingertip bruises).
  - With imprint of hand or implement.
- *Fractures*: no fracture in isolation is pathognomonic of child abuse. Features of concern include:
  - Fractures inconsistent with the developmental stage of the child or where there is an inadequate explanation as to cause.
  - Multiple fractures of different ages.
- Features which may indicate *neglect* such as:
  - Inappropriate or dirty clothing.
  - Failure to thrive.
  - Developmental impairment.
  - Behavioural difficulties.
  - Failure to attend medical or therapy appointments.
  - Lack of compliance with treatment.
- Features which may indicate *factitious or induced illness (FII)*
  - Inconsistent or unexplained symptoms or clinical findings (perplexing presentations).
  - Exaggeration of symptoms and over-medicalization.

Principles of management of suspected abuse or neglect

- The child's welfare is paramount. In particular, the child's best interests over-ride other considerations such as confidentiality and the carer's interests.
- Discuss concerns with senior colleagues or the lead or designated professional for child protection.
- Record history and observations carefully.
- If you have concerns that a child may be suffering, or may be likely to suffer, significant harm you have a responsibility to refer to children's social care so that a multi-agency assessment can take place.

Further reading

Cardiff Child Protection Systematic Review Group. *Bruising*. Available at: ✍ http://www.core-info. cardiff.ac.uk.

Cardiff Child Protection Systematic Review Group. *Fractures*. Available at: ✍ http://www.core-info. cardiff.ac.uk.

GMC. *Protecting Children and young people: The responsibilities of all doctors.* GMC, 2012. Available at: ℘ http://www.gmc-uk.org/guidance.

HM Government Department for children, schools and families. *Working together to safeguard children: A guide to inter-agency working to safeguard and promote the welfare of children.* London: DfE, 2015. Available at ℘ http://www.gov.uk/government/publications

Radford L, Corral S, Bradley C, et al. *Child Abuse and Neglect in the UK today.* NSPCC, 2011. Available at ℘ http://www.nspcc.org.uk/globalassets/documents/research-reports/child-abuse-neglect-uk-today-research-report.pdf; ℘ http://www.nspcc.org.uk/globalassets/documents/research-reports/child-abuse-neglect-uk-today-research-report.pdf

RCPCH. *Child Protection Companion 2013, 2nd Edition.* RCPCH, 2013. Available at ℘ http://www.rcpch.ac.uk/child-protection-publications

Malignancy and musculoskeletal presentations

- In childhood malignancies, it is estimated that up to 2/3 of children have musculoskeletal manifestations at initial presentation.
- Bone pain, myalgia, and articular symptoms such as arthritis and arthralgia are all well described.
- Malignancy can occasionally present with arthritis, mimicking JIA and should be excluded in all children with musculoskeletal complaints to avoid diagnostic delay.
- An incorrect diagnosis of JIA and resulting pre-treatment with corticosteroids or cytotoxic agents such as methotrexate (MTX) may cause difficulty with bone marrow interpretation, precipitate tumour lysis syndrome, and may even lead to a poor response to chemotherapeutic agents.
- It is reported that neoplasia accounts for less than 1% of referrals to paediatric rheumatology services. The majority of these malignancies are accounted for by leukaemias and lymphomas, but occasionally such musculoskeletal findings may occur as a result of solid tumours.

Leukaemia

- Leukaemia is by far the commonest form of cancer in children, accounting for 30% of all childhood malignancies, with acute lymphoblastic leukaemia (ALL) representing the majority.
- Arthritis is noted in >25% at presentation. Large joints are more frequently involved than small joints and an oligoarticular course more commonly reported than a polyarticular course. Knee or hip are most commonly involved in 36% and 34% respectively.
- Distinguishing ALL from JIA can be difficult. Clinical and laboratory features that may help discriminate ALL from JIA are outlined in Box 2.1.
- ALL with MSK involvement is associated with a longer delay to diagnosis (almost twice as long than those with no MSK features).
- Children with ALL and joint or bone disease often report intense continuous pain that is often out of context with clinical findings.
  - Affected children typically have exquisite tenderness across the metaphysis of the surrounding bones of the swollen joints.
- Progressive anaemia is the most common haematological change, with changes in platelet count and white cell counts (WCCs) less frequently seen.
- It is imperative to be aware that a normal/low WCC and normal blood film can be seen, especially in the early stages of ALL, and may remain normal for weeks and months after onset of joint symptoms.
- The pathognomonic leukaemic cells or blast cells are typically absent at the onset of the disease.
- Systemic features such as daily fever and hepatosplenomegaly can occur with all types of neoplasia and can mimic childhood rheumatic diseases such as systemic onset JIA and connective tissue disorders.

Box 2.1 Red flags! Features suggestive of malignancy rather than JIA

- Severe metaphyseal tenderness or other non-articular bone pain.
- Intense continuous pain and immobility.
- Nocturnal pain (especially if unilateral).
- Back pain.
- Absence of early morning stiffness.
- Low/normal WCC; low/normal platelet count; dropping Hb; normal serum ferritin with systemic features (rash, fever).
- Arthritis with raised LDH levels*.
- Abnormal blood film (not always present).
- Radiological findings of metaphyseal radiolucent bands, periosteal reaction, sclerotic and osteolytic lesions.
- Presence of abnormal blood count and nocturnal pain has a sensitivity and specificity 85% for ALL.

* Raised LDH alone has a low sensitivity in distinguishing JIA from ALL.

Investigations

- Routine blood tests including: FBC and blood film, routine clinical chemistry (U&Es, LFTs, bone biochemistry), ESR, CRP.
- Serum LDH, uric acid.
- Plain film X-rays (Fig. 2.1).
- Bone marrow aspirate and trephine.

Management

- With the initiation of appropriate treatment for ALL, the associated arthritis will usually quickly resolve.
- The use of analgesia in the form of NSAIDs and supportive measures from physiotherapy and occupational therapy is beneficial particularly in the acute state of the illness, and can be particularly useful symptomatically whilst investigations are completed and definitive treatment started.

Lymphoma

- Musculoskeletal symptoms in association with lymphoma are less commonly seen than with ALL.
- Bone pain is the commonest feature described and a true arthritis is rarely seen.
- Non-Hodgkin and Hodgkin lymphomas can cause bone pain as a result of direct invasion of the cortex or marrow by the tumour leading to bone infarction.
- Other causes of bone pain result from hypertrophic osteoarthropathy that stimulates an acute and painful periostitis.
- Lymphomas need in particular to be excluded in those with suspected systemic onset JIA, as many overlapping clinical features exist such as arthralgia, fever, malaise, splenomegaly, and lymphadenopathy.

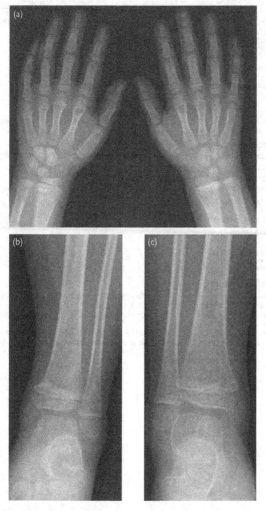

Fig. 2.1 X-ray images of ALL. The bones are osteopenic. There is periosteal reaction along both distal radius and ulna (a). There is patchy metaphyseal sclerosis and lucency of both wrists (a), also at both ankle joints (b, c). Faint periosteal reaction is visible along the lateral distal tibia (c).

- The lymphadenopathy in lymphomas is often described as matted and may be more rubbery than that of systemic onset JIA, although these are not reliable distinguishing features.
- Abdominal/thoracic imaging (US/CT scan).
- Lymph node biopsy: *lymph node removal by excision is preferred over needle biopsy, and should be performed in all patients where possible.*

Neuroblastoma

- The commonest solid tumour in toddlers and also the commonest tumours to occur outside the CNS in children are neuroblastomas.
- As 75% of children have metastatic disease including bone involvement at diagnosis, musculoskeletal symptoms (in particular bone pain) are frequently reported.
- Back pain in any young child or toddler is a cause for alarm and urinary catecholamines and catecholamine metabolites (VMA and HVA) are warranted in addition to imaging such as MRI.
- Lytic lesions may be visible on plain film x-ray as well as the other red flags outlined in Box 2.1.

Osteoid osteoma

See ➲ Bone tumours, pp. 59–61.

Osteosarcoma

See ➲ Bone tumours, pp. 59–61.

Further reading

Barbosa CM, Hilario MO, Terreri MT, et al. Musculoskeletal manifestations at the onset of acute leukaemias in childhood. *J Pediatr (Rio J)* 2002; **78**:481–4.

Cabral DA, Tucker LB. Malignancies in children who initially present with rheumatic complaints. *J Pediatr* 1999; **134**:53–7.

Robazzi TC, Mendonca N, Silva LR, et al. Osteoarticular manifestations as initial presentation of acute leukemias in children and adolescents in Bahia, Brazil. *J Pediatr Hematol Oncol* 2007;**29**:622–62.

Brix N, Hasle H et al. Arthritis as presenting manifestation of acute lymphoblastic leukemia in children. *Arch Dis Child* 2015;**100**:821–825.

Bone tumours

Presentation

Bone tumours (benign or malignant) can present with unexplained pain and swelling. Malignant bone tumours are rare but life threatening and early detection is important. The following clinical features may be present:

- Pain—worse at night but can fluctuate.
- Swelling—initially soft-tissue oedema; later bony enlargement and soft tissue extension.
- Coincidental injury. Not causative but may bring attention to swelling.
- Cachexia and weight-loss.
- Pathological fracture through the lesion (5–10%).
- Rarely, symptoms of metastases to lung. Shortness of breath, chest pain, haemoptysis.

Principles of investigation and management

- Patients with suspicious lesions should be referred urgently to a specialist bone tumour MDT, as per NICE guidelines, for biopsy (which requires careful planning) and further treatment. *Referral should not wait for further imaging investigations.*
- Blood tests may show raised inflammatory markers (but not always), serum alkaline phosphatase or lactate dehydrogenase (LDH).
- Imaging:
  - Plain x-ray is mandatory and detects most primary bone tumours. A normal x-ray does not exclude a bone tumour. Soft tissue tumours can show calcification or bone involvement.
  - The long bone and above the joint should be included in x-ray.
  - MRI—delineates local extent of tumour, and associated soft tissue mass, involvement of critical anatomical structures, skip lesions within long bones, and allows biopsy planning.
  - CT chest and whole body isotope bone scans are used to stage malignant primary bone and soft tissue tumours. Metastases occur most frequently in the lungs and rarely in the lymph nodes.
  - US—helpful screening investigation for soft tissue masses, can confirm a diagnosis of benign lipoma or vascular malformation, and may also show intralesional calcification, e.g. in synovial sarcomas.
- Biopsies provide a histological diagnosis and tumour grading; they should be performed by or after discussion with the surgical team who will perform the definitive resection.
- Staging systems depend on the diagnosis, histological grade of the tumour, size of the tumour, and the presence or absence of metastases. Staging determines future management.

Malignant bone tumours (Fig. 2.2)

Most common malignant bone tumours are osteosarcoma (55%) and Ewing's sarcoma (35%). Chondrosarcoma is extremely rare in children.

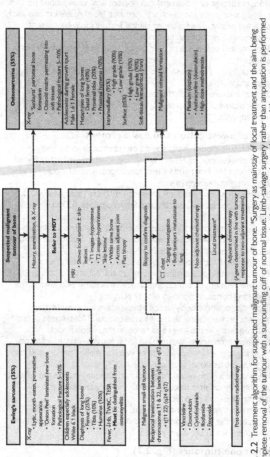

Fig. 2.2 Treatment algorithm for suspected malignant tumour of bone. *Surgery as mainstay of local treatment and the aim being complete removal of the tumour with a surrounding cuff of normal tissue. Limb-salvage surgery rather than amputation is performed in 90% of cases. Major long-bone defects are most often reconstructed with massive endoprostheses, and these can extend to accommodate for growth in children. Radiotherapy can be used as an adjunct to surgery in Ewing's sarcoma (either pre or post operatively), or as the sole local treatment if surgical resection is not feasible. Where available, patients should be enrolled in clinical trials.

Note: It is important to consider clinical trials opportunities for all patients.

Benign bone tumours

Benign bone tumours are more common than malignant lesions. However, urgent investigation and referral to an MDT must be initiated for any suspicious lesion. See Fig 2.3.

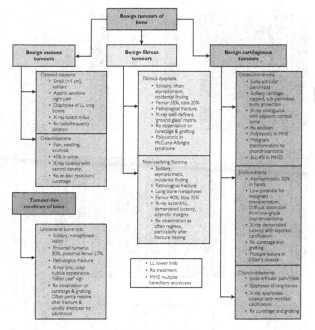

Fig. 2.3 Treatment algorithm for benign tumours of bone.

Soft-tissue sarcomas

See Fig 2.4.

- Although most soft tissue masses are benign, the following are 'red flags' suggestive of malignancy:
  - Lump increasing in size, lump deep to fascia, lump >5cm diameter.
  - Pain, often worse at night.
  - Lump recurring after previous excision.
- Paediatric soft tissue sarcomas are usually classified as rhabdomyosarcomas or non-rhabdomyosarcomas.
- Non-rhabdomyosarcomas are a rare but heterogenous group of tumours in children. Chemotherapy is usually given for malignant tumours.

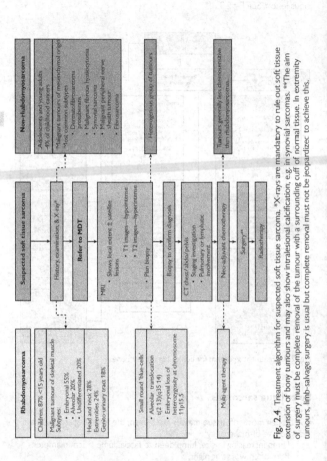

Fig. 2.4 Treatment algorithm for suspected soft tissue sarcoma. *X-rays are mandatory to rule out soft tissue extension of bony tumours and may also show intralesional calcification, e.g. in synovial sarcomas. **The aim of surgery must be complete removal of the tumour with a surrounding cuff of normal tissue. In extremity tumours, limb-salvage surgery is usual but complete removal must not be jeopardized to achieve this.

Content within the figure:

Suspected soft tissue sarcoma

History, examination, & X-ray*

Refer to MDT

MRI
• Shows local extent ± satellite lesions
  • T1 images—hypointense
  • T2 images—hyperintense
• Plan biopsy

Biopsy to confirm diagnosis

CT chest/abdo/pelvis
• Staging investigation
  • Pulmonary or lymphatic involvement

Neo-adjuvant chemotherapy

Surgery**

Radiotherapy

Rhabdomyosarcoma
Children: 87% <15 years old
Malignant tumour of skeletal muscle
Subtypes:
• Embryonal 55%
• Alveolar 20%
• Undifferentiated 20%
Head and neck 28%
Extremities 24%
Genito-urinary tract 18%

• Small round 'blue-cells'
• Alveolar translocation t(2 13)(q35 14)
• Embryonal loss of heterozygosity at chromosome 11p15.5

Multi-agent therapy

Non-rhabdomyosarcoma
Adolescents and young adults
9% of childhood cancers
*Malignant tumours of mesenchymal origin
*Most common subtypes
• Dermatofibrosarcoma protuberans
• Malignant fibrous histiocytoma
• Synovial sarcoma
• Malignant peripheral nerve sheath tumour
• Fibrosarcoma

Heterogeneous group of tumours

Tumours generally less chemosensitive than rhabdomyosarcomas.

Bone and joint infections

Septic arthritis and osteomyelitis

Incidence is 2–10 per 100,000 in the general childhood population.

Bacterial infection of the bone or joint should be suspected in infants or children with acute onset of:
- Fever.
- Unexplained limp (see ➲ The limping child, pp. 78–81) and/or abnormal posture/gait and/or reluctance to use the limb, inability to weight bear, and complete or partial limitation of movement on examination.
- Musculoskeletal pain ± presence of local bone or joint tenderness, bone or joint swelling, erythema ('hot, swollen, joint'), or pain on passive motion of the joint.

- Septic arthritis and osteomyelitis may occur separately or together, may affect 1 or many joints, and the clinical presentation depends on the organism and host immunity. Infants may not appear unwell, and may not always have a high fever. Careful comprehensive examination must be undertaken by a clinician experienced in the assessment of joints.
- Prognosis: usually good unless the diagnosis is delayed.

Septic arthritis

- Septic arthritis is an infectious arthritis of a synovial joint, and is a *medical emergency*.
- The frequency is highest in young children; 50% of all cases present in first 2 yrs of life with a greater tendency in boys (2:1). Most common joints (75%) affected in lower limb (knee >hip >ankle). Approximately 25% infections affecting the upper limbs.
- Bacteria may reach the joint:
  - through haematogenous spread (most common route for bacterial joint infection).
  - by direct penetration (e.g. through the skin).
  - or by local spread from an adjacent infected site.
- Neonates and infants are at high risk of *septic arthritis* developing from osteomyelitis, as infection can spread easily from the metaphysis via the patent transepiphyseal vessels.
- In certain regions, particularly in Europe and the Middle East, *Kingella kingae* has become one of the most common pathogens. The rising incidence is mostly attributable to progressive PCR techniques used for its detection. *Kingella* produces milder infections, is responsive to antibiotics, and tends to affect the cartilaginous epiphyses.

Most common pathogens for both septic arthritis and osteomyelitis
- <12 months old: *Staphylococcus aureus*, Group B *Streptococcus*, Gram-negative bacilli.
- 1–5yrs: *Staphylococcus aureus*, Group A *Streptococcus*, *Streptococcus pneumoniae*, *Haemophilus influenzae*, *Enterobacter* (osteomyelitis).
- 5–12yrs: *Staphylococcus aureus*, Group A *Streptococcus*.
- 12–18yrs: *Staphylococcus aureus*, *Neisseria gonorrhoea*.

Osteomyelitis

- Osteomyelitis is infection of bone.
- The frequency of osteomyelitis is greatest in infants. 1/3 of all cases occur in the first 2 years of life. Half of all cases occur by 5 years of age. Boys >girls (2:1)
- Often preceded by history of trauma in the affected extremity.
- Infection is usually seen in the metaphyseal region of bones.
- Most infections are spread via the haematogenous route from a 1° site of entry (e.g. respiratory, ear, nose, or throat, skin). Infection may also occur by direct inoculation (open fractures, penetrating wounds) or local extension from adjacent sites.
- In the neonate or infant *transepiphyseal* vessels are patent and infection may spread to the adjacent joint causing a septic arthritis.
- Organisms are not always isolated. The yield for bacterial growth from synovial fluid and bone aspirate is usually poor.

Types of osteomyelitis
- Acute.
- Subacute (2–3 weeks' duration).
- Chronic: may develop sequestrum and involucrum.
- *Bone abscesses* may develop with surrounding thick fibrous tissue and sclerotic bone (Brodie's abscess).
- Chronic recurrent multifocal osteomyelitis (CRMO, see ➔ Chronic recurrent multifocal osteomyelitis, pp. 313–15).

General principles of management for bone and joint infections

- Prompt diagnosis, adequate and urgent washout, and drainage of joint is required followed by immediate institution of appropriate antibiotics are important to optimize outcome.
- Assessment and management should involve on-call teams for paediatrics, orthopaedics, and microbiology and be guided by local policy for clinical service and antibiotic use. Consideration of antibiotics to cover MRSA or Panton–Valentine leukocidin (PVL) producing *Staphylococcus aureus* may be warranted in certain clinical situations. Special requests to look for the gene encoding PVL *S. aureus* can be made when samples are sent for tissue diagnosis.
- Early referral to orthopaedic team for consideration of irrigation and debridement of the affected joint, and drainage of any associated osteomyelitis. Joint washout and drainage generally always requires a general anaesthetic. Orthopaedic opinion should be sought early to clarify if an aspiration of bone or bone biopsy should be taken, *before* instituting IV antibiotics.
- Empirical IV antibiotics (penicillin and cephalosporin) while awaiting cultures. General current practice is IV antibiotics for up to 3 weeks (until inflammatory markers normalize), followed by oral antibiotics for

a total of 4–6 weeks. There is no evidence comparing long versus short courses of antibiotics.

- Recent trends in the UK show an increased incidence of community-associated methicillin-resistant *S. aureus* (CA-MRSA). As a result many antimicrobial policies in many hospitals for septic arthritis now include clindamycin which has good action against CA-MRSA.
- Appropriate analgesia and anti-inflammatory medication is required. The affected joint should be rested until there is clinical improvement and pain has settled.
- Early physiotherapy assessment is important to guide mobilization as appropriate.
- Investigations:
  - Joint aspiration with Gram-stain microscopy and culture of synovial fluid. (Consider mycobacterial infection; see ➜ Tuberculosis and mycobacterial disease, pp. 384–90.)
  - Inoculating blood culture bottles directly with synovial fluid improves yield and may be helpful for isolating certain bacteria.
  - PCR on synovial fluid or of synovial tissue may be useful if other cultures have been negative.
  - Blood cultures (ideally, 3 sets over 3 days, always worthwhile; repeat blood cultures if reinserting a cannula in a child).
  - FBC, ESR, CRP can be helpful in the assessment; for bacterial infections, expect WCC to be raised with neutrophilia, and moderately raised CRP. CRP is a better predictor than ESR for acute infection. If high at beginning as a baseline marker, they may be helpful with assessment of progress (resolution towards normal indicating improvement); however, blood tests are *not* diagnostic of septic arthritis, they can only guide management with assessment of the clinical situation.
- Imaging:
  - X-ray—may be normal initially; may show fluid or soft tissue swelling; or widened joint space. Bony changes may not be evident for 14–21 days.
  - Ultrasound scan joint—may show effusion and can guide joint aspiration.
  - MRI—useful if diagnosis unclear or osteomyelitis suspected. Sensitive to early changes and very useful in suspected vertebral osteomyelitis.
  - Radionuclide bone scan (showing ↑ uptake) can be useful if MRI unavailable.

Pointers towards septic arthritis

Kocher proposed clinical prediction scores based on 4 independent factors to differentiate septic arthritis from transient synovitis (Box 2.2).

Box 2.2 Four factors used to predict septic arthritis
- Fever >38.5°C.
- Non-weight-bearing or pain with passive motion of the joint.
- ESR: >40mm/h.
- WCC: >12 × 10^9.

Probability of septic arthritis with the number of predictors present:

Number of factors	Probability
0	<0.2%
1	3.0%
2	40.0%
3	93.1%
4	99.6%

Reproduced with permission from Kocher MS, Zurakowski D, Kasser JR Differentiating between septic arthritis and transient synovitis of the hip in children: an evidence-based clinical prediction algorithm *Journal of Joint and Bone Surgery,* Volume 01, Issue 12, pp. 1002–70, Copyright © 1999 Wolters Kluwer Health.

Reactive arthritis
- Definition—reactive arthritis is an aseptic acute inflammatory arthritis occurring with, or following, an intercurrent infection, without evidence of the causative organism in the joint. Should be suspected where >1 joint affected and clinical presentation includes potential source of extra-articular infection.
- The infectious agent responsible for triggering the arthritis is generally outside the joint. For agents commonly associated with reactive arthritis, see Table 2.1.
- Reactive arthritis can occur at any age. Reactive arthritis typically follows 7–10 days after an episode of gastroenteritis (young children), typically involves lower limb large joints (knee>ankle >hip) and there is an association of this type of arthritis with HLA B-27 positivity. Acute phase reactants are usually raised (often very high), blood cultures and autoantibodies are negative and the diagnosis may rest on serology or urethral or stool cultures.
- In adolescents, it is important to differentiate reactive arthritis (following an episode of sexually acquired urethritis from gonococcal arthritis or *Chlamydia* infection. Reiter's disease/syndrome is former terminology used to describe the triad of urethritis, conjunctivitis, and arthritis. Patients may have multiple infections (*Chlamydia*, Gonococcus, and HIV).

Investigations in suspected reactive arthritis:
- Acute phase reactants.
- Cultures:
  - Blood.
  - Stool (*Shigella, Salmonella, Yersinia, Campylobacter*).
  - Urethral (Gonococcus [Gram negative], *Chlamydia*).
  - Synovial fluid (Gram stain and culture).
  - Throat swab (*Streptococcus*).

Table 2.1 Pathogens associated with arthritis

Type	Organism	Organism associated with condition		
		Septic arthritis	Osteomyelitis	Reactive arthritis
Bacteria	Staphylococcus aureus	√	√	
	Streptococcus spp	√	√	√
	Group A	√	√	
	(Group B Strep in neonate)	√	√	
	Streptococcus pneumoniae	√	√	√
	Salmonella			√
	Shigella			√
	Campylobacter			√
	Neisseria meningitidis, N. gonorrhoeae	√	√	√
	Brucella melitensis, canis	√	√	
	Chlamydia			√
	Mycoplasma pneumoniae (Ureaplasma)	√		√
Mycobacteria	Mycobacterium tuberculosis (see ⊃ Tuberculosis and mycobacterial disease, pp. 384–90)	√	√	
Atypical mycobacteria*	Mycobacterium avium complex	√		
	Mycobacterium malmoense (see ⊃ Tuberculosis and mycobacterial disease, pp. 384–90)	√		
Spirochaete	Borrelia burgdorferi (see ⊃ Lyme disease pp. 400–4)	√		√
Viruses	Parvovirus B19			√
	Rubella			√
Protozoa	Toxoplasma*			√
	Giardiasis			√
Helminths	Toxocara	√		√
	Dracunculus			√
	Schistosoma	√		√
Fungi*	Histoplasma	√		√
	Cryptococcus	√		

* In the immunosuppressed patient (see ⊃ Tuberculosis and mycobacterial disease, pp. 384–90).

- Serology:
  - *Salmonella, Yersinia, Campylobacter.*
  - ASOT and anti-DNAseB (streptococcal infection) see Tables 2.1 and 2.9.
- HLA B27.
- Management involves establishing a diagnosis and excluding infection, symptoms control with NSAIDS, analgesia, and early physiotherapy involvement. Intra-articular steroid injection will be helpful with persistent arthritis (and once septic arthritis excluded).

Gonococcal arthritis

- Gonococcal arthritis may present as a septic arthritis associated with fever, rigors, skin lesions (macular rash, pustules, or blisters), tenosynovitis, and polyarthritis.
- The knee is the most commonly affected joint, but any joint may be involved.
- If suspected, Gram stain, and culture of synovial fluid, blood cultures, and any exudative lesions will be useful. The possibility of sexual abuse should be considered in a child with gonococcal arthritis.

Further reading

Frank G, Mahoney HM, Eppes SC. Musculoskeletal infections in children. *Pediatr Clin North Am* 2005; **52**(4):1083–6, ix.

Mathews CJ, Kingsley G, Field M, et al. Management of septic arthritis: a systematic review. *Ann Rheum Dis* 2007; **66**(4):440–5.

Infections in the immunocompromised

Background

- Chronic inflammatory diseases are managed with a combination of immunosuppressive and anti-inflammatory agents, including steroids, disease modifying anti-rheumatic drugs (DMARDs) and recent novel biological agents, having significant impact on symptom relief and quality of life.
- However, in order to reduce inflammation, they inhibit innate and adaptive immune pathways, making patients increasingly susceptible to both serious and opportunistic infections.
- Although the benefits usually outweigh the risks, infectious complications need to be minimized by careful assessment prior to their commencement and close monitoring whilst on them.

- *Serious infection:* infection requiring treatment with IV antimicrobial therapy, needing hospitalization, or causing death.
- *Opportunistic infection:* infection caused by microorganisms with a limited pathogenic capacity under ordinary circumstances, but able to cause serious disease in the immunocompromised host.

At-risk populations

A lack of high-quality epidemiological data limits our current knowledge about the relative risks (RR) of serious and opportunistic infections in children receiving immunosuppressive and anti-inflammatory regimens. In addition, it is difficult to determine the relative contribution of the underlying disease itself, comorbidities, and other immunosuppressive co-medication. The following statements are consensus derived:

Corticosteroids

- Immunosuppressive if >2mg/kg given for over 1 week or 1mg/kg for over 4 weeks.
- Mechanism of action via multiple mechanisms that are not yet fully understood, involving phospholipase A2 inhibitory proteins and lipocortins, which control the biosynthesis of potent mediators of inflammation such as prostaglandins and leukotrienes. Cause broad cellular and humoral immunosuppression, resulting in susceptibility to viral, bacterial, and fungal infections.
- Infection risk increases with higher doses and longer duration of treatment.
  - It is important to use the lowest dose for shortest duration.

DMARDs

- The infection risk increases when DMARDs are used in combination and/or neutropenia occurs.
- Numerous case reports of opportunistic infections:
- *Pneumocystis jiroveci* pneumonia, reactivation of viruses (EBV, CMV, HSV, VZV).
- In descending order, the risk of infection is greatest with cyclophosphamide (RR 2.3)>corticosteroids (RR 1.63)>azathioprine (RR 1.52)>MTX (RR 1.30)>cyclosporine/mycophenolate mofetil (MMF).

Novel biological agents
- Various agents, including TNF-A inhibitors, IL-1 and IL-6 antagonists, T-cell co-stimulation modulators (CTLA-4 fusion proteins), and anti-CD20 agents are increasingly used (see ⊃ Biologic therapies for paediatric rheumatological diseases, pp. 448–54). The well-defined mode of action of these agents allows potential infectious complications to be anticipated (Table 2.2).
  - The RR of infection associated with these agents is unknown in children although adult epidemiological data suggest higher rates of infection with novel biological agents compared to DMARDs. In descending order the risk is thought to be greatest with TNF-α inhibitors (RR 1.52)> IL-1R/IL-6R antagonists/anti-CD20 agents > T cell co-stimulation modulators.
  - Standard-dose (OR 1.31) and high-dose (OR 1.90) biological drugs (with or without traditional DMARDs) are associated with an increase in serious infections compared with traditional DMARDs, although low-dose biological drugs are not (0.93).
  - The risk is highest in the 1st year of treatment
  - Infections include TB reactivation/infection (see ⊃Tuberculosis and mycobacterial disease, pp. 384–90), fungal infections, severe pyogenic bacterial infections, PJP, virus reactivation.

Strategies for managing severe and opportunistic infections
See Fig 2.5.
- Fever—may arise from infection or be caused by the underlying inflammatory pathology itself.
- Clinical presentation of infection may be altered by underlying disease/immunomodulatory therapy.
- Opportunistic infections—hard to recognize by virtue of their rare presentation but can cause significant morbidity and mortality.

Screening
- Prior to starting immunosuppressive therapy, patients should be screened for latent infections, especially TB as per local guidelines. Treat active or latent TB prior to starting immunosuppressive therapy (see ⊃Tuberculosis and mycobacterial disease, pp. 384–90.)
- Thorough history to evaluate TB risk, varicella immunity, immunization status, and future travel plans; clinical examination and investigations to exclude active infections, including dental status, VZV serology, and FBC to exclude neutropenia or lymphopenia.

Vaccination
- Ideally vaccinate >4 weeks prior to commencing immunosuppressive therapy.

Varicella:
  - If varicella antibody status negative.
  - Consider vaccinating 1st-degree family members (history and/or serologically negative).

Table 2.2 The infectious complications and organisms associated with novel biological agents

Drug	TNF-α inhibitors	IL-1 antagonists	Anti-CD20 agents	T cell costimulation modulators	IL-6 antagonists
Most commonly used	Etanercept Infliximab Adalimumab	Anakinra Rilonacept Canakinumab	Rituximab	Abatacept	Tocilizumab
Infectious complications	Pneumonia UTI URTI incl. sinusitis Skin + soft tissue infections Musculoskeletal infections	URTI Pneumonia Cellulitis	Pneumonia UTI URTI Shingles	URTI inc. Sinusitis Pneumonia Septicaemia Skin+soft tissue inf.	URTI Gastroenteritis
Organisms	M. tuberculosis NTM Salmonella spp. Listeria Nocardia Candida Aspergillus Histoplasma Coccidioides Blastomyces Cryptococcus Hepatitis B VZV CMV Toxoplasma PJP	Bacteria ?VZV	Bacteria including Staphylococcus and Pseudomonas Enterovirus Hepatitis B Hepatitis C JC virus (risk of PML) VZV	VZV HSV Aspergillus Candida	EBV PJP

TNF, tumour necrosis factor; UTI, urinary tract infection; URTI, upper respiratory tract infection; NTM, non-tuberculous mycobacteria; VZV, varicella zoster virus; CMV, cytomegalovirus; EBV, Epstein–Barr virus; PJP, Pneumocystis jirovec pneumonia; PML, progressive multifocal leukoencephalopathy

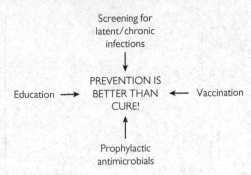

Fig. 2.5 Prevention of infection.

Pneumococcus:
- Ensure vaccination with Prevenar-13 as per the recommended child-hood schedule.

Influenza:
- Influenza vaccination is recommended annually in the autumn.
- Avoid live vaccines; rest of childhood immunization schedule should be followed.
  - Live vaccines can be given once off steroid treatment for >3 months or other immunosuppression for >6 months.
- Give zoster immunoglobulin (ZIG) if significant exposure to chickenpox in non-immune patients, up to 7 days post-exposure. Immunoglobulin if significant contact with measles, irrespective of antibody status.

Prophylactic antimicrobials
Prophylaxis should be considered in patients who are neutropenic, lympho-penic, or live in an 'endemic' area (e.g. *Histoplasma*). Seek specialist paedi-atric infectious diseases advice.

Education
- Avoid foods associated with *Listeria* and *Salmonella* infection (unpasteurized milk, soft cheeses and undercooked eggs and meat). Avoid visits to zoo/animal farms.
- Ensure that parents recognize the early signs of infection and understand that urgent medical assessment is required (see ⊃ Biologic therapies for paediatric rheumatological diseases, pp. 448–54 and ⊃The role of the clinical nurse specialist, pp. 420–2).

The approach to the immunocompromised child presenting with fever

- Fever may be the only sign of serious infection, especially in the child with neutropenia.
  - *Beware*: TNF-α and IL-1/IL-6 inhibitors may 'mask' fever and an inflammatory response (i.e. CRP may be normal or only mildly elevated).
- Serious bacterial infections, invasive fungal infections, and disseminated viral infections must be distinguished from self-limiting viral infections.
  - Empirical treatment is often initiated until this distinction is made.
- The profile of infection (organism, severity) varies with the immunosuppressive therapy being used (especially for combinations).
  - The highest risk is in haematopoietic stem cell transplantation.
- The algorithm in Fig. 2.6 provides an approach for managing the immunocompromised child presenting with fever.

Important notes

Children with persistent musculoskeletal pain should have the following work-up considered:
- Complete/FBC with differential.
- Acute phase reactants (ESR, CRP).
- Routine serum chemistries (including creatinine, liver, and muscle enzymes).
- Urinalysis.
- Imaging studies (plain x-rays of involved area, other studies as indicated in the algorithm(s)).
- Testing for mycobacterial infection.

Caveats

- Minor trauma and infections are common in children and may not necessarily be related to the diagnosis.
- Consider malignancy and non-accidental injury (child abuse) as alternative diagnosis.

Further reading

RCPCH. Immunisation against infectious disease—'The Green Book', 2013; Best Practice Guidelines, Immunisation of the Immunocompromised Child. London: RCPCH, 2002. Available at: ℘ http://www.RCPCH.ac.uk/guidelines.

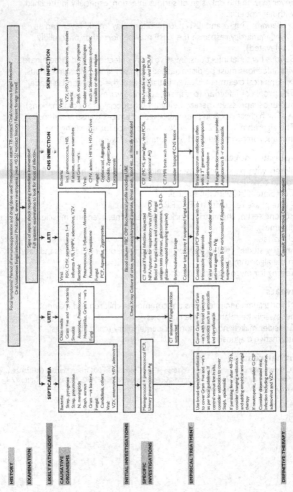

HISTORY
Focal symptoms? Period of immunosuppression and drug (dose used) Immunosuppression state? TB contact? Immunisation state? Oral/cutaneous fungal infections? Oral/cutaneous fungal infections? Prolonged, severe neutropenia (neut <0.5)? Mucositis history? Recent foreign travel?

EXAMINATION
Signs of septic shock requiring immediate intervention?
Full systematic examination to look for focus of infection.

LIKELY PATHOLOGY | SEPTICAEMIA | URTI | LRTI | CNS INFECTION | SKIN INFECTION

CAUSATIVE ORGANISMS

SEPTICAEMIA
Bacterial:
Strep. pyogenes
Strep. pneumoniae
N. meningitidis
Staph. aureus
Gram –ve bacteria
Fungal:
Candidiasis, others
Viral:
VZV, enterovirus, HSV, adenovirus

URTI
Otitis media
Gram +ve and –ve bacteria
Sinusitis:
Anaerobes, Pneumococcus,
Anaerobes, Pneumococcus,
Haemophilus, Gram's –ve's
Fungi

LRTI
Viral:
Incl. CMV, parainfluenza 1–4
influenza A/B, HMPV, adenovirus, VZV
Bacterial:
Pneumococcus, H. influenzae, Moraxella
Pseudomonas, Mycoplasma
Fungal:
PCP, Aspergillus, Zygomycetes

CNS INFECTION
Bacterial:
Incl. pneumococcus, HiB
If abscess, consider anaerobes
and Gram –ve's
Viral:
CMV, adeno-, HHV6, HSV, JC virus
Fungal:
Cryptococcal, Aspergillus
Candida, Zygomycetes
Protozoa:
Toxoplasmosis

SKIN INFECTION
Viral:
VZV, HSV, HHV6, adenovirus, measles
Bacterial:
Staph. aureus and Strep. pyogenes
Consider non-infective pathologies
such as Stevens–Johnson syndrome,
vasculitis or disease relapse

INITIAL INVESTIGATIONS
Blood culture• FBC, CRP, Biochemical profile including U&E
Check X-ray Culture of urine, sputum, nasopharyngeal aspirate, throat swab, stool etc. as clinically indicated

SPECIFIC INVESTIGATIONS

SEPTICAEMIA
Meningococcal ± pneumococcal PCR
Urinary pneumococcal Ag

URTI
CT sinuses if fungal infection
suspected

LRTI
CT chest if fungal infection suspected
NPA/sputum for respiratory virus (IF/PCR)
Blood for fungal culture and consider fungal
antigen tests (mannan, galactomannan, 1,3-ß-D-
glucan—repeated sampling required)
Bronchoalveolar lavage
Consider lung biopsy if suspected fungal lesion

CNS INFECTION
CSF (PCR's, protozoa, viral PCR's
cryptococcal Ag)
CT /MRI brain with contrast
Consider biopsy of CNS lesion

SKIN INFECTION
Skin/vesicle scrapings for
bacterial C+S, viral PCR/IF
Consider skin biopsy

EMPIRICAL TREATMENT

SEPTICAEMIA
Use broad-spectrum antibiotics
to cover Gram +ve and –ve's
as per local guidelines. If
central venous catheter in situ,
consider antibiotics to cover
Staph. epidermidis
If persisting fever after 48–72h,
consider changing antibiotics
and adding empirical anti-fungal
therapy
If neutropenic, consider G-CSF
Consider disseminated viral
infection including enterovirus,
adenovirus and VZV.

URTI
Cover Gram +ve and Gram
–ve's with broad spectrum
antibiotics such as amoxicillin
and ciprofloxacin

LRTI
Consider empirical PCP treatment with co-
trimoxazole and steroids
If viral aetiology confirmed, consider specific
anti-viral agent +/– IVIg
Amphotericin B for voriconazole if Aspergillus
suspected.

CNS INFECTION
Broad-spectrum antibiotics often
with a 3rd generation cephalosporin
+/– metronidazole
If fungal infection suspected, consider
Amphotericin B or voriconazole

DEFINITIVE THERAPY
Consult with Infectious Diseases colleagues

Fig. 2.6 The approach to the immunocompromised child presenting with fever.

Fractures in children and adolescents

See Tables 2.3–2.5.

Excluding fractures as a cause of pain

- Check for a history of injury, e.g. witnessed fall, pain immediately after fall.
  - Be alert for potential of NAI (see ❷ Musculoskeletal presentations and non-accidental injury, pp. 52–4)
  - Be alert for fragility fractures (see ❷ Metabolic bone diseases, pp. 358–61)
- In school age children and older, accurate palpation to determine site of pain, e.g. periarticular versus shaft of long bones, supracondylar humerus versus epicondyles, distal radius versus scaphoid.
- Imaging appropriately—focal x-rays are better than whole, long-bone x-rays. Ultrasound scan and bone scan are not useful for detection of acute fractures. In young children with unossified epiphyses, an arthrogram under general anaesthesia is useful to exclude displaced intra-articular fractures.
- Interpret radiographs appropriately for the age—fractures can be confused with physes (growth plates), e.g. is the physis at the site of tenderness? Compare with normal age specific radiographs and x-ray contralateral limb for comparison.
- Growth arrest and subsequent deformity are most common following direct physeal trauma.
- The rate of complications is dependent on the type of fracture, the actual physis involved and the age of the patient (Fig. 2.7).
- Salter-Harris type IV and V fractures are more likely to cause bone bridge formation than types I–III (Fig. 2.8).
- The distal femur and proximal tibia are the most susceptible physeal plates to develop bone bridges following trauma.
- Peripheral growth arrest usually causes angular deformity and the management depends on the extent of the bone bridge. Whereas, central growth arrests usually cause leg-length discrepancy and 50% of the physeal plate may be resected and still allow continued longitudinal growth.

Table 2.3 Fractures in children: epidemiology

Age groups (yr)	Incidence number per 1000 children per year	Common mechanisms	Common fractures (prevalence %)*	
0–1 (infants and pre-walkers)	3.6	Non accidental injury (NAI)	Clavicle	22.2
		Fall below bed height	Distal humerus	22.2
			Distal radius	11.1
			Radius & ulna shaft	11.1
			Tibia	8.9
2–4 (pre-school)	12.9	Fall below bed height	Distal humerus	22.0
		NAI	Distal radius	21.3
		Falls down stairs	Clavicle	15.0
			Radius & ulna shaft	9.5
			Finger phalanges	7.1
5–11 (school children)	23.2	Fall below bed height	Distal radius	40.3
		Sport	Finger phalanges	14.4
		Blunt trauma	Distal humerus	7.5
		Falls down stairs	Radius & ulna shaft	5.9
		Trauma (road traffic accident [RTA])	Metacarpus	5.3
12–16 (adolescents)	26.6	Sports	Distal radius	28.0
		Fights	Finger phalanges	20.3
		Blunt trauma	Metacarpus	14.3
		RTA	Clavicle	7.0
		Fall below bed height	Metatarsus	5.3

* Rennie L, Court-Brown CM, Mok JY, et al. The epidemiology of fractures in children. *Injury* 2007; **38**(8):913–22.

Table 2.4 Fractures in children: management

Principles of fracture management	Objectives	Options (depends on fracture site, rehabilitation requirements and surgeon's preference)
Reduction	Restores alignment and function	*Closed reduction*: general anaesthetic or local anaesthetic manipulation
	Reduces pain	*Open reduction*: especially for intra-articular fractures.
Immobilization	Maintains alignment (after reduction)	*Non operative*: casts/splints
	Reduces pain	*Operative*: percutaneous wires, plate & screws, intramedullary fixation, external fixation
Rehabilitation	Restores strength, range of motion and function	Mobilization Gradual return to activity Physiotherapy

Table 2.5 Fractures in children and adults: comparison of complications

Differences	Adult	Child
Angular deformity	Due to malunion at fracture	Due to malunion or eccentric physeal injury <50%. Depends on age of child and site of fracture.
Shortening	Due to bone loss	Due to bone loss or central physeal injury >50%. Depends on age of child and site of fracture
Healing time	Longer	Shorter due to cellular periosteum
Fragility fractures	Due to osteoporosis	Osteogenesis imperfecta or rickets—check for short stature, family history, serum calcium and PTH

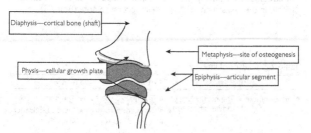

Fig. 2.7 Sites of fracture

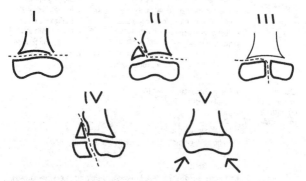

Fig. 2.8 Salter and Harris classification of fractures

Reproduced with permission from Salter, RB, and Harris, WR. Injuries involving the epiphyseal plate. *Journal of Bone and Joint Surgery*, Volume 45, Issue 3, pp. 487–622, Copyright © 1963 Wolters Kluwer Health.

The limping child

- Limping is a symptom and not a diagnosis. Acute limping invariably results from pain and the antalgic (painful) gait refers to the child minimizing weight bearing on the sore limb, with a shortened stance phase and increasing the swing phase of the gait cycle (see ➔ The gait cycle and abnormal gait patterns, p. 11). When assessing gait in the young child, especially the preschool age, it is important to be aware of the normal process of gait development, normal variants, and age-related gait changes (see ➔ Chapter 1. p. 1).
- Epidemiological studies are sparse—in one study children with an acute limp accounted for <2% of all paediatric emergency department attendances, although this may well be more common in the primary care setting.
- The age of the child is most helpful in establishing a differential diagnosis (Table 2.6). Trauma is the commonest cause of limping and in the case of atraumatic limp, many will resolve spontaneously. However common pitfalls in the assessment of limp are important to note (Box 2.3).

Table 2.6 Causes of limp by age

	0–3 yrs	4–10 yrs	11–16 yrs
Most common	• Trauma (including toddler's fracture)	• Trauma • Transient synovitis • Perthes' disease	• Trauma • Osgood–Schlatter disease
Conditions requiring urgent intervention	• Osteomyelitis • Septic arthritis • NAI • Malignancy (e.g. neuroblastoma) • Testicular torsion • Inguinal hernia	• Osteomyelitis • Septic arthritis • NAI • Malignant disease (e.g. acute lymphocytic leukaemia) • Testicular torsion • Appendicitis • Inguinal hernia	• Osteomyelitis • Septic arthritis • Slipped upper femoral epiphysis • Malignancy (e.g. bone tumours) • Testicular torsion • Appendicitis • Inguinal hernia
Other important conditions to consider	• Developmental dysplasia of the hip • JIA	• JIA	• JIA
	• Metabolic (e.g. rickets) • Haematological disease (e.g. sickle cell anaemia) • Reactive arthritis • Lyme arthritis • Multisystem diseases (e.g. juvenile systemic lupus erythematosus, juvenile dermatomyositis)		

Box 2.3 Common pitfalls observed in the assessment of the limping child

- Ascribing limp to trauma or hypermobility and overlooking features that suggest other causes.
- The concept of referred pain (e.g. from the abdomen [and testes in boys], back, or chest and hip pathology manifesting as knee pain).
- Think beyond the hip (!) and examine the child comprehensively.
- Classical clinical features of sepsis may be masked in the immunosuppressed child.
- Mycobacterial infection can be easily missed.
- Synovial fluid may be sterile in partially treated septic arthritis.
- Labelling children with daytime symptoms as having 'growing pains'.
- Medically unexplained limp or physical symptoms warrant specific management and referral (i.e. discharge without a diagnosis and follow-up plan is not advised).
- The blood film may be normal in children with malignancy.
- Radiographs are often normal in children with early sepsis or arthritis.
- Acute phase reactants may be normal in children with arthritis.
- RF is usually negative in children with arthritis.
- ANA and RF may be false positives in children without inflammatory joint or muscle disease.
- Pathology in the joint or muscle or bone

- Most cases of limp are an *acquired* abnormality of gait. However, in the child who has 'always had a limp' from initial weight bearing it is important to consider a 'missed' diagnosis of developmental dysplasia of the hip (DDH) or neurological conditions such as cerebral palsy. Furthermore, limping typically affects one leg but in some instances *bilateral* involvement can occur (e.g. Perthes' disease, DDH, slipped capital femoral epiphysis) and makes clinical assessment particularly difficult. See ➡ Hip pain and hip problems in children and adolescents, pp. 111–18.
- It is important to assess limping children very carefully for 'red flags' suggestive of potentially life-threatening causes (including sepsis, malignancy, and NAI) which although uncommon, can lead to long-term morbidity or mortality. Such causes must therefore be considered, actively excluded, and not missed (Table 2.7).
- The discrimination between septic arthritis and reactive arthritis (transient synovitis) at the hip is a common clinical scenario. Kocher's clinical prediction rules (see Box 2.2) can be helpful but should not replace experienced clinical judgement (see also ➡ Chapter 6, p. 383 and ➡ Hip pain and hip problems in children and adolescents, pp. 111–18). Caution is warranted when limp is attributed to reactive arthritis as the prevalence of viral infections within childhood is high, and such reports may be coincidental.

Table 2.7 The limping child and features that suggest severe life-threatening conditions

Malignancy	Non-accidental injury	Sepsis
• Night pain	• Delay in seeking medical attention	• Complete non-weight bearing
• Pain severe and non-remitting	• Changeable history inconsistent with pattern of injury	• Pseudo-paralysis of limb
• Bone pain	• Explanation of injury incongruent with developmental stage of child	• Any attempt to passively move the limb is resisted and causes extreme distress
• Pallor	• Repeated presentations	• Pain severe and non-remitting
• Bruising	• Unwitnessed injury	• Limb held in a position which accommodates joint volume due to effusion
• Lymphadenopathy	• Patterns of injury suggestive of NAI (e.g. bruising over soft tissue areas, multiple bruises, bruises that carry the imprint of an implement)	• Night pain and waking
• Hepatosplenomegaly		• Fever
• Anaemia, thrombocytopenia	• Distinctive burns, e.g. round cigarette burn, forced immersion burn	• Immunocompromised child—due to 1° disease or medications
• Systemic symptoms (lethargy, weight loss, night sweats, fever)	• Complete non-weight bearing with occult fracture	• Back pain in the unwell child
• Complete non-weight bearing	• Type of fracture, e.g. metaphyseal	
• Back pain in the unwell child	• Multiple injuries	
• Weight loss	• Unkempt appearance and poor hygiene	

- It is also worth remembering that children with established conditions, such as JIA or cerebral palsy, can develop acute limp from causes such as slipped upper femoral epiphysis (SUFE) or Perthes' disease. Septic arthritis can occur although is a rare complication post intra-articular steroid injection in JIA management, but must be considered in the era of increasingly immunosuppressive treatments (see ➔ Infections in the immunocompromised, pp. 69–73).
- Evidence-based clinical practice guidelines have been implemented in some emergency departments to assist in the management of children with limp, with the aim of improving patient care, reducing the overall time spent in hospital, the need for unnecessary laboratory investigations and ensuring that appropriate investigations or referrals are carried out.
- It is important that children presenting with a limp are followed-up with clear instructions (e.g. parent information leaflet) on when to re-seek medical attention. Children with persistent, intermittent or unexplained limp warrant further assessment to establish the diagnosis and prompt referral to paediatric rheumatology is suggested.
- Suggested approaches to the limping child (according to presence or absence of fever) are given (Figs. 2.9 and 2.10).

Indications for urgent assessment of limp

- The very young (under 3 years of age).
- The ill and febrile.
- The non-weight bearing.
- Children with painful restricted hip movements.
- The child who is immunosuppressed.
- Essentially when septic arthritis, osteomyelitis, fractures, NAI, SUFE and malignancy are suspected.

Further reading

Fischer SU, Beattie TF. The limping child: epidemiology, assessment and outcome. *J Bone Joint Surg* 1999;**81B**:1029–34.

Kocher MS, Mandiga R, Zurakowski D, et al. Validation of a clinical prediction rule for the differentiation between septic arthritis and transient synovitis of the hip in children. *J Bone Joint Surgery of Am* 2004;**86A**(8):1629–35.

McCanny PJ1, McCoy S, Grant T, Walsh S, O'Sullivan R. Implementation of an evidence based guideline reduces blood tests and length of stay for the limping child in a paediatric emergency department. *Emerg Med J* 2013;**30**(1):19–23.

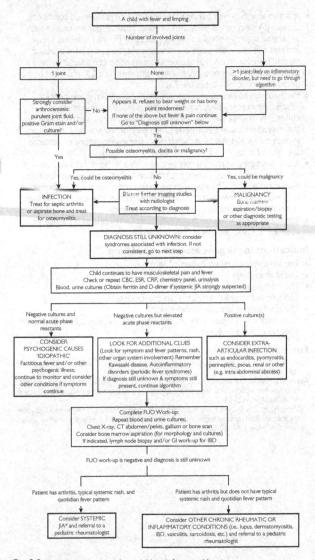

Fig. 2.9 Treatment algorithm for a child with fever and limping
Adapted with permission from Y Kimura. Common presenting problems. In: Szer IS, Kimura Y, Malleson PN, and Southwood T (eds). *Arthritis in Children and Adolescents: Juvenile Idiopathic Arthritis.* Oxford: Oxford University Press, Copyright © 2006 Oxford University Press.

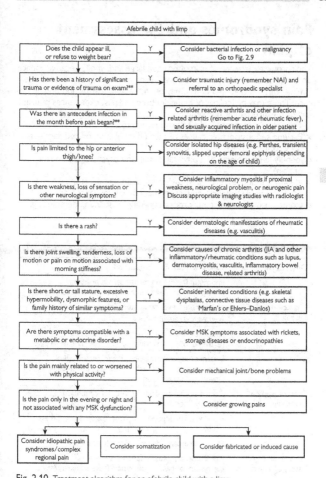

Fig. 2.10 Treatment algorithm for an afebrile child with a limp

Adapted with permission from Y Kimura. Common presenting problems. In: Szer IS, Kimura Y, Malleson PN, and Southwood T (eds.). *Arthritis in Children and Adolescents: Juvenile Idiopathic Arthritis.* Oxford: Oxford University Press, Copyright © 2006 Oxford University Press.

Pain syndromes and the assessment of pain

The chronic experience of pain often has a large and wholly negative impact on the physical and psychological well-being of a young person and their family. Both the child and family may be distressed, fearful, and hoping for cure. There may be feelings of being doubted and past experiences of failed and pain-exacerbating interventions.

The pain assessment (Table 2.8) should aim to:
- Exclude serious possible causes of pain (identification of 'red flags'—see ⟶ Chapter 1, p. 8).
- Identify key problems (the physical, social, and psychological impact of pain).
- Identify a treatment plan (acknowledging aetiological factors, environmental stressors and factors that convey resilience), and
- Commence the therapeutic process, building trust and understanding.

Table 2.8 History: important areas to cover in the assessment of pain

Onset of pain	When/where/how pain started
	Important factors in the history, e.g. preceding infection, trauma, operation, or persisting disease
Characteristics of the pain	Nature/site/severity/variationGetting better/worse Aggravators/ameliorators
	Specific symptoms, e.g. paraesthesia, allodynia (extreme hypersensitivity), skin changes, nocturnal pain
Other symptoms	Systemic/abdominal/genito-urinary/neurological symptoms, e.g. fever, rash, weight loss, appetite change, fatigue, change in mood
Effect of pain on daily living	Sleep disturbance, daytime naps, concentration/memory/mood
	Activity: on bad/good days, school attendance, fitness, hobbies
	Effects on independence and family dynamics
Past and family history of illness	Past illness/operations; family history of illness or pain, e.g. history of painful conditions/fatigue/anxiety/sleep disturbance
Family, emotional, and social circumstances	Family environment/occupations/changes since onset of pain, e.g. any stressors in school, family or peer groups

Examination

Full examination at the beginning may prevent repetition and unnecessary investigations later. Any concerns regarding the diagnosis should be followed-up at this point, avoiding delays that can lead to a worsening of fear, pain symptoms, and associated disability.

Assessing the impact of pain

The history will outline the impact that the pain is having on the individual and their family (e.g. effect on sleep, mood, appetite and fitness, disruption to schooling, social isolation, loss of independence, and widespread family disruption, including financial hardship).

Assessment tools

- *Visual analogue scale (VAS)*—a simple tool for measurement of pain severity as perceived by the child or carer; useful for assessing pain intensity experienced; patients mark their level of pain on a continuous scale from 0 to 10.
- *Faces pain scale*—pictures of faces depicting expressions showing various levels of a pain response; often used in younger children.
- *Bath Adolescent Pain Questionnaire & Bath Adolescent Pain Questionnaire for Parent*— two multidisciplinary tools developed specifically for use in measuring the impact of pain on adolescents with chronic pain and their parents.

Clinical features associated with chronic pain conditions

Pain may start in a localized area with an associated avoidance of movement, and may lead to radiation to other areas of the body, increased pain intensity, muscle spasms, abnormal posture, reduced fitness, and pain-associated anxiety. Effects on other body systems include:

- Hypersensitivity or allodynia—unbearable pain on minimal contact; heightened fear of being touched.
- Thermodysregulation—cool and mottled or red and hot skin, especially limbs; abnormal perception of temperature.
- Autonomic dysfunction—sympathetic nervous system stimulation by continuous pain and anxiety signals.
- Musculoskeletal disequilibrium—changes to gait and resting postures of the trunk and limbs; muscle and tendon tightening; altered mechanical load associated with adaptive, protective positioning.

Recognized pain conditions

The most common chronic pain conditions reviewed in paediatric rheumatology settings are:

- *Diffuse idiopathic musculoskeletal pain (juvenile fibromyalgia):* generalized pain, often with gradual onset and may follow a period of illness or hypermobility. Fatigue, poor sleep, and low mood are often prominent.
- *Chronic pain related to hypermobility:* ligamentous laxity of joints presenting in association with diffuse pain conditions such as lower-limb. With arthralgia, anterior knee pain, and back pain; not all hypermobile individuals will be symptomatic.
- *Complex regional pain syndrome (CRPS):* see ➔ Complex regional pain syndrome, pp. 86–7.

- *Chronic back pain* (see ➲ Back pain in children and adolescents, pp. 105–7): low back pain common in adolescence; may be associated with posture, load bearing, and sedentary activity.
- *Persistent joint pain following previous or controlled inflammation*: the degree of disabling pain does not always mirror inflammatory joint activity; environmental and cognitive behavioural factors influence the experience of pain.

Principles of management

- The focus is on symptom management and psychosocial rehabilitation rather than cure.
- Education—to support the rationale for rehabilitation: understand how the body works to maintain pain that is no longer useful, challenge misconceptions of pain always signifying pathology and reduce pain-associated fear.
- Pharmacotherapy—simple analgesics can be tried; gabapentin and pregabalin may be helpful in neuropathic pain, as well as amitriptyline; medication should be used alongside multidisciplinary therapy. Medicine review is often an essential task in this population. Polypharmacy, risk of dosing and combination errors, and confusion over the utility of previously and currently prescribed medication is common. Drug withdrawal, detoxification, and replacement should be carefully managed.
- Physical therapy—early intensive physiotherapy is the treatment of choice to accelerate mobilization; psychological support is important.
- Psychological therapy—should ideally be delivered by a paediatric psychologist who may use therapies such as cognitive-behavioural therapy, acceptance and mindfulness to help the young person and family move forward with rehabilitation, and support engagement with normal life activities.

Complex regional pain syndrome

CRPS type I (CRPS I) is a potentially incapacitating syndrome which can occur after a minor injury or operation to a limb. CRPS I has an impact on all tissues and can impair all functions of that extremity, possibly resulting in severe impairment and therapy-resistant pain. In children it is seen more commonly in adolescent girls and not infrequently in young people who are premorbidly very physically active and able. Much academic attention to this condition is targeting the neurophysiological changes that are now evident and the mechanisms of central sensitization.

Clinical features

In children the lower limb is more commonly involved than the upper limb. The pain is usually out of proportion to the inciting event and accompanied by allodynia.

The International Association for the Study of Pain (IASP) has diagnostic criteria for adults with CRPS but not children. Although these diagnostic criteria hold true for children and adolescents, it is widely believed that the dystrophic changes and long-term disability are less common when compared with adults. Occasionally >1 limb may be affected at presentation. It is not unusual for a hand or other leg to develop CRPS months after a leg has been affected.

Features commonly seen in CRPS

- Unexplained diffuse pain (although occasionally very localized).
- Difference in skin colour in relation to the healthy symmetrical limb.
- Oedema (may be transient).
- Difference in skin temperature in relation to the healthy symmetrical limb.
- Limited range of movement and impaired function.
- Worsening of symptoms during exercise.

Rehabilitation

- Key to rehabilitation is reversing the unusual positioning of the limb and returning children to a more active lifestyle while the pain, altered proprioception, and thermodysregulation are still present. Many young people find gentle physical therapy intolerable and continue to hold the affected limb in a fixed position and this further ↑ pain-associated disability with heightening anxiety and low mood.
- Medical therapies are limited but, in addition to regular analgesics, gabapentin and pregabalin may help neuropathic pain. Amitriptyline may have a specific role to help the burning sensation. The true efficacy of these treatments in CRPS is unknown; the consensus is that they are to be used only as an adjunct with ongoing physical and psychological therapy. Other interventions (e.g. pain-relieving blocks/topical patches) are still used albeit with little evidence for their effect.
- Early recognition of CRPS is key. At this stage multidisciplinary input including pain education, targeted physical rehabilitation, psychological support, and analgesia should be instigated. In the majority the condition becomes less bothersome with children returning to normal activities, often leading to complete cessation of symptoms. A few continue to have long-term problems with escalating pain associated disability.

The role of the psychologist in the multidisciplinary team

- Persistent pain brings distress, fear, disability, adult attention, and changes to the usual family functioning. Young people with chronic pain report sleep disturbance, disordered mood, appetite disruption, low feelings, social isolation, and unwelcome dependency on parents. When maintained, these factors perpetuate pain and disability.
- Routines of normal schooling can become unmanageable and further strained by interpersonal problems in explaining confusing problems. School absence commonly occurs, further removing the child from their normal social environment. This contributes to the impact on their developmental trajectory, especially around adolescence: usually a time of change, experimentation, social maturation, and development of independence.

- Parental stress is also significant—parents experience distress and conflict in parenting their child. They report struggling to cure and comfort their child, recognizing that the desire to protect may be counterproductive.

Delivering psychological support

It is important that psychological support is integrated in the overall management of patients with chronic pain as early as possible. Once the diagnosis is made the emphasis can move from investigation and cure to symptom management, functional improvement, and psychosocial rehabilitation. This should be delivered by all members of the MDT with a consistent approach.

Components of psychological intervention

- Exploring difficult thoughts and emotions related to pain and the impact of pain on life.
- Maintaining engagement in rehabilitation by understanding values.
- Pain education and activity management.
- Communication and managing social interactions with friends and teachers.
- Parenting approaches to enable parents to support their child in their rehabilitation.
- Goal setting and return to age appropriate activities including school.

Key principles

- Disengagement from the pursuit of pain relief and engagement with normal life activities.
- Focus on goals that are important to the individual child.
- Exercise and physical therapy is key to the rehabilitation of young people with persistent pain and psychological support is crucial to address fear of damage, worries about return to activities, develop strategies for engagement in activity in the presence of ongoing pain.
- Work with parents as a core part of the parents in the rehabilitation process.

Specific psychological therapies

Acceptance and commitment therapy, cognitive behavioural therapy, mindfulness, motivational interviewing and family therapy.

Further reading

Clinch J, Eccleston C. Chronic musculoskeletal pain in children: assessment and management. *Rheumatology* 2009;48:466–74.

Eccleston C, Jordan A, McCracken LM, et al. The Bath Adolescent Pain Questionnaire (BAPQ): development and preliminary psychometric evaluation of an instrument to assess the impact of chronic pain on adolescents. *Pain* 2005;118:263–70

Growing pains

Overview

- A 'lay term' encompassing non-specific musculoskeletal pains commonly experienced by many healthy young children (with equal gender ratio), characterized by poorly localized aches and pains in the calves, shins, feet, and ankles, usually relieved with massage or simple analgesics, and often predictable to occur later in the day, evenings, and after periods of activity.
- The cause is unknown but there is no clear association with growth (thus the term is a misnomer). Children with growing pains often have features of hypermobility although not all hypermobile children have pain; the causal association of hypermobility with pain in children remains controversial. There is often a family history of growing pains.
- There is no specific test to positively confirm the diagnosis and clinical assessment is integral to excluding potential causes of MSK pains. (See ⊋ Chapter 1, pp. 2–3).
  - The 'rules' (red flags) of growing pains (Box 2.4) are important— where the clinical pattern 'does not fit' these rules, further investigation is required.
  - The history should focus on the pattern, predictability, and site of pain—it is important to probe for indicators of concern (Box 2.5).
  - Physical examination requires a comprehensive MSK examination (see ⊋ Chapter 1, pp. 2–3) and general examination.
  - Nocturnal pain is common in growing pains—concern is warranted if night waking is becoming more frequent, unremitting, or localized to one site. Response to NSAIDS is common but (benign) bone tumours need to be considered (see ⊋ Bone tumours, pp. 59–61).

Management

- Investigation is not needed unless concern has been raised (Box 2.4). Investigations are summarized in Box 2.5.
- Reassurance and explanation is paramount:
  - Growing pains are likely to improve as the child gets older.
  - Advice on footwear (supportive and well fitting); trainers with arch supports are ideal (note shoelaces are best tied and 'Velcro' fastened firmly). Specialist orthotics rarely needed.
  - Given the predictability of pains and to prevent night waking, analgesics before physical activities or at bedtime may be helpful.
- It is important to address parental concerns and give clear instructions when to seek medical attention again (e.g. limping, joint swelling, asymmetrical involvement 1 leg being affected or pains elsewhere (e.g. fingers), or daytime symptoms, systemically unwell avoidance of previously enjoyed activities).
- A parent information leaflet is available: ⅋ http://www.arthritisresearchuk.org/files/6541_20022010162934.pdf.

Box 2.4 The 'rules' of growing pains

'Rules' of growing pains
- Pains never present at the start of the day after waking.
- Child doesn't limp.
- Physical activities not limited by symptoms.
- Pains symmetrical in lower limbs and not limited to joints.
- Physical examination normal (joint hypermobility may or may not be detected).
- Systemically well and major motor milestones normal.
- Age range 3–12yr.

Indications for concern
- Abnormal growth (height and weight).
- Abnormal developmental milestones:
  - *Delay* (especially major motor skills) suggestive of neurological disease or metabolic bone disease or
  - *Regression* of achieved motor milestones (consider inflammatory joint or muscle disease).
- Impaired functional ability (ask about play, sport, schoolwork, 'clumsiness').
- Limping (intermittent or persistent).
- Morning symptoms (other than tiredness after disturbed sleep) or mood changes may suggest inflammatory arthritis.
- Widespread pain (such as upper limbs and back).
- School absenteeism.

Box 2.5 Investigations that may be indicated
- FBC (and film), acute phase reactants (ESR, CRP).
- Biochemistry (bone biochemistry and vitamin D) to exclude metabolic bone disease including osteomalacia (see ➔ Metabolic bone diseases, pp. 358–61).
- Thyroid function, muscle enzymes to exclude inflammatory muscle disease (see ➔ Juvenile dermatomyositis, pp. 280–7).
- X-ray of legs (hips with frog views) to exclude hip pathology, e.g. Perthes disease (see Table 2.13).
- Radioisotope bone scan to exclude local hot spots (e.g. osteoid osteoma, occult fracture)—see ➔ Bone tumours, pp. 59–61.

Further reading
Foster HE, Boyd D, Jandial S. *Growing Pains. A Practical Guide for Primary Care.* ARC, 2008. Available at: Ⓙ http://www.arthritisresearchuk.org/files/6541_20022010162934.pdf.

The child with recurrent fever

Background

- Paediatricians are often faced with a child presenting with fever.
- The differential diagnosis is broad and includes infectious, oncologic, and inflammatory causes.
- Recurrent fever, a fairly common scenario, may be associated with rather different conditions.
- Although recurrent fever is the presenting symptom of several serious illnesses, in many cases no defined aetiology can be found despite exhaustive investigations.
- Assessment of a child with recurrent fever must consider clinical, serological, and sometimes genetic clues that may allow identification of the underlying cause, thus facilitating appropriate management.
- Patients with recurrent fever often come to the clinic during their symptom-free periods, making the diagnostic task difficult. Thus, history taking and review of abnormalities in laboratory tests become important sources of critical information in order to generate a differential diagnosis.

Definitions

- *Recurrent fever* may be defined as 3 or more episodes of fever in a 6-month period, with no defined medical illness explaining the fevers and with an interval of at least 7 days between febrile episodes.
  - Such (apparently) symptom-free intervals may show either 'clock-work' or irregular periodicity which may last weeks to months.
- *Periodic fever* is a type of recurrent fever with a regular (and often predictable) interval between febrile episodes.
  - PFAPA syndrome (periodic fever, aphthous stomatitis, pharyngitis and cervical adenopathy), an idiopathic inflammatory disorder, is the leading cause of periodic fever in children.
- Other polygenic and monogenic syndromes usually have less regular symptom-free intervals.

Assessment

- A simple framework within which the clinician can consider the various differential diagnoses for recurrent fever is:
  - Does the child have an under active immune system (immunodeficiency with infection)?
  - Does the child have an over active immune system causing sterile inflammation (autoinflammatory disease or autoimmunity)?
  - Or 'a bit of both': immunodeficiency with immune dysregulation, an increasingly recognized scenario?

Thus, approaching the differential diagnosis of a child with recurrent fever includes:

- extensive history taking and detailed analysis of symptoms.
- demographic setting (ethnicity, age of onset of symptoms).
- family history (of autoimmune diseases, autoinflammatory disorders, AA amyloidosis and/or renal failure).

- Enquiring about characteristics of the fever episodes:
  - potential triggers.
  - prodrome.
  - periodicity.
  - magnitude of fever.
  - duration of individual febrile episodes.
  - duration of intervals.
  - alleviating factors.
  - associated symptoms.
  - response to treatment(s).
- Physical examination may be noncontributory if the patient is seen when well.
- Abnormalities in weight and height should alert about chronic conditions.
- During febrile episodes careful examination of skin, musculoskeletal system, eyes, mucosae, abdomen (presence of organomegaly), and virtually any organ system can yield relevant information.
- Initial laboratory tests are needed to confirm or exclude infection and/or inflammation.
- Repetition of testing may be required to identify the presence of inflammatory markers as a consistent feature of the episodes, and their normalization in-between febrile episodes.
- Exclusion of both usual and unusual infections is often needed.

Initial workup may include:
- complete blood count (CBC) with differential white cell count.
- ESR and CRP.
- hepatic enzymes.
- Albumin.
- immunoglobulins including IgA, and more contentiously IgD as high levels are common in mevalonate kinase deficiency (MKD), although this finding is neither specific or sensitive for this monogenic autoinflammatory disease.
- bacterial cultures of urine and blood.
- infectious disease serology (seek expert advice, (Table 2.9)).
- uric acid, lactate dehydrogenase, and urine vanillylmandelic acid (abnormalities may indicate the presence of malignancy).
- Iron studies including ferritin (to consider the possibility of evolving haemophagocytic lymphohistiocytosis or macrophage activation syndrome, see ➔ Chapter 4: Macrophage activation syndrome pp. 321–4).
- A basic autoimmune profile.

Points to consider for subsequent specialist workup:
- In patients with an elevated ESR and CRP these tests should be repeated during a symptom-free interval to establish whether these normalize or not.
- Advanced laboratory tests should be employed when a specific diagnosis is suspected (e.g. autoantibodies and C3/C4 for SLE and other autoimmune conditions; immunophenotype for immunodeficiencies, etc).

- Certain markers can be helpful in the setting of a probable
  autoinflammatory condition. This context points of note are:
  - Serum amyloid A (SAA) is not specific for autoinflammatory disease
    and may also be elevated in infection.
  - Urine mevalonate excretion is elevated during crises in MKD, but
    requires specific laboratory expertise to detect reliably.
  - Ferritin levels are usually modestly elevated in active SJIA, but much
    higher in MAS.
  - S100A8/9 and S100A12 are usually elevated in most autoinflamma-
    tory disorders in the active phase, and are not routinely available in
    most laboratories.
  - Molecular genetic analyses may confirm/or exclude the diagnosis of
    several autoinflammatory disorders: increasingly, next-generation
    sequencing offers the possibility of targeted gene panels that allow
    simultaneous screening of many genes for a fraction of the cost of
    conventional Sanger sequencing. Seek expert advice.

Differential diagnosis

- Infection (with or without immunodeficiency)
  - repeated, common infections in infancy.
  - urinary tract infection.
  - sinopulmonary infection.
  - occult dental infection.
  - viral (EBV, Parvovirus, or other virus) infection.
  - bacterial (brucellosis, borreliosis, mycobacterial) infection.
  - infections in immunodeficiencies.
  - insufficiently treated infection.
  - malaria.
- Malignancy
  - lymphoma.
  - leukemia.
  - other.
- Non-infectious inflammatory diseases (autoimmune and
  autoinflammatory diseases).
  - autoimmune diseases (e.g. SLE).
  - monogenic (see ➔ Chapter 4 on autoinflammatory diseases,
    pp. 303–12) and polygenic autoinflammatory diseases (including sys-
    temic juvenile arthritis, inflammatory bowel disease, Behçet's disease,
    and PFAPA. See Box 2.6).
- Cyclic neutropenia.
- Benign hyperthermia.
- Factitious fever.
- Drug fever.

Management

- Explanation of symptoms and reassurance, where appropriate.
- Referral to a subspecialist (rheumatologist, ID specialist, immunologist,
  oncologist).
- Genetic counselling (monogenic diseases).
- Specific management of the underlying disease: see Table 2.9 and
  Table 2.10.

Box 2.6 Diagnostic criteria for PFAPA (periodic fever, aphthous stomatitis, pharyngitis and cervical adenopathy) syndrome

- Regularly recurring fevers with an early age of onset (< 5 years of age).
- Symptoms in the absence of upper respiratory tract infection with at least one of the following:
  - aphthous stomatitis
  - cervical lymphadenopathy
  - pharyngitis.
- Exclusion of cyclic neutropenia.
- Completely asymptomatic interval between episodes.
- Normal growth and development.

Table 2.9 Differential diagnosis for recurrent fevers in the young

	Immunodeficiency	SLE	Autoinflammatory	Malignancy	CN	Factitious	Benign	Self-limited infections in a healthy child	Drug fever
Age of onset	Infancy	Puberty	Early childhood, adolescence	1–4yr; puberty	Infancy, early childhood	Variable	Variable	Infancy	Variable
Duration of episodes	Days to weeks	Days to weeks	Days to weeks	Days to weeks	3–10 days	Days	Days	Days	Days to weeks
Associated symptoms	Diarrhoea, weight loss, failure to thrive, slow response to ATB, protracted course of common infections. Hospitalizations often needed	Weight loss, exanthema, MSK	Variable	Weight loss, anaemia, bone pain	Mouth ulcers, gingivitis, cervical adenitis	None	None	The expected according to trigger (e.g. EBV), Exathema, adenitis	Sometimes mouth ulcers and rash
Duration of interval between episodes	Variable	Variable	Variable	Variable	21 days	Variable	Variable	Variable	
Symptoms between episodes	Yes	Yes	Variable	Yes	None	None	None	None	
Triggers	Infection	Infection, stress	Stress, immunizations						Drug (ATB, anticonvulsant)
Family history	Commonly present	Sometimes present	Commonly present	None	Sometimes present	None	None	None	
Useful investigations	CBC, IgG, IgA, IgM, immunophenotype	ANA, anti-DNA, complement	CBC, CRP	LDH, uric acid, bone scan, CT	CBC 2–3 times a week for 6 weeks	Regular, supervised temperature measurement	Exclusion of illness	Cultures, serologies	Eosinophils, discontinuation of drug

Table 2.10 Causes of recurrent fevers in children

	FCAS	MWS	NOMID	MKD	FMF
Age of onset	Infancy	Infancy	Neonatal/infancy	Infancy/childhood	Childhood, adolescence
Typical duration of episodes	12–24hr after exposure	12hr to days	Continuously ill	4–6 days	12–72hr
Associated symptoms	Urticarial rash, arthralgia, conjunctivitis	Urticarial rash, conjunctivitis, hearing loss, arthralgia/arthritis	Urticarial rash, conjunctivitis, organomegaly, hypertrophic arthropathy, papilledema, hearing loss, progressive CNS impairment	Cervical adenitis, abdominal pain, vomiting, diarrhoea, arthritis, rash	Serositis, abdominal/chest pain, arthritis, rash
Duration of interval between episodes	Variable	Variable	Variable	4–6 weeks	Months
Symptoms between episodes	None	Deafness	Continuously ill	None or constitutional	Excertional leg pain in a minority
Triggers	Cold	Cold, stress, trauma		Vaccines, trauma	Stress, menses, physical activity
Useful investigations	*NLRP3* genetic screening	*NLRP3* genetic screening	*NLRP3* genetic screening	IgA, urine mevalonate; *MVK* genetic screening	*MEFV* genetic screening
Effective therapies	IL-1 blockade	IL-1 blockade	IL-1 blockade	NSAIDs, corticosteroids, IL-1 blockade, TNF antagonists, IL-6 blockade	Colchicine IL-1 blockade

TRAPS	PFAPA	SJIA	CRMO	IBD	Behcet's
Childhood	<5yr	Early childhood	Childhood, adolescence	Childhood, adolescence	Childhood, adolescence
1–2 weeks	4–5 days	Days to weeks	Variable	Variable	Variable
Muscle pain, erythematous rash, conjunctivitis, periorbital oedema, abdominal pain	Aphthous stomatitis, pharyngitis, cervical adenitis (abdominal pain and headaches may occur)	Evanescent rash, arthritis, organomegaly, serositis	Bone pain, pustulosis (IBD may coexist)	Abdominal pain, diarrhoea, uveitis, oral ulcers, arthritis, erythema nodosum	Aphthous stomatitis, arthritis, genital ulcers, uveitis, meningitis, diarrhoea, papulopustular lesions (IBD may coexist)
Weeks to months	3–6 weeks	Weeks to months	Variable	Weeks to months	Months
None or constitutional	None	None or constitutional	None or constitutional	None or constitutional	None or constitutional
Stress, menses, trauma	Stress	Infections	Trauma	Stress	Trauma
TNFRSF1A genetic screening	Normalization of CRP in between attacks	Ferritin	Bone scan, whole body MRI	Faecal calprotectin; Bowel biopsy	Pathergy test, HLA B51
Corticosteroids, IL-1 blockade, TNF antagonists	Prednisolone (on the first day to abort attack), tonsillectomy	IL-1 blockade, IL-6 blockade	NSAIDs, pamidronate, TNF antagonists	Mesalazine, corticosteroids, TNF antagonists	Colchicine, azathioprine, TNF antagonists

Table 2.9 Differential diagnosis for recurrent fevers in the young. SLE: systemic lupus erythematosus; MSK: musculo-skeletal; CBC: complete blood count; CRP: C reactive protein; CT: computer tomography; CN: cyclic neutropenia; ATB: antibiotics.

Table 2.10 Features and management of autoinflammatory disease. FCAS: familial cold autoinflammatory syndrome; MWS: Muckle Wells Syndrome; NOMID: neonatal onset multisystemic inflammatory disease; MKD: mevalonate kinase deficiency; FMF: familial Mediterranean fever; TRAPS: TNF receptor associated periodic syndrome; PFAPA: periodic fever aphthous ulceration pharyngitis and adenitis; SJIA: systemic juvenile idiopathic arthritis; CRMO: chronic relapsing multifocal osteomyelitis; IBD: inflammatory bowel disease.

Further reading

Russo RA, Brogan PA. Monogenic autoinflammatory diseases. *Rheumatology (Oxford)*. 2014;53: 1927–39.

Pyrexia of unknown origin

Definition

Essentially this is a term for persistent or recurrent pyrexia that persists for longer than you would expect from a self-limiting viral illness (e.g. 5 days), has not responded to empirical antibiotics (if thought needed), and has evaded diagnosis from reasonable 1st-line history, examination, and investigation.

One useful working definition of pyrexia of unknown origin (PUO) is: pyrexia >38.0°C on several occasions, >3 weeks' duration of illness, and failure to reach diagnosis despite 1 week of inpatient investigations.

Key points

- Always consider incomplete Kawasaki disease, especially if faced with an irritable young child with fever ± other suggestive history, signs, or suggestive blood results (see ➜ Kawasaki disease, pp. 190–5). Omitting early treatment of this can ↑ risk of significant coronary artery aneurysms.
- In the immunosuppressed child (e.g. neonate, neutropenic, HIV+ve, on immunosuppressive treatment, or 1° immunodeficiency), different causes (especially infections, e.g. fungal, *Cryptosporidium*) are more likely and treatment against relevant possible infection should be given alongside investigation.
- Antibiotics have often been tried and no benefit seen, especially in young children.
- 1st-line investigation usually includes:
  - Blood cultures when pyrexial.
  - Urine microscopy and culture.
  - Chest x-ray (CXR).
  - Cerebrospinal fluid (CSF) microscopy, culture, and PCR analysis for HSV.

Assessment

The approach includes investing time in carefully reviewing the history including:

- Detailed review of all systems including rashes, weight loss, bowel symptoms, joint symptoms, mouth ulcers.
- Foreign travel, history of tick / insect bites.
- Health of family members recently and family history of unexplained fever.
- Pets and their health.
- Drug and medication history.
- Hobbies (e.g. camping/trekking), swimming in lakes or rivers, and especially recently.
- Sexual history when relevant.

Detailed examination of all systems and repeated examination including:

- Examining skin for rashes, especially when pyrexial.
- Lymphadenopathy.
- Mouth for ulcers.

- Auscultation of heart sounds.
- Assessment of hands for features of endocarditis and nailfold capillaries.
- Abdomen and testes for any tenderness/swelling.
- Joints for any evidence of arthritis.
- Routine fundoscopy and consider requesting slit lamp examination by ophthalmologist to look for uveitis/other intraocular pathology.
- Eyes, lips, palms, soles, perineum (peeling is often overlooked at this site), neck, and trunk for features of Kawasaki disease: remember that clinical signs can present sequentially, may be subtle and can only last a few days.

Investigation and management

- Further investigations follow-up on clues found from the history, examination and initial test results. Table 2.11 includes the more common causes (focus being for a patient in the UK) and clues that should guide investigations, although this is not an exhaustive list.
- Foreign travel will raise the chances of different infections linked to the area visited.
- There are a few paediatric cohort studies published describing the ultimate diagnoses, but all are very dependent on local population and pathway of referral to the cohort.
- Management depends on the proven or strongly suspected diagnosis.

Consider consulting other specialties

- Infectious diseases.
- Haematology/oncology.
- Gastroenterology.
- Endocrinology.
- Interventional radiology.

Prognosis

- 5–15% remain undiagnosed even after extensive evaluation.
- No evidence to support prolonged hospitalization if patient stable and whose work-up is unrevealing.
- Further outpatient care should include close follow-up procedures, open access for reassessment and systematic re-evaluation to guide further outpatient investigation.

Table 2.11 Causes and relevant investigations for PUO

Diagnosis	Suggestive features	Useful investigations
a) Localized bacterial infections		
Abscess, e.g. abdominal, pelvic	Localizing symptoms	Imaging, e.g. USS, CT, MRI, white cell scan
Endocarditis	New murmur, haematuria, splinter haemorrhages, Janeway lesions, Roth's spots	Repeated blood cultures, transthoracic echocardiogram; consider trans-oesophageal echocardiogram (seek expert advice)
Septic arthritis	Localizing symptoms and signs	Imaging, e.g. US, MRI, joint aspiration
Osteomyelitis	Localizing symptoms	Plain x-ray (although insensitive especially early), bone scan, MRI
Sinusitis/ mastoiditis	Localized pain/tenderness	CT with contrast
b) Other infections		
EBV, CMV	Lymphadenopathy	IgM against EBV/CMV, PCR testing of blood
Cat scratch disease	Lymphadenopathy. Contact with cats	Serology (*Bartonella*). Lymph node biopsy
Tuberculosis	Family or contact history, travel, night sweats	CXR, Mantoux, Quantiferon TB test, specific culture, 16s ribosomal PCR of lesional tissue or fluid
HIV	Recurrent infections, maternal ill-health, sexually active or other risk factors	Blood HIV PCR
HHV6	Rash, febrile convulsion, aseptic meningitis	PCR of blood and CSF
Brucellosis	Farming community, hepatosplenomegaly	Serology (*Brucella*). Specific culture of urine + blood
Campylobacter, Salmonella, Shigella, or *Yersinia*	Diarrhoea	Repeated stool microscopy and culture.
Hepatitis	Jaundice, abdominal pain, diarrhoea	Serology for HAV, HBV, HCV
Leptospirosis	Farming/river contact, headache, myalgia then headache	Serology (*Leptospira*)
Malaria	Travel to endemic area in preceding months	Repeated blood films
Lyme disease	Rash, tick bite, aseptic meningitis, arthritis	Serology (*Borrelia*)

Table 2.11 Contd.

Diagnosis	Suggestive features	Useful investigations
c) Post-infectious		
Acute rheumatic fever	Recent pharyngitis, carditis, Duckett Jones criteria	Throat swab, ASOT/ anti-DNAase B, ECG, echocardiogram
Post streptococcal reactive arthritis	Recent pharyngitis, fleeting arthritis	Throat swab, ASOT/ anti-DNAase B
Other reactive arthritis	Arthritis, urethritis, conjunctivitis, recent infection	HLA B27 status, stool culture, urethral swab including *Chlamydia* culture/ PCR and gonorrhoea microscopy/culture
d) Malignancy		
Leukaemia	Anaemia, cytopenia (including platelet count inappropriately low or normal for raised inflammatory markers), night pain	Blood film, flow cytometry of peripheral lymphocytes, bone marrow aspirate
Lymphoma	Lymphadenopathy, weight loss, night sweats	LDH, abdominal US, lymph node biopsy
Neuroblastoma	Mass, anaemia	Urine VMA and HVA: creatinine ratio, abdominal US
Wilm's tumour	Abdominal pain and mass, haematuria	Abdominal US
e) Autoimmune/auto-inflammatory		
Systemic juvenile idiopathic arthritis	Typical rash with daily pyrexia, arthritis (may be later), lymphadenopathy, mild splenomegaly	Ferritin, abdominal US.
Kawasaki disease	Irritable (with sterile CSF), eye and mouth changes, rash, lymphadenopathy, peeling skin	Echocardiogram. NB a normal result does not exclude Kawasaki disease. Abdominal US (hydrops gall bladder).
SLE	Rash, arthralgia, low mood and lethargy, Lymphopenia, cytopenia, proteinuria. Varied presentation incl. hepatitis, psychosis.	ANA screen, ENA Abs, dsDNA antibodies, ACL and lupus anticoagulant, C3 and C4, renal biopsy if significant nephritis. Raised ESR, but normal CRP (if no infection).
Juvenile dermatomyositis	Typical rashes, abnormal nailfold capillaries, proximal muscle weakness	CK, LDH, MRI thigh muscles—see ➔ Juvenile dermatomyositis, pp. 280–7

Table 2.11 Contd.

Diagnosis	Suggestive features	Useful investigations
Periodic fever syndromes (see ➔ pp. 303–12)	Chronic episodic fever, well in between, with stereotyped clinical features, otherwise thriving	Acute phase response when well and soon after onset, gene mutation analysis
CINCA/CAPS	Neonatal onset, irritable, rash, arthritis	Gene mutation analysis. See ➔ Cryopyrin associated periodic syndrome (CAPS), p. 309
Sarcoidosis	Arthritis, rash, uveitis, chest disease (hilar lymphadenopathy ± interstitial lung disease)	Serum ACE, CXR, serum calcium, consider lesional tissue biopsy. See ➔ Sarcoidosis, pp. 316–20
Vasculitis	Rash, renal concerns, arthritis, ENT, respiratory or cerebral concerns, testicular +/ or abdominal pain, many other potential multi-systemic features	Skin biopsy, selective visceral digital subtraction arteriography, ANCA
Inflammatory bowel disease	Diarrhoea and/or nausea, weight loss, mouth ulcers	Faecal calprotectin, upper and lower GI endoscopy, MRI bowel, labelled white cell scan
Thyrotoxicosis	Weight loss, tremor, sweating, tachycardia	Thyroid function tests (including T_3 if strongly suspect, as well as TSH and T_4), thyroid autoantibodies
f) Miscellaneous		
Factitious	Not recorded in hospital by others	Careful observation in hospital. Consider child protection proceedings to arrange supervised access by parents / carers
Drug-induced fever	Suggestive history	Stop suspected drug(s)
Kikuchi disease	Lymphadenopathy progressing to necrotizing lymphadenitis (especially cervical), leukopenia Asian origin especially; observed particularly in SLE	Lymph node biopsy
Castleman's disease	'Giant lymph node hypertrophy', unifocal or multicentric	HHV8 serology and/or PCR, lymph node excision biopsy. FDG PET-CT scan, serum cytokine analysis (esp. IL-6) if available

Further reading

Cogulu O, Koturoglu G, Kurugol Z, et al. Evaluation of 80 children with prolonged fever. *Pediatr Int* 2003;45:564–9.

Joshi N, Rajeshwari K, Dubey AP, et al. Clinical spectrum of fever of unknown origin among Indian children. *Ann Trop Paediatr* 2008;28:261–6.

Pasic S, Minic A, Djuric P, et al. Fever of unknown origin in 185 paediatric patients: a single-centre experience. *Acta Paediatr* 2006;95:463–6.

Back pain in children and adolescents

Epidemiological studies report back pain in children to be more common than previously thought, with a higher prevalence of non-specific lower back pain as the child matures. Recent meta-analysis showed a mean point prevalence of 12% and mean lifetime prevalence of 40%. A detailed history and examination identifying red flag symptoms (Table 2.12) and signs (Table 2.13) should point towards appropriate investigation and diagnosis of pathological causes.

Table 2.12 'Red flag' symptoms in back pain

Examination	Red flag symptoms
Age of child	<4yr
Chronicity	>4 weeks, persistent and worsening
Site	Cervical spine, point tenderness
Exacerbating factors	Hyperextension
Diurnal variation	Worse at night, early morning stiffness
Systemic features	Pyrexia, weight loss, malaise
Neurological symptoms	Altered bladder and bowel function, paresthesia, headaches
Past medical or family history	Systemic disease, e.g. JIA, sickle cell, TB, (see ➔ Tuberculosis and mycobacterial disease, pp. 384–90), neurofibromatosis
Drug history	Pain unresponsive to analgesia,* chronic steroid use
Social activities	History of trauma or foreign travel, interference with function. Lifestyle and psychological factors should also be enquired about (e.g. bullying at school)

* Benign osteoid osteoma pain often responds well to NSAID therapy.

Table 2.13 'Red flag' signs in back pain

Examination	Red flag signs
Cardiovascular	Tachycardia
Respiratory	Reduced air entry, mediastinal shift
Gastrointestinal	Abdominal mass
Neurological	Altered power, tone, reflexes, sensation
Musculoskeletal	Altered normal spine curvature or gait. Scoliosis (especially if painful). Vertebral/intervertebral tenderness
Systemic	Pyrexia, lymphadenopathy
Dermatological	Rash, easy bruising/bleeding, café au lait patches, infected skin, midline skin lesions

Back examination

(See ➔ pREMS, pp. 23–7.)
- Look: observe posture and gait (evidence of kyphosis, loss of lumbar lordosis, scoliosis- and if present assess whether fixed or postural), pelvic tilt, shoulder asymmetry, leg-length discrepancy.
- Feel: palpate spine for point tenderness, muscle spasm. Palpate sacroiliac joints.
- Move: range of spinal movement (forward/lateral flexion, extension, rotation), and hyperextension on one leg ('stork test': for lumbar spondylosis—standing on one leg and bringing back into lumbar extension elicits pain ipsilateral to the pars interarticularis lesion).
  - Also examine hips, test straight leg raise with dorsiflexion of foot and assess hamstring length.
- Measure/other: leg-length discrepancy, neurological assessment.

Investigation

If no red flags, imaging unlikely to be helpful. If investigation clinically indicated, do not be reassured by a normal x-ray. MRI, CT, bone scan or SPECT may be needed.

Muscular pain

Common causes include poor posture, hypermobility, leg-length discrepancy, idiopathic scoliosis, asymmetrical load bearing (e.g. schoolbag on one shoulder). No need for imaging (refer scoliosis to scoliosis service). Treatment—advice, analgesia, physiotherapy.

Spondylosis

A bony defect in the pars articularis, analogous to a stress fracture, commonest L4, L5.
- The commonest identifiable cause of low back pain in young athletes, often boys who participate in sports involving repetitive hyperextension and rotational spinal loading, e.g. gymnastics, weight lifting, cricket. Pain may radiate to buttocks.
- If bilateral may progress to *spondylolisthesis*; the forward slip of one vertebra on the vertebra below—usually L5/S1. May compress nerve roots. More common in females during adolescent growth spurt.
- One-legged hyperextension test (stork test—see above) may be positive. A lumbosacral step may be palpated. Hamstrings often tight with increased popliteal angle.
- The defect may be seen on standing PA/lateral x-ray. If x-rays normal but clinical suspicion high, arrange localized MRI or CT (discuss with radiology).
- Management includes review by orthopaedic surgeon—rest, analgesia, physiotherapy. Indications for bracing and/or surgery include a slip of >50% vertebral body width, progressive changes, neurological deficit present.

Scheuermann's disease (juvenile kyphosis)

Often a coincidental finding on x-ray and considered a normal variant of unknown aetiology. May be associated with mild/moderate pain, onset around puberty.

- Kyphotic deformity of thoracic or thoracolumbar spine which does not disappear on lying supine or with hyperextension. Fixed kyphosis is 40° Cobb angle or more, with pain at apex of kyphosis or lower lumbar spine.
- X-ray criterion—>5° anterior wedging of at least 3 adjacent vertebral bodies. In addition there may be irregularity and flattening of vertebral end plates, narrowed disc spaces, Schmorl's nodes (extrusion of disc substance through the vertebral end plate).
- If pain is severe, consider whether other pathology is present.
- Management—analgesia. Symptoms usually resolve with skeletal maturity, but surgical intervention may be required if curvature >70°, refractory pain or neurological deficit.

Disc degeneration

This is present in a significant number (16–26%) of 10–19 yr-olds. May be asymptomatic but pain more likely if *disc prolapse* is present.
- May present with sciatica and/or have positive straight leg raise or dermatomal numbness.
- MRI if suspect disc herniation.
- Management: rest, analgesia, NSAIDs, physiotherapy. Conservative management is less successful than in adults and surgery may be required (e.g. severe pain, progressive neurology).

Tumours—benign/malignant

- Consider if painful scoliosis, persistent or night pain, progressive pain/ disability.
- 6–25% patients with leukaemia present with back pain along with pallor, anorexia, fever, bruising.
- X-ray then MRI, CT or bone scan (discuss with radiology), ± bloods: FBC and film, CRP, LDH, urine catecholamines, and abdominal US.

Osteoporosis

See → Metabolic bone diseases, pp. 358–61.

Idiopathic pain syndrome (see → Pain syndromes and the assessment of pain, pp. 84–8), *infective causes* (discitis, osteomyelitis etc) (see → pp. 63–8) and *inflammatory disorders* (spondyloarthropathies) are discussed elsewhere.

It is also important to remember the possibility of *referred pain* (e.g. from abdomen, chest, or renal causes).

Further reading

Houghton KM. Review for the generalist: evaluation of low back pain in children and adolescents. Pediatric *Rheumatology* 2010;8:28 (open access): ℘ http://www.ped-rheum.com/content/pdf/ 1546-0096-8-28.pdf.

Scoliosis

Scoliosis is a 3-dimensional deformity in which the spine deviates from the midline in the coronal plane by >10° and the affected vertebrae rotate maximally at the apex of the curve. The curve may be single or double (Fig. 2.11).

Causes

- Non-structural: postural/compensatory.
- Transient: sciatic/hysterical/inflammatory/infection.
- Structural:
  - Idiopathic (most common)
  - Congenital, e.g. hemivertebrae
  - Neuromuscular, e.g. muscular dystrophies, cerebral palsy
  - Syndromic, e.g. Marfan's, Rett's
  - Neurofibromatosis-related
  - Trauma
  - Tumour (intra- or extraspinal)
  - Leg length discrepancy

Idiopathic scoliosis

- 80% are idiopathic and classified according to age of onset:
  - Early onset <7 yrs.
  - Late onset 7–18 yrs.
- More common in adolescents than juveniles, more common in females:
  - Thoracic curves are usually to the right.

Symptoms

Idiopathic scoliosis is not associated with significant pain and may present with asymmetry of shoulders, trunk skin creases, leg length discrepancy, or clothes not hanging properly. Often found incidentally. School screening programmes are not deemed cost-effective. A painful scoliosis or with neurological involvement suggest an underlying serious cause ('red flag' for urgent referral).

Examination

(see ➲ pREMS, pp. 23–7)

- 'Look'—observe standing posture. Is the head in the midline, is there shoulder asymmetry, are the iliac crests level?
  - Observe in forward flexion from behind and from the side—is there a single or double curve, is the curve to right or left, is a rib hump visible, are there skin changes (e.g. cafe au lait spots suggestive of neurofibromatosis or hairy patches/sacral dimpling suggestive of spinal dysraphism)?
- 'Feel'—is there spinal tenderness?
- 'Move'—does the curve correct on lateral flexion, sitting, or is it fixed?
- 'Measure/other'—is there leg-length discrepancy? Is there neurological deficit? Is there pes cavus?

Red flags (for urgent referral)

Pain, neurological signs (root or cord compression).

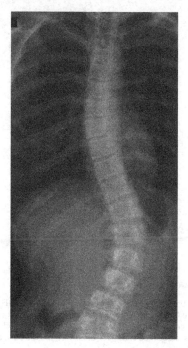

Fig. 2.11 X-ray of patient with idiopathic scoliosis. A right thoracic and left lumbar curve is seen.

Management

- If red flags, refer urgently to scoliosis service.
- If idiopathic scoliosis likely, refer to local scoliosis service for further assessment.
- Treatment options depend on severity and include casting (under 2 yrs old) or bracing, until stopped growing to prevent progression. If severe, surgical interventions including growth modulation devices such as magnetic growth rods in <10yrs, or spinal fusion in adolescents when spine stopped growing.

Investigations

- AP and lateral x-rays of the whole spine should be taken standing in a standardized way.
  - The Cobb angle is determined by identifying the vertebrae at the upper and lower end of the curve, with greatest tilt to concavity of curve and drawing a line along the upper and lower end plates accordingly.

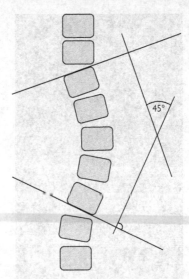

Fig. 2.12 Cobb angle.

- The Cobb angle is the angle between these two lines (Fig. 2.12). Note: the Cobb angle correlates poorly with overall cosmetic appearance which may be affected by number, size, and location of curves, associated chest wall deformity, muscle bulk, and fat distribution.
- MRI and isotope bone scan are required with a painful scoliosis—bone scan may detect osteoid osteomas which can be missed on MRI.
- MRI required with presence of red flags. It is reported that left-hand thoracic curves have a high incidence of neural axis abnormalities (e.g. Arnold Chiari malformation). Albeit a contentious observation, MRI is advised with left-hand thoracic curves.
- Pulmonary function tests are necessary in significant thoracic scoliosis; impact on cardiovascular function is low unless the curve is large with Cobb angle >100°.

Prognosis
Worse prognosis and greater likelihood of progression:
- Large curves, thoracic and double 1° curves.
- Earlier onset pre-skeletal maturation as scoliosis progresses through pubertal growth phases.
- In adolescent idiopathic scoliosis, the Risser grade (degree of fusion of the iliac apophysis reflecting skeletal age) can be used with the Cobb angle to give an estimate of the chance of progression in a population.
  - Risser grade 0–1: curves 20–29° have >65% risk of progression.
  - Risser grade 2–4: curves 20–29° have > 20% risk of progression.

Hip pain and hip problems in children and adolescents

- Hip problems in children and adolescents can present with pain, limp (see ➲ pp. 78–81), deformity, inability to bear weight or as part of a systemic illness. Early diagnosis and appropriate treatment are paramount to avoid permanent damage.
- Children are optimally managed by an experienced MDT including orthopaedics, rheumatology, and infectious diseases as indicated, especially before invasive procedures are contemplated. Alleviation of pain should be given due importance from the start and throughout the investigation phase.
- The clinical assessment is integral to making a diagnosis and the differential diagnosis is broad but may be differentiated by age (see Tables 2.14–2.16 with more detail given in relevant chapters). *Red flags* (see ➲ p. 80) for septic arthritis, osteomyelitis, malignancy, and NAI are vital to consider and exclude. Investigations should be tailored to the most likely differential diagnoses based on the clinical assessment.
- Key features in the clinical assessment include:
  - History: onset and symptom duration, characteristics of pain, morning stiffness, functional impairment, presence of other joints affected, fever and associated systemic symptoms, coexistent medical conditions, and identification of precipitating factors including trauma. *Note that trauma is common in the young child and a common error to explain musculoskeletal presentations which can be due to other causes.*
  - Hip problems can present with subtle or vague symptoms, e.g. irritability, crying during hip abduction such as nappy-change, or as delay/regression, of motor milestones in children. Hip pain can be localized to the groin or referred to the thigh or knee. Pain felt at the pelvic brim should not be confused with hip pain.
- Physical examination:
  - Presence of fever and systemic features of any concurrent illness. Examine all joints (the pGALS screen is useful—see ➲ pGALS, pp. 18–22), assess gait and check for limb shortening. Pain on passive movements, specifically internal rotation, suggests hip pathology—note that the position that allows for maximal intracapsular volume and resultant comfort in the presence of an effusion, is that of external rotation, flexion, and abduction.
  - Pathology elsewhere (e.g. abdomen, spine, sacroiliac joint, nerves) can mimic hip problems and this requires diligent exclusion.
- Other differential diagnoses across all age groups:
  - JIA from late infancy: monoarthritis of hip is uncommon, but does occur.
  - Infection-related arthritis: reactive arthritis (*Yersinia, Salmonella, Shigella, Campylobacter,* and *Chlamydia* in adolescents); post-streptococcal arthritis; TB arthritis, gonococcal arthritis in adolescents—see ➲ p. 68. Rarer bacteria: *Mycoplasma, Borrelia burgdorferi* (Lyme disease), *Brucella.*

Table 2.14 Differential diagnosis of hip pathology by age: age group: 0–4 years

	Developmental dysplasia of hip	Transient synovitis	Septic arthritis/ osteomyelitis (see p. 63)	Malignancy (see pp. 55–3)	Trauma
Demographics	♀>♂ 1–5 per 1000 (True dislocation)	♂>♀ 1–2 per 1000	Slightly more common in boys 5–10 per 100000	Generally more common in boys	Commonest cause in general—beware not all causes of hip pain are trauma related!
Patho-physiology	Disruption of normal relation between femoral head & acetabulum	Idiopathic self-limiting synovial inflammation	Haematogenous spread most often, direct extension less common. Staph. aureus most common pathogen overall. Consider Group B Strep. & Gram-ve bacilli in neonates. Others: TB, rarer bacteria	Bone marrow infiltration-leukaemia, metastatic tumour (neuroblastoma), 1° bone tumours and soft tissue tumours (such as rhabdomyosarcoma) are rare	Green-stick fractures common in toddlers Consider NAI
Predisposing factors & associations	Family history Breech Oligohydramnios Neuromuscular disease	Viral or bacterial illness Minor trauma	Immunosuppression Trauma Sickle-cell disease Interventional procedures in neonates especially preterms	Congenital:Down's, Bloom's, Fanconi's syndromes	Bone mineralization disorders (see pp. 358–61) Social history in NAI
Clinical features	Hip click/clunk Can present later in infancy, asymmetry of skin creases Shortening of limb	Pain + limp ± Most common cause of hip pain in children excluding trauma	Fever, pain++, inability to bear weight, restriction of joint movement, other systemic signs	Severe/nocturnal pain, inability to weight-bear, bony tenderness ±, Systemic—fever, anaemia, weight loss	Pain, inability to weight bear, local tenderness, local bruising ±

Diagnosis	Clinical (neonatal screening)—Ortolani & Barlow test, MSUS 4–6 months of age X-ray—for late presentation MRI—for complications	Blood tests can be abnormal Radiology might show effusion (MSUS and MRI)	USS useful to show effusion, MRI for osteomyelitis/abscess Inflammatory markers are often high. Joint aspiration—gold standard A high index of suspicion is required for diagnosis (Kochers prediction rule; see ➡ p. 66)	Radiology for site & extent—MRI/CT, bone scan may show 'hotspots' FBC/bone marrow to exclude leukaemia Urinary catecholamines-screening for neuroblastoma Bone biopsy—definitive histological diagnosis
				History for mechanism of injury Imaging—x-ray usually suffices MRI for detailed evaluation & to exclude other causes
Treatment	Abduction brace Closed reduction Open surgical reduction Acetabuloplasty	Symptomatic NSAIDs	Arthroscopic/open drainage ± joint lavage Antibiotics—in general, IV followed by oral, although duration is not clearly defined	Modality dependent on pathology: chemotherapy, radiotherapy, surgical resection
				Orthopaedic management Pain relief Management of NAI
Course & complications	Good outcome if early identification & treatment Persistent dysplasia Avascular necrosis (2° to treatment)	Usually resolves within 2 weeks Recurrence risk of 15%, usually within 6 months—unclear if associated with subsequent development of Perthes' disease	Increase in intra-articular pressure I compromised blood supply & avascular necrosis Joint destruction can occur without prompt or adequate treatment	Prognosis dependent on staging Poor prognosis in advanced malignant disease
				Excellent prognosis with early treatment Prognosis for NAI is dependent on coexisting injuries and chronic impact

see ➡ p. 66

Table 2.15 Differential diagnosis of hip pathology by age: age group: 4–8 years

	Perthes' disease(Legg–Calve–Perthes)	Septic arthritis and osteomyelitis	Tumours/malignancy	Transient synovitis
Demographics	♂>♀ 5–15 per 100,000	See Table 2.12 and ⊕ Bone and joint infections, pp. 63–8	See Table 2.12 and ⊕ Bone tumours, pp. 59–61 Frequency of bone tumours increases with age	Less common as age advances after 4–6yr
Patho-physiology	Idiopathic avascular necrosis of femoral epiphysis	Septic arthritis diminishes in frequency after 2yr of age—however should be excluded	Benign bone tumours: • Osteochondroma—most common • Osteoid osteoma—pain dramatically responsive to NSAIDs	
Predisposing factors & associations	Epiphyseal dysplasia Hypothyroidism Delayed bone age Caucasians Coagulation abnormalities			
Clinical features	Pain ±, limp worsening with exercise Bilateral in 10–15%		Malignant bone tumours: • Osteosarcoma most common—associa ion with previous irradiation • Ewing's sarcoma 2nd most common—commmcner in white boys, diaphyseal in contrast to most 1° bone tumours which are metaphyseal	
Diagnosis	Clinical: restriction of internal rotation and abduction X-ray, MRI, bone scintigraphy			
Treatment	NSAIDs Restriction of activity/immobilization Surgery: osteotomy, augmentation plasty			
Course & complications	Treatment does not halt natural course Bad prognosis if older age at onset & greater extent of femoral head involvement Deformity of femoral head in severe cases Long term—early osteoarthritis			

Table 2.16 Differential diagnosis of hip pathology by age group: 8–16 yrs

	Slipped capital femoral epiphysis (SCFE)	Trauma	Tumour/malignancy	Infection	Avascular necrosis or osteonecrosis
Demographics	♂ > ♀ 1–3 per 100,000	♂ > ♀	Refer to Tables 2.12 and 2.13 Benign tumours can arise from bone, cartilage, fibrous tissue or soft tissues Benign tumours such as osteoid osteoma, and malignant tumours such as osteosarcoma and Ewing's sarcoma are more common in this age group As in all age groups, it is important to consider malignancy not arising primarily from the bone, e.g. leukaemia	Refer to Tables 2.12 and 2.13 Amongst other pathogens, also consider Gonococcus and Chlamydia in sexually active adolescents Gonococcal arthritis can lead to early joint destruction if not identified in time	♂ = ♀

Table 2.16 Contd.

	Slipped capital femoral epiphysis (SCFE)	Trauma	Tumours/malignancy	Infection	Avascular necrosis or osteonecrosis
Pathophysiology	Posterior & inferior displacement of epiphysis (2° to displacement of proximal femoral metaphysis) Classification: • Acute/chronic/ acute-on-chronic • Stable/unstable • Radiographic • Preslip, Grade I, II, III	Sports-related injuries: Ligamentous injuries Avulsion injuries—due to inherent weakness across open epiphysis Apophyseal injuries and apophysitis—chronic overuse and repetitive muscle contractions Stress fractures—chronic repetitive microtrauma Transient demineralization of hip Post-traumatic chondrolysis of hip			Circulatory compromise can be 1° or 2° to causes listed below Bilateral occurrence in 50%, if not associated with trauma
Predisposing factors & associations	Overweight or obese (but can also occur in thin patients) Hypothyroidism Growth hormone deficiency Exposure to radiation Afro-Caribbeans	High-impact sports Chronic or repeated microtrauma/sustained overuse Inherent bone mineralization problems			Drugs—steroids, LMW heparin Haemoglobinopathies Coagulopathies Skeletal dysplasias Infections—HIV, *Meningococcus* Inflammatory bowel disease, trauma, malignancy, vasculitis/ JIA, orthopaedic (previous DH, SCFE, Perthe's)

Clinical features	Pain +, limp +, Inability to walk in unstable variety Presentation with knee pain or limp alone leads to delayed diagnosis Bilateral in 20–40%	Pain, restriction of movement, localized swelling/bruising ±; presence of hernia in 'sportsman's hernia (a type of imminent direct hernia that can cause chronic groin pain in athletes) Sudden pain following intense physical activity typical of acute chondrolysis	Insidious onset of pain which typically occurs with standing or walking ↓ abduction and rotation on examination Limp is a late finding
Diagnosis	X-ray: • AP—'Klein's line' (a line drawn along the superior femoral neck should normally intersect a portion of the femoral head) • Frog lateral view MRI—useful in 'pre-slip' stage	Typical history X-ray MRI Hip arthroscopy for isolated labral tears, loose bodies	Low index of suspicion if associated risk factors MRI—most sensitive for early diagnosis
Treatment	Surgical: early in situ stabilization by screw fixation Unstable SCFE is an orthopaedic emergency	Orthopaedic management Pain relief	Medical: pain relief, bisphosphonates Surgical: core decompression and bone grafting
Course & complications	Bad prognosis if ↑ severity of slippage and delay in diagnosis Complications: • Avascular necrosis • Acute chondrolysis Long-term—early osteoarthritis	Consider pain syndromes if not getting better with conventional treatment after excluding important differentials	Femoral head collapse can occur if diagnosis is delayed, in which case total hip replacement might be needed Fractures can occur as a complication of surgery

- Congenital / genetic causes—epiphyseal dysplasia (see ⮕ pp. 362–70), metabolic storage disorders (e.g. Gaucher's (see ⮕ pp. 332–7), CACP (Camptodactyly, Arthropathy, Coxa vara, Pericarditis) syndrome (varus hip alignment usually detected on radiological examination) etc.
- Malignancy—1° bone tumours, benign and malignant (see ⮕ pp. 55–8)—referred pain from the spine, abdomen or pelvis (including retrocaecal appendicitis) may present with hip pain.
- Osteoarthritis—1° (rare in the absence of predisposing conditions such as skeletal dysplasia (see ⮕ pp. 362–70) and 2° to pre-existing hip disease.
- Chronic idiopathic pain syndromes (see ⮕ pp. 84–8) need careful exclusion of organic pathology.

Further reading

Fabry G. Clinical practice: the hip from birth to adolescence. *Eur J Pediatr* 2010;169(2):143–8.
Gill KG. Pediatric hip: Pearls and pitfalls. *Semin Musculoskelet Radiol* 2013;17(3):328–338
Houghton KM. Review for the generalist: evaluation of pediatric hip pain. *Pediatr Rheumatol Online J* 2009;7:10.

Knee pain in children and adolescents

Pain in and around the knee joint is very common and often recovers spontaneously. More persistent knee pain may indicate a specific condition as described in the following section. *It is always important to consider referred pain from the hip or thigh especially when there are no abnormal findings on knee examination.*

Causes

See Table 2.17.

Mechanical

Anterior knee pain/patellofemoral pain:

- Pain at the front of the knee, made worse by inactivity, stair climbing, or any activity involving bending the knee. Often aggravated by sport. Common at time of growth spurts.
- Genu valgum, hypermobility, femoral torsion, and pronated feet contribute to anterior knee pain.
- Management:
  - Optimizing strength of pelvifemoral musculature.*
  - Optimizing balance between quadriceps and hamstrings.
  - Optimizing strength between individual components of quadriceps muscle bellies.
  - Improving proprioception.
  - Consideration of foot orthoses.
    - —Note: non-participation in PE/sport does not influence rate of recovery so participation is strongly encouraged where possible.
- Chondromalacia patellae:
  - This term is a misnomer and source of confusion. The presence of 'soft cartilage' is not correlated with patellar pain.
  - If anterior knee pain then see earlier in this list.
- Patella dislocation:
  - The patella commonly tilts and glides toward the lateral aspect of the knee—the patella may slip and stay there—'dislocation'— although slips which sublux and return to the anatomically correct position are more common.
  - Several anatomical conditions can precipitate recurrent dislocation— flat patella, patella alta, shallow femoral trochlea, femoral torsion, loose medial structures, general joint laxity.
  - Management: optimizing strength of pelvifemoral musculature, reduction of patella, and knee immobilized. For recurrent dislocation—arthroscopic lateral release of lateral retinaculum or stabilization of the patella.
- Osgood–Schlatter's disease:
  - Caused by repetitive microtrauma to the tibial tubercle apophysis, usually in jumping sports (overuse traction apophysitis).

---

* Optimizing hip abductors strength helps to support the knee whilst a tight iliotibial band can pull the patella laterally exacerbating maltracking along the femoral groove.

Table 2.17 Summary of causes of mechanical knee pain

	Symptoms	Signs	Management	Orthopaedic referral
Patellofemoral pain	Pain
Worse with activity	Genu valgum
Hypermobility
Tibial torsion
Pronated forefeet	Physiotherapy
Activity modification	No
Patella dislocation	Pain	Dislocated patella	Reduction of patella
Mobilization	Yes if recurrent dislocation
Osgood-Schlatter	Pain on activity	Pain on resisted extension	Ice
Activity modification	No
Sinding-Larsen-Johansson	Pain lower pole patella	Tender lower pole patella
Worse on extension	Ice
Physiotherapy
Activity modification	No
Plica syndrome	Pain on flexion	May be tenderness	NSAID, I/A steroids, activity modification	No
Osteochondritis	Pain, Locking
Weakness	May be normal	Analgesics	Yes
Loose body	Pain, Locking
Giving way
Swelling	May be normal
Tenderness, effusion,
↓ extension	NSAIDs	Yes—arthroscopic removal of loose body
Haemarthrosis	Pain
Swelling (soon after injury)	Large, tense effusion
Hamstring spasm	Aspiration to confirm	Yes
Fat pad impingement	Pain, swelling
↓ movement	Pain when knee flexed suddenly	NSAIDS, physiotherapy	No

- Symptoms—often low-grade ache and inflammation around tibial tuberosity, associated with activity. Pain relieved by rest.
- Signs—pain reproduced by resisted extension from 90° of flexion.
- Imaging –x-ray usually normal. US/MRI may show fragmented apophysis.
- Management—ice for pain, activity modification, i.e. encourage swimming and cycling and avoid jumping. Symptoms are self-limiting.
- Sinding–Larsen and Johansson syndrome:
  - Caused by repetitive microtrauma at the insertion of patellar tendon onto lower patella pole (overuse traction apophysitis). Often seen in conjunction with over pronated feet.
  - Symptoms—pain and tenderness precipitated by overstraining or trauma.
  - Signs—slightly swollen, warm tender bump. Pain worse on resisted extension.
  - Imaging—US/MRI may show fragmented lower pole of patella. Helpful to monitor disease course.
  - Management—initially ice, stretching, and strengthening exercises. Avoid running, jumping, squatting activities. Usually resolves in 3–6 months.
- Plica syndrome:
  - Result of remnant fetal tissue in the knee. When knee flexed plica is exposed to injury and becomes inflamed.
  - Can be confused with meniscal tears or patellar tendonitis.
  - Imaging—MRI often not helpful. Often seen on arthroscopic examination.
  - Management—NSAIDs, intra-articular cortisone, activity modification.
- Osteochondritis dissecans:
  - Focal area of detached or semi-detached subchondral bone with hyaline articular cartilage on top. Common cause of loose body within the knee. ♂:♀=3:1.
  - History of trauma in approx 40%.
  - Symptoms—initially pain, then locking and weakness.
  - Signs—may be normal.
  - Imaging—x-ray, MRI, or arthroscopy can be used to confirm diagnosis.
  - Management—referral to Orthopaedics. Fix bone fragments in place or remove if loose.
- Loose body:
  - Can be fibrinous (i.e. inflammation), cartilaginous (i.e. meniscal tear), or osteocartilaginous (i.e. osteochrondritis dissecans).
  - Presents with knee, pain, intermittent locking, the joint may 'give way' and signs of tenderness, soft tissue swelling, joint effusion may be present and extension may be limited.
  - Imaging—x-ray may demonstrate larger lesions. US/MRI and arthroscopy can confirm diagnosis.
  - Management—for small lesions NSAIDs may be helpful but in general loose bodies need to be removed by arthroscopy.

- Haemarthrosis:
  - In ~80% cases, this follows a twisting injury to the knee, i.e. anterior cruciate ligament rupture with pain and swelling (often large) <15 to 30min of injury with large tense knee effusion, often hamstring spasm and severe limitation of movement.
  - Imaging—x-ray, MRI, or arthroscopy to confirm underlying injury.
  - Management—aspiration to confirm. Referral to Orthopaedics.
- Fat pad impingement syndrome:
  - Traumatic and inflammatory changes in the infrapatellar fat pad.
  - Symptoms—pain, swelling, restricted movement, and symptoms may be chronic and infrapatellar. Pain is present when the flexed knee is extended suddenly.
  - Imaging—MRI, acute findings of ↑ fluid and chronic findings similar to scarring after arthroscopy. Arthroscopy doesn't visualize the fat pad well.
  - Management—NSAIDs if inflammation persistent, quadriceps strengthening or taping may be helpful.
- Iliotibial band* or tensor fascia lata (TFL) problems can present with knee pain or pain may be higher up thigh.

Inflammatory

- Septic arthritis or osteomyelitis (see ➔ p. 63 and p. 64).
- Juvenile idiopathic arthritis (see ➔ p. 131).
- Reactive arthritis (see ➔ pp. 66–8).
- The presence of red flag symptoms (fever, chills, weight loss) indicate urgent referral.

Tumours

- Benign—osteochondromas can occur in femur or tibia resulting in knee pain. Often not painful and don't require surgery. Osteoid osteomas may occur and need referral to paediatric orthopaedics/local bone tumour service.
- Malignant—osteosarcoma (commonly around the knee) and Ewing's sarcoma (involves long bones of leg or pelvis). Need urgent referral to paediatric orthopaedics/local bone tumour service (see ➔ pp. 59–61).

Foot and ankle problems

Flexible flat feet

- Clinical—considered 'normal' in many children (see ➲ Normal variants and podiatry, ➲ pp. 9–10):
  - By 8yrs, few children have flat feet.
  - Absence of arch when standing flat, but arches apparent when stand on tip-toe or big toes passively dorsiflexed.
  - More common in hypermobile children—typically symptomless (present with parental anxiety).
- Management—reassurance and footwear advice, most do not benefit from insoles/physiotherapy input.
- Red flag—failure of arch to return on tip-toe standing implies rigid flat feet: consider tarsal coalition or arthritis at sub-talar joint (see ➲ p. 143).

Tarsal coalition

- Definition:
  - Failure of segmentation of tarsal bones, typically calcaneonavicular or talocalcaneal joints.
  - May be cartilaginous/fibrous (and therefore missed on x-ray).
- Clinical:
  - Painful feet, non-flexible flat feet (50% bilateral).
  - Typically presents in adolescents (4>5).
- Management—orthotics, NSAIDs, in extreme cases, surgery is required.

Pes cavus

- Clinical:
  - A normal variant (see ➲ pp. 9–10).
  - 'High arches' and may associate with persistent tip-toe gait.
  - May be asymptomatic or present with pain (2° to metatarsal compression) or clumsy walking.
  - Consider neurological/neuromuscular abnormalities, e.g. spina bifida, Charcot–Marie–Tooth, Friedreich's ataxia, or metabolic storage diseases (see ➲ pp. 332–7).
- Management:
  - Typically no treatment is needed.
  - May require insoles/orthoses and refer for surgery if pain is severe.

Metatarsus adductus

- Clinical:
  - A normal variant (see ➲ pp. 9–10).
  - Causes in-toeing (medial deviation of foot); can be familial or positional.
- Management—tends to correct with wearing shoes, rarely needs treatment (such as serial casting, splints).

Rocker bottom feet

- (= congential convex pes valgus = congenital vertical talus)

- Clinical:
  - Usually detected in newborn, talus dislocated, pointing downwards.
  - Associated with neurological problems but often idiopathic.
- Management—casting is little use if foot not flexible and surgery may be required.

Congenital talipes equinovarus

- (=clubfoot)
- Clinical:
  - Usually detected in newborn, foot held pointing down (equino) and folded in (varus).
  - Structural abnormality (as opposed to positional talipes which resolved with physio).
- Management:
  - Casting (Ponseti method) is current treatment of choice.
  - May need surgery.

Intoeing

- Clinical:
- Normal variant (see ➲ pp. 9–10 Normal variants).
  - Usually a result of a rotational deformity of long bones rather than an abnormality in the foot (most often due to femoral anteversion (90%) or tibial torsion):
    —Assess patella position with child standing feet pointing forwards—if patella pointing straight, then rotational deformity is distal, if pointing medially, rotational deformity is proximal).
    —Assess thigh–foot angle (see ➲ Clinical skills, p. 1).

Achilles tendonitis

- Clinical:
  - Typically an overuse injury in sporty children.
  - Rare in those <14yrs, pain with activity, especially jumping.
- Management:
  - Rest, ice, compress, elevate (RICE).
  - Modify activity/stretching exercises/physiotherapy/orthoses (gel heel cup).
  - NSAIDs.
  - *Never* inject steroids (this weakens the tendon, risking rupture).

Sever's disease (similar to apophysitis at other sites)

- Definition—apophysitis of os calcis at insertion of Achilles tendon.
- Clinical:
  - Typically occurs before skeleton matures, as a result of either rapid growth or excessive activity.
  - Usually children 7–14yrs old and present with pain increasing with activity.
- Management: similar to Achilles tendonitis.

Plantar fasciitis

- Clinical:
  - Inflammation of plantar fascia, usually from repeat microtrauma.
  - Heel pain, worse with ↑ activity (or impact to ground).
  - Differential diagnosis: includes JIA (enthesitis-related arthritis)
  - See **→** JIA, p. 143.
- Management—similar to Achilles tendonitis.

Osteochondroses

(also see **→** Osteochondroses, pp. 371–4)
- Occur in growing skeleton, with disruption of blood supply due to recurrent insult.
- Kohlers's disease:
  - Osteochondrosis of navicular bone.
  - Typically 5–9yr-olds with midfoot pain, swelling, (can be bilateral).
  - X-ray: ↑ sclerosis of navicular bone.
  - Management—as for Achilles tendonitis.
- Freiberg's disease:
  - Osteonecrosis of 2nd or 3rd metatarsal head.
  - Typically adolescent girls, increasing forefoot pain and focal tenderness over head of affected head.
  - Management—RICE, modify activity/footwear, surgery in extremes.

Arthritis

- Can affect any joint in ankle/foot especially if swollen or restricted in range of movement.
- Need to consider septic/reactive/JIA (see **→** pp. 63–8):
  - Septic—febrile, unwell child, extreme reluctance to move joint, raised acute inflammatory markers (esp. CRP), other markers of sepsis—see **→** Infection, pp. 69–73.
  - Reactive—recent history URTI or GI upset (and sexually acquired infection in the adolescent)—see **→** Infection, pp. 69–73.
  - JIA: see **→** Chapter 3, p. 131.

Joint hypermobility

Background

- The normal range of motion of joints is variable, with children possessing an inherently greater range than adults, and females greater than males.
- The prevalence of joint hypermobility (JH) in children has been variously reported between 2.3% and 64% dependent on the age, ethnicity, and defining criteria used.
- The majority of these children are asymptomatic, and many use their hypermobility to advantage, e.g. ballet dancers and gymnasts who are hypermobile appear to be at less risk of injury, and musicians benefit from a wide hand span.
- Conversely, some children and young people suffer symptoms, presumed to be due to their hypermobility, and in this case the condition is called symptomatic hypermobility (SH), previously called 'joint hypermobility syndrome' (JHS). Musculoskeletal pain is the commonest symptom and hypermobility (defined as >=6/9 in this study) at 14 yrs has been reported to increase the risk of shoulder, knee, ankle/foot pain at age 18 (OR 1.68–1.83) (Tobias et al. 2013). However symptoms do not appear to be correlated with the number of joints involved or the degree of hypermobility.
- Various other symptoms have been attributed to JH including delayed motor milestones and poor motor competence, relating to impaired joint proprioception (resulting in falls and co-ordination difficulties). Some children with JH may also present with non musculoskeletal symptoms including chronic constipation, abdominal pain, irritable bowel syndrome, urinary dysfunction, and anxiety. There is currently no population-based evidence to support an association. Several large school population studies in Turkey and Sweden have looked for any association of hypermobility using Beighton >4, with any of the many reported symptoms (including musculoskeletal pain), and found none, other than pes planus. Thus any purported relationship with these symptoms is controversial; but a recent study suggests that children with hypermobility syndrome have a lower quality of life relating to pain, fatigue, and stress incontinence compared to healthy peers (Pacey et al. 2015).
- The degree of hypermobility reduces with age and in most children their musculoskeletal pain will reduce as joints become more stable.

Definition

- There are no validated scoring systems for hypermobility in children.
- The Beighton score is recognized for defining hypermobility in adults (with a score of ≥ 4/9) and the modified Brighton score for adult JHS, but neither is validated in children.
- Indeed, 26.5% of healthy Dutch children (n=773) aged 4–9yrs scored 4, and 5.3% aged 10–12yrs. Thus Beighton scoring defines a quarter of all children <10yrs of age as hypermobile.
- In a large UK cohort study (n=6022) of 14-year-old children 27.5% of girls and 10.6% of boys were deemed hypermobile using a score of ≥4

on the Beighton scale, with 4.6% scoring ≥6. In addition, 45% of girls and 29% of boys had hypermobile fingers. Some have argued that ≥6 should define hypermobility in children, but this has not been formally validated.

- Other scoring systems have been described for children (e.g. Bulbena) but none are sufficiently well validated to be in widespread use.
- Ehlers–Danlos Syndrome (EDS) hypermobility type is used interchangeably with JHS but its distinction from other forms of EDS (which can be genetically identified) should be clearly stated to families, and the authors do not recommend its use.
- *Pragmatic definition of SH in the paediatric population*—a child or young person with musculoskeletal pain and signs of hypermobility, with no other cause found for their symptoms.

The 9-point Beighton scoring system for joint hypermobility (4 points defines hypermobility in adults, but 5 and 6 have been suggested for children)

Scoring 1 point each side
- Passive dorsiflexion of the 5th MCP joint to 90°.
- Apposition of thumb to volar forearm.
- Hyperextension of the elbow >10°.
- Hyperextension of the knee >10°.

Scoring 1 point
- Touch palms to floor with knees straight.

Epidemiology

- There is a greater range of joint mobility in Asians than sub-Saharan Africans, who are more mobile than Caucasians. Girls affected more commonly than boys.
- A significant proportion of new referrals to paediatric rheumatology clinics have non inflammatory-musculoskeletal pain (with or without hypermobility).

Pathophysiology

- Unknown.
- The lack of clear diagnostic criteria mean that there is significant heterogeneity in any described cohort with SH. Sub grouping into different phenotypes may be helpful.
- There is no genetic or other test.
- Genes encoding collagens and collagen-modifying enzymes may be good candidates for those manifesting signs at the more severe end of the spectrum. Adult studies suggest abnormality in collagen bundle structure on skin biopsy but significantly more work is required.
- Biomechanical imbalance is most likely to be the cause of pain, exacerbated by weakness, but this is unproven.
- Biopsychosocial factors are thought to contribute to the degree of difficulty the child or young person experiences. There has been no correlation found between degree of hypermobility and severity of symptoms reported.

Clinical presentation

Symptoms

- The child has joint pain during or after activity. Typically they complain of pain in lower limbs after walking just short distances and this is commonly manifested when walking to and from school.
- Pain occurring in the evening after an active day, again typically in the lower limbs (see ➲ Anterior knee pain, pp. 119–22).
- Occasional joint swelling, lasting a few days only.
- Stiffness can be reported but this is muscular in nature and needs to be differentiated from the joint stiffness of inflammatory conditions.
- Handwriting difficulties.
- Joint dislocation/subluxation—less common.
- 'Clicking' and 'cracking' of joints.
- Frequent 'sprained ankles'.
- Back pain, anterior knee pain, and TMJ dysfunction may be reported.
- Fatigue and generalized pain can occur in a small number of children and young people with SH, with a presentation similar to chronic pain syndromes (see below).

Family history

Frequently 1st-degree relatives are also described as having lax joints or being 'double jointed'.

Past history

- There is some evidence that JH is linked with delayed motor development and the mean age of first walking may be later (15 months).
- Described as clumsy, poor motor competence, and some have a diagnosis of developmental coordination disorder.
- Constipation, urinary tract infections, stress incontinence, other urinary dysfunction.
- Non-specific abdominal pain, headaches, and generalized pain sometimes reported
- Presence of obesity has been linked to increased prediction of musculoskeletal pain in adolescence in those who are hypermobile in childhood.

Examination

- Height and weight show normal growth.
- Normal examination of cardiovascular, respiratory, and abdominal systems. Neurological examination reveals normal muscle bulk, strength, and reflexes.
- Musculoskeletal examination shows increased range of joint movement. Pes planus with calcaneo valgus, i.e. a mobile flat foot (arch forms when child stands on tip-toe) and valgus heel position are common. Paradoxically tight hamstrings are often found (see ➲ Anterior knee pain, pp. 119–22).
- Normal skin elasticity, absence of scarring, normal dentition and palate. Bruising may be more commonly seen.

Differential diagnoses

SH is primarily a clinical diagnosis dependent on typical clinical history and physical signs. The following differentials should be considered and ruled out clinically or by investigation:

- Known heritable connective tissue disorder (see ⊃ Heritable connective tissue disorders, pp. 375–81), e.g.:
  - Ehlers–Danlos syndrome (other than the hypermobility type)—look for skin hyperextensibility, bruising, tissue paper scarring.
  - Marfan syndrome—marfanoid habitus, cardiovascular or ocular involvement.
  - Osteogenesis imperfecta—blue sclerae, short stature, multiple fractures, and hearing loss.
- Juvenile idiopathic arthritis (see ⊃ JIA, p. 131).
- Pain syndromes: diffuse idiopathic pain syndrome; localized idiopathic pain syndrome; fibromyalgia (see ⊃ Pain syndromes, pp. 84–8).
- Malignancy: leukaemia; Ewing's sarcoma; osteosarcoma.
- Congenital disorders associated with hypermobility: Down syndrome, Klinefelter's, Williams' syndrome, Stickler's syndrome; fragile X, autistic spectrum disorders; skeletal dysplasias (pseudoachondroplasia) and metabolic disorders such as homocystinuria.

Management

- In the majority of mild cases, all that is required is a diagnosis with explanation of the condition, reassurance that serious pathology has been excluded and written information (see ⊃ Patient information, p. 130).
- The child and family need to know that there are no long-term consequences (the link with later osteoarthritis is as yet unproven). Most children improve with age. Most children will not have any of the reported associated problems.
- Escalation of analgesia is common, but universally unhelpful and should be avoided.
- Supportive footwear is often beneficial (e.g. trainers —fastened properly, and supportive boots). The evidence for orthotics is poor, but these could be tested in the individual child (parents can obtain 'off the shelf' orthoses in the first instance).
- A physiotherapy assessment is often helpful to assess the biomechanics and advise stretches and muscle strengthening exercises.
- More severe cases may benefit from more regular physiotherapy both generalized and targeted, and occupational therapy may help with handwriting and manual dexterity.
- Qualitative evidence suggests intensive MDT is beneficial for most patients but requires good parental supervision, time practical exercises, and clear evidence of benefit seen by the patient
- If there are particular problems with generalized pain resulting in fatigue, reduced activities, and school absence, cognitive behavioural therapy with graded physical exercise and goal setting may benefit the child/ young person.
- It is recommended that if additional symptoms are presented, appropriate investigations and management / referral are undertaken.

Idiopathic nocturnal leg pain

Common, benign condition, otherwise known as 'growing pains' characterized by intermittent lower limb pain at night with symptom-free intervals of days, weeks or months. There is a reported association with hypermobility. See ➔ Growing pains, pp. 89–90.

Patient information

- The Hypermobility Syndrome Association website for kids and teens ℅ http://teens.hypermobility.org/index.php.
- Arthritis Research UK patient information leaflet: ℅ http://www.arthritisresearchuk.org/arthritis_information/arthritis_types__symptoms/joint_hypermobility.aspx

Further reading

Birt L, Pheil M, MacGregor AJ, et al. Adherence to home physiotherapy treatment in children and young people with joint hypermobility: A qualitative report of family perspectives on acceptability and efficacy. Musculoskeletal Care 2011;12(1):56–61.

Kemp S, Roberts I, Gamble C, et al. A randomised comparative trial of generalised vs targeted physiotherapy in the management of childhood hypermobility. Rheumatology 2010; 49:315–25.

Tobias JH, Deere K, Palmer S, et al. Joint hypermobility is a risk factor for musculoskeletal pain during adolescence: findings of a prospective cohort study. Arthritis Rheum 2013;65:1107–15.

Pacey V, Adams RD, Tofts V et al. Joint hypermobility syndrome subclassification in paediatrics: a factor analytic approach Arch Dis Child 2015;100(1): 8–13.

Pacey V, Tofts L, Wesley A et al. Joint hypermobility syndrome: a review for clinicians. J Paediatr Child Health 2015; 51(4):373–80.

van der Giessen LJ, Liekens D, Rutgers KJ. Validation of Beighton score and prevalence of connective tissue signs in 773 Dutch children. J Rheumatol 2001;28(12):2726–30.

Juvenile idiopathic arthritis

Genetics and JIA: HLA and non-HLA/MHC associations with subtypes of JIA

Association studies in JIA

The association study is the standard methodology used in the search for genetic risk factors for JIA. There are a number of issues regarding study design that the clinician must be aware of, to understand and put into context the genetic findings to date for JIA (Fig. 3.1).

Genetic risk factors identified to date for JIA

Human leucocyte antigen (HLA)

The major histocompatibility complex (MHC) is the most consistently associated locus in JIA.

Multiple HLA class I and class II associations exist with JIA, with each ILAR subtype having a specific pattern of HLA associations, although it should be noted that there are also overlapping associations, particularly between oligoarthritis and RF−ve polyarthritis. HLA-DRB1*11 conferred the strongest risk in systemic JIA (sJIA).

Non-HLA/MHC loci

The candidate gene approach has previously been the main strategy used in the search for JIA susceptibility loci to date but large-scale mapping studies are now being performed. Most studies investigated association of regions known to be associated with other autoimmune diseases for association with JIA. Many regions show modest association but not all were replicated in independent cohorts. Only two non-HLA regions reached genome-wide significance (PTPN22 and PTPN2).

Some association studies performed in the past for JIA have suffered from inadequate sample sizes.

There have been three genome wide association study (GWAS) for JIA as a whole published to date. One identified the association of the VTCN1 (B7-Homolog 4 [B7-H4]) gene with JIA and was validated in an independent dataset. The second identified c3orf130/CD80 on chromosome 3 and IL15, and was validated in an independent dataset. The third identified CXCR4 on chromosome 2. None of these regions identified by GWAS reach genome-wide significance.

The largest study to date in JIA was published in 2013: a consortium of researchers brought together a sample size of 2816 cases with oligoarticular and RF−ve polyarticular JIA and 13,056 healthy controls. These were genotyped in a custom designed microarray, Immunochip. It confirmed 3 regions that have previously reached genome-wide significance threshold and identified 14 new loci, most notably a number of genes in the IL2 pathway. It also identified 11 regions at a suggestive significance threshold. These are highlighted in Table 3.1.

A recent investigation meta-analysis of paediatric onset autoimmune diseases, confirmed association with PTPN22, ANKRD55, IL2/IL21, and IL2RA in JIA and identified a novel locus for JIA, ANKRD30A. Large-scale GWAS and meta-analysis are still required in JIA to identify novel regions for the subtypes.

Subgroup-specific associations

There is an issue with association analysis by JIA subtype in that, for many JIA case cohorts, it results in small sample sizes that often are not sufficiently

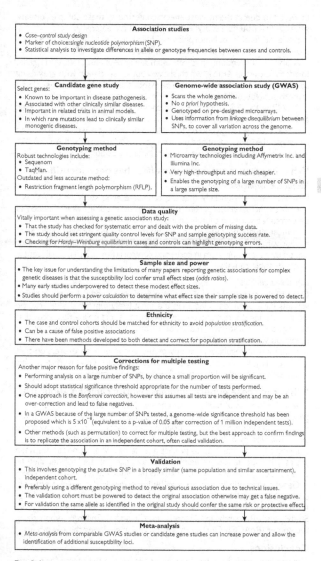

Association studies
- *Case–control study* design
- Marker of choice: *single nucleotide polymorphism* (SNP).
- Statistical analysis to investigate differences in allele or genotype frequencies between cases and controls.

Candidate gene study
Select genes:
- Known to be important in disease pathogenesis.
- Associated with other clinically similar diseases.
- Important in related traits in animal models.
- In which rare mutations lead to clinically similar monogenic diseases.

Genome-wide association study (GWAS)
- Scans the whole genome.
- No *a priori* hypothesis.
- Genotyped on pre-designed microarrays.
- Uses information from *linkage disequilibrium* between SNPs, to cover all variation across the genome.

Genotyping method
Robust technologies include:
- Sequenom
- TaqMan
Outdated and less accurate method:
- Restriction fragment length polymorphism (RFLP).

Genotyping method
- Microarray technologies including Affymetrix Inc. and Illumina Inc.
- Very high-throughput and much cheaper.
- Enables the genotyping of a large number of SNPs in a large sample size.

Data quality
Vitally important when assessing a genetic association study:
- That the study has checked for systematic error and dealt with the problem of missing data.
- The study should set stringent quality control levels for SNP and sample genotyping success rate.
- Checking for *Hardy–Weinberg equilibrium* in cases and controls can highlight genotyping errors.

Sample size and power
- The key issue for understanding the limitations of many papers reporting genetic associations for complex genetic diseases is that the susceptibility loci confer small effect sizes (*odds ratios*).
- Many early studies underpowered to detect these modest effect sizes.
- Studies should perform a *power calculation* to determine what effect size their sample size is powered to detect.

Ethnicity
- The case and control cohorts should be matched for ethnicity to avoid *population stratification*.
- Can be a cause of false positive associations.
- There have been methods developed to both detect and correct for population stratification.

Corrections for multiple testing
Another major reason for false positive findings:
- Performing analysis on a large number of SNPs, by chance a small proportion will be significant.
- Should adopt statistical significance threshold appropriate for the number of tests performed.
- One approach is the *Bonferroni correction*, however this assumes all tests are independent and may be an over-correction and lead to false negatives.
- In a GWAS because of the large number of SNPs tested, a genome-wide significance threshold has been proposed which is 5×10^{-8} (equivalent to a p-value of 0.05 after correction of 1 million independent tests).
- Other methods (such as permutation) to correct for multiple testing, but the best approach to confirm findings is to replicate the association in an independent cohort, often called validation.

Validation
- This involves genotyping the putative SNP in a broadly similar (same population and similar ascertainment), independent cohort.
- Preferably using a different genotyping method to reveal spurious association due to technical issues.
- The validation cohort must be powered to detect the original association otherwise may get a false negative.
- For validation the same allele as identified in the original study should confer the same risk or protective effect.

Meta-analysis
- *Meta-analysis* from comparable GWAS studies or candidate gene studies can increase power and allow the identification of additional susceptibility loci.

Fig. 3.1 Association studies.

powered to detect the modest effects conferred by these complex disease genes. A few potential subtype specific effects are emerging:

Single nucleotide polymorphisms (SNPs) in the *IL1 ligand* cluster, *IL1 receptor* cluster and *IL6* promoter show association with sJIA.

A SNP in the endoplasmic reticulum aminopeptidase 1 (*ERAP1*) gene, formerly known as *ARTS1*, which shows robust association with ankylosing spondylitis (AS) has been shown to be associated with the enthesitis-related arthritis subtype of JIA.

A SNP in the *IL23* receptor gene shows association with the psoriatic arthritis subtype of JIA.

More recently a large GWAS for sJIA has been performed, which focused initially on the MHC, identified the strongest association with HLA-DRB1*11 and its defining amino acid residue glutamate at position 58.

What happens once a genetic effect has been identified?

Resequencing/fine-mapping

In most cases it is unlikely that the candidate gene study or GWAS will identify the actual *causal variant*, but they do detect SNPs which happen to be correlated with the causal variant.

In most situations it will be important to screen the whole region for all genetic variation, possibly by resequencing, and then fine-mapping the association by genotyping them in cases and controls (Box 3.1). This will identify all the possible causal variants.

Functional analysis

Once all the statistical analysis has been performed and the putative causal variants have been identified then the most likely functional SNPs can be identified using the multiple computational tools and online resources that are available. These give information from multiple independent experiments on what role the SNP may have biologically, for example, whether the SNP lies in regulatory regions of the genome, is an expression-trait locus (eQTL), lies in transcription factor binding site. This prioritizes SNPs for investigation and guides future functional experiments.

What can these genetic findings tell the clinician about JIA?

They will inform us of the important pathways involved in JIA disease pathogenesis. We are already seeing strong evidence to suggest a vital role for the IL-2 pathway in JIA and other autoimmune diseases. Once we know more about the biology of JIA, we may identify novel therapeutic targets.

Eventually they may help us predict disease risk. We are not at this stage yet as it is important to remember that for many of the loci identified to date the actual causative genetic variants have not yet been clearly defined.

Genetic susceptibility factors may be important in determining not only susceptibility to JIA but also to a child's disease outcome. Prospective, long-term outcome studies, such as the CAPS (Childhood Arthritis Prospective Study) and Research in Arthritis in Canadian Children emphasizing Outcomes (ReACCh-Out) study, will be vital in exploring this hypothesis.

Conclusions

The last few years there has been great progress in the search for genetic risk factors for JIA, with many confirmed associations. Much larger sample sizes will need to be collected to enable more powerful analysis of the specific subtypes of JIA.

Table 3.1 Non-MHC regions reaching genome wide significant association with JIA and its subtypes

Gene Region	Chr	SNP	Bestp-value	Study population	Subtypes	Reference	Previous evidence for association
PTPN22	1	rs6679677	3.19×10^{-25}	US, UK & Germany	O, RF-P	Hinks et al., 2013	Yes
STAT4	2	rs10174238	1.28×10^{-13}	US, UK & Germany	O, RF-P	Hinks et al., 2013	Yes
PTPN2	18	rs2847293	1.44×10^{-12}	US, UK & Germany	O, RF-P	Hinks et al., 2013	Yes
ANKRD55	5	rs71624419	4.40×10^{-11}	US, UK & Germany	O, RF-P	Hinks et al., 2013	No
IL2/IL21	4	rs1479924	6.24×10^{-11}	US, UK & Germany	O, RF-P	Hinks et al., 2013	Yes
ANKRD30A	10	rs7100025	8.4×10^{-11}	US, Aus, Nor	All JIA	Li et al., 2015	No
TYK2	19	rs34536443	1×10^{-10}	US, UK & Germany	O, RF-P	Hinks et al., 2013	No
IL2RA	10	rs7909519	8×10^{-10}	US, UK & Germany	O, RF-P	Hinks et al., 2013	Yes
SH2B3/ATXN2	12	rs3184504	2.60×10^{-09}	US, UK & Germany	O, RF-P	Hinks et al., 2013	Yes
ERAP2/LNPEP	5	rs27290	7.5×10^{-09}	US, UK & Germany	O, RF-P	Hinks et al., 2013	No
UBE2L3	22	rs2266959	6.2×10^{-09}	US, UK & Germany	O, RF-P	Hinks et al., 2013	No
C5orf56/IRF1	5	rs4705862	1.02×10^{-08}	US, UK & Germany	O, RF-P	Hinks et al., 2013	No
RUNX1	21	rs9979383	1.06×10^{-08}	US, UK & Germany	O, RF-P	Hinks et al., 2013	No
IL2RB	22	rs2284033	1.55×10^{-08}	US, UK & Germany	O, RF-P	Hinks et al., 2013	No
ATP8B2/IL6R	1	rs11265608	2.75×10^{-08}	US, UK & Germany	O, RF-P	Hinks et al., 2013	No
FAS	10	rs7069750	2.93×10^{-08}	US, UK & Germany	O, RF-P	Hinks et al., 2013	No
ZFP36L1	14	rs12433551	1.59×10^{-08}	US, UK & Germany	O, RF-P	Hinks et al., 2013	No

Chr=chromosome. O=oligoarticular JIA, RF-P=RF negative polyarticular JIA. Aus=Australia, Nor=Norway

Box 3.1 Definitions often used in clinical genetics

Allele

Alternative form of a genetic locus; a single allele for each locus is inherited from each parent.

Association study

Investigation of correlation between a genetic variant and disease/trait.

Candidate gene

A gene for which there is evidence for a possible role in the disease or trait that is under investigation.

Case–control design

An association study design which compares group of individuals (cases) that are selected for the phenotype of interest with a group not ascertained for the phenotype (controls).

Causal variant

The actual disease causing variant. This may be a non-synonymous coding SNP which has a significant effect on the protein, or it can affect expression of the gene, causing upregulation or downregulation of the protein.

Genome wide association study (GWAS)

Association study performed for a dense array of SNPs, which capture a substantial proportion of common variation in the genome, genotyped in disease cases and ethnically matched controls.

Genome wide significance

A threshold for claiming robust association ($p < 5 \times 10^{-8}$) to correct for the multiple testing of SNPs for association in GWAS. Generally accepted as the threshold to claim association with disease.

Genotype

The combination of each allele inherited from each parent forms a person's genotype for a SNP.

Haplotype

A combination of alleles at a region (locus) on a chromosome that are transmitted together.

Hardy–Weinberg equilibrium (HWE)

A theoretical relationship between genotype and allele frequencies, for a SNP, that is found in a stable population. In the context of genetic association studies, deviations from HWE can be used to highlight genotyping errors.

Immunochip

An Illumina microarray which enabled cost-effective replication of autoimmune GWAS hits and fine-mapping of 186 established autoimmune loci, including the HLA region.

Box 3.1 Contd.

Imputation

The statistical inference of unknown genotypes, using a reference panel genotyped in a larger set of markers. It enables the investigation of untyped SNPs for association with disease.

Linkage analysis

Mapping of genes, by typing genetic variants, in families to identify regions that are associated with a disease or trait within a pedigree more often than expected by chance.

Linkage disequilibrium

Combinations of alleles or genetic markers which occur together more or less frequently in a population than would be expected from a random formation of haplotypes from alleles based on their frequencies.

Meta-analysis

A method of combining results across genetic studies. It can involve the combination of p-values or, more commonly, effect sizes. It can lead to increased statistical power, give more precise estimates of effect size, and also allows assessment of consistency and heterogeneity of association across different study populations.

Minor allele frequency (MAF)

The frequency of a SNP's less frequent allele in a given population.

Odds ratio (OR)

A measurement of association that is commonly used in case–control studies. It is defined as the odds of exposure to the susceptible genetic variant in cases compared with the odds of exposure in controls. If the odds ratio is >1, then the genetic variant is associated with disease.

Population stratification

This is caused by systematic differences in allele frequencies between sub-populations in a population possibly due to different ancestry; if these subgroups also have a difference in prevalence of the disease or trait studied that it can lead to false positive associations.

Power calculation

Assessment of how many samples must be collected and analysed in order to achieve sufficient power to detect the hypothesized effect. After conducting a study, power analysis can also shed light on negative results by indicating whether the study was underpowered, or what the smallest detectable effect size would be given the actual sample size.

Single nucleotide polymorphism (SNP)

DNA sequence variations that occur when a single nucleotide (A, T, C, or G) in the genome sequence is altered.

Further reading

Finkel TH, Li J, Wei Z, et al. Variants in CXCR4 associate with juvenile idiopathic arthritis susceptibility. *BMC Med Genet* 2016:17:24

Hinks A, Cobb J, Marion MC, et al. Dense genotyping of immune-related disease regions identifies 14 new susceptibility loci for juvenile idiopathic arthritis. *Nat Genet* 2013:45(6):664–669.

Hinks A, Barton A, Shephard N, et al. Identification of a novel susceptibility locus for juvenile idiopathic arthritis by genome-wide association analysis. *Arthritis Rheum* 2009:60:258–63.

Li YR, Li J, Zhao SD, et al. Meta-analysis of shared genetic architecture across ten pediatric autoimmune diseases. *Nat Med* 2015:21:1018–27.

Moncrieffe H, Prahalad S, Thompson SD. Genetics of juvenile idiopathic arthritis: new tools bring new approaches. *Curr Opin Rheumatol* 2014:26:579–584.

Ombrello MJ, Remmers EF, Tachmazidou I, et al. HLA-DRB1*11 and variants of the MHC class II locus are strong risk factors for systemic juvenile idiopathic arthritis. *PNAS* 2015: 112:15970–5.

Thompson SD, Marion MC, Sudman M, et al. Genome-wide association analysis of juvenile idiopathic arthritis identifies a new susceptibility locus at chromosomal region 3q13. *Arthritis Rheum* 2012:64:2781–91.

Aetiology of juvenile idiopathic arthritis

Pathogenesis

- JIA is an autoimmune disorder; the immune system fails to distinguish between self and non-self and attacks synovium (membrane lining of the joint), leading to arthritis. Synovium becomes thickened, highly vascular and infiltrated with T cells, macrophages, dendritic cells, B cells, and NK cells, and secretes an inflammatory exudate (causing joint effusions).
- Persistence of inflammation: cells are recruited into the joint by attaching to upregulated adhesion molecules on inflamed endothelium (inner layer of blood vessels). Resident fibroblasts (synoviocytes) and recruited immune cells secrete high levels of chemokines, which attract further inflammatory cells, and angiogenic factors (e.g. VEGF) causing highly vascular proliferation of synovium.
- T cells are ↑ in synovium and synovial fluid and secrete several potent cytokines (see Table 3.2), leading to cartilage and bony damage. T cells secreting IL-17 (Th17 cells) are heavily implicated in psoriatic- and enthesitis-related arthritis. Remission in JIA is linked with high levels of synovial regulatory T cells (specialised T cells which counter inflammation).
- B cells are ↓ in synovial fluid, but circulating B cells secrete cytokines and activate T cells. Specialized B cells, plasma cells, secrete auto-antibodies (rheumatoid factor (RF) and anti-cyclic citrullinated protein (CCP), and ANA) associated with specific disease sub-types but are not thought to be directly pathogenic.
- sJIA has similar features with other auto-inflammatory disorders (see ➲ Chapter 4: autoinflammatory diseases, pp. 303–12); high levels of IL-1β and IL-6 cause systemic inflammatory features and growth retardation. Macrophage activation syndrome (MAS) is associated with a defect in NK cell function, which prevents NK cells from killing activated lymphocytes and macrophages (see Chapter 4 on Macrophage activation syndrome, pp. 321–4).

Genetics

(see also ➲ genetics of JIA, pp. 132–8)

- JIA is linked with several genetic polymorphisms (variations in the genetic code), but each only contributes a small risk of developing the disease.
- Genes linked with JIA include:
  - Human Leukocyte Antigens (HLA, system of immune recognition, expressed on almost all cells): HLA-B27 is strongly associated with ERA; A*02 with oligoarthritis; and DRB1*11, DQB1 with rheumatoid factor (RF)–ve polyarthritis; DR4 with RF+ polyarthritis (as in adult RA).
  - Cytokine/chemokine-related genes: IL-10 with oligoarthritis; IL-6 with sJIA; and IL-23 receptor, CCL5, and TNFα with psoriatic arthritis.
  - Immune-associated genes: PTPN22, TRAF1, STAT4, and CD25 are important in the control of T cell activation; mutations of MUNC13-4 and perforin in sJIA may be important in the development of MAS in select patients, but usually MAS in sJIA occurs without evidence of any monogenic cause.

Table 3.2 Summary of cytokines and inflammatory mediators important in JIA

Cytokine/Mediator	Cell	Pathology
TNFα	Monocytes, T, B cells, PMN, mast cells, fibroblasts	Activates monocytes and neutrophils Damages cartilage ↑ Endothelial cell adhesion molecules Inhibits regulatory T cells
IL-1β	Monocytes, fibroblasts	Activates osteoclasts (bone damage) Fibroblast cytokine, chemokine release ↑ Endothelial cell adhesion molecules
IL-17	T cells (Th17), mast cells	Chemokine release (recruit PMN) Cartilage damage Activates osteoclasts Synergizes with TNFα and IL-1β
IL-6	Monocytes, fibroblasts, B cells	B cell activation Inhibits regulatory T cells Growth retardation Acute phase response and anaemia
IFNγ	T cells (Th1, CD8, NK cells)	Activates monocytes ↑ Endothelial cell adhesion molecules May assist recruitment of Th17 cells Important in the pathogenesis of MAS
MRP8/14 (inflammatory mediator important in sJIA)	Monocytes, PMN	Activates monocytes, Promotes pathological CD8+ T cells Secretion of IL-1β ↑ Endothelial cell adhesion molecules

Environment
- Infection: There is no clear infectious trigger for JIA. DNA from several bacteria and viruses including parvovirus B19 have been detected in JIA serum and joints, but are of uncertain significance.
- Family conditions: High parental income and being an only child are associated with JIA which relates to the hygiene hypothesis (lack of early childhood infection increases the risks of autoimmunity). Fetal exposure to smoking may increase the risk of JIA in girls.

Classification of JIA

Background

Historically, nomenclature and criteria had developed independently in Europe and North America. This hampered research and did not allow comparisons between publications. To address this, a Classification Taskforce of the Paediatric Standing Committee of International League of Associations for Rheumatology (ILAR) developed consensus criteria under an umbrella term Juvenile Idiopathic Arthritis (JIA).

The primary aim of the ILAR proposals for classification JIA was to delineate, for research purposes, relatively homogeneous, mutually exclusive categories of idiopathic childhood arthritis based on predominant clinical and laboratory features.

It is anticipated that the proposed classification will undergo further revision in order to correct anomalies, and in response to new information. Classification subtypes were last updated in 2001.

General definition of JIA

Juvenile idiopathic arthritis is arthritis of unknown aetiology that begins before the 16th birthday and persists for at least 6 weeks; other known conditions are excluded.

JIA subtypes

Seven subtypes of JIA are recognized in the current classification system. These are summarized in Table 3.3. Each subtype requires the presence of certain features (inclusion criteria) and the absence of others (exclusion criteria) during the first 6 months of the condition.

Table 3.3 Summary of ILAR classification of JIA

JIA subtype	Features	Exclusions
Systemic onset	Arthritis > 1 joint, with/preceded by fever (daily fever > 3 days) of at least 2 weeks' duration + > 1 of:	A,B,C,D
	Non-fixed erythematous rash; Generalized lymphadenopathy; Hepatomegaly +/or splenomegaly; Serositis	
Oligoarthritis	Arthritis 1–4 joints in 1st 6 months. Subcategories:	A,B,C,D,E
	Persistent: persists, 1–4 joints ; Extended: > 4 joints after 1st 6 months	
Polyarthritis RF−ve	Arthritis ≥ 5 joints during 1st 6 months; RF negative.	A,B,C,D,E
Polyarthritis RF+ve	Arthritis ≥ 5 joints during 1st 6 months of disease	A,B,C,E
	> 2 RF +, > 3 months apart during 1st 6 months of disease	

Table 3.3 Contd.

JIA subtype	Features	Exclusions
Psoriatic arthritis	Arthritis and psoriasis, or arthritis + > 2:	B,C,D,E
	Dactylitis; nail pitting / onycholysis; Psoriasis in 1st- degree relative	
Enthesitis related arthritis	Arthritis and enthesitis, or arthritis / enthesitis + > 2:	A,D,E
	Sacroiliac joint tenderness +/or inflammatory lumbosacral pain, currently or historically; HLA-B27 antigen; Onset in a male > 6 years old; Acute symptomatic anterior uveitis; Family history (1st degree relative) of any of the following: Ankylosing spondylitis, enthesitis related arthritis, sacroiliitis with inflammatory bowel disease, Reiter's syndrome, acute anterior uveitis	
Undifferentiated arthritis	Arthritis that fulfils criteria in no category or > 2 categories	

Exclusion criteria:

A. Psoriasis or a history of psoriasis in the patient or first degree relative.

B. Arthritis in an HLA-B27 positive male beginning after the 6th birthday.

C. Ankylosing spondylitis, enthesitis related arthritis, sacroiliitis with inflammatory bowel disease, Reiter's syndrome, or acute anterior uveitis, or a history of one of these disorders in a first-degree relative.

D. The presence of IgM rheumatoid factor on at least 2 occasions at least 3 months apart.

E. The presence of systemic JIA in the patient. The application of exclusions is indicated under each category, and may change as new data become available.

Further reading

Petty, R.E. et al. International League of Associations for Rheumatology classification of juvenile idiopathic arthritis: second revision, Edmonton, 2001. *J Rheumatol* 2004;31:390–2.

JIA subtypes and their clinical presentations

- JIA is the most common form of chronic inflammatory joint disease in children and adolescents. It is defined as persistent joint inflammation (of >6 weeks duration) with onset before 16 yrs of age in the absence of infection or any other defined cause.
  - 95% of children with JIA have a disease that is clinically and immuno-genetically distinct from RA in adults.
  - Newly presenting JIA is one of the commonest physically disabling conditions of childhood, with a prevalence of approximately 1 in 1000 children, (i.e. the same as diabetes or epilepsy) and amounting to over 12,000 affected children in the UK.
  - JIA is a heterogeneous group of conditions and clinical presentation varies with the disease subtype (Table 3.4). There are at least 7 different subtypes of JIA. The classification is essentially clinical and based on the number of joints affected in the first 6 months, the presence or absence of RF, HLA B27 tissue type, systemic features (such as fever or rash), and other extra-articular features (such as psoriasis or enthesitis).
  - Uveitis is an important complication of JIA and affects at least 1/3 of children; the highest risk is young children, females and those that carry antinuclear factor (see ➜ Uveitis screening pp. 148–51).
- JIA is essentially a clinical diagnosis and one of exclusion with a wide differential diagnosis (see ➜ Clinical skills p. 1):
  - Classically a joint affected by arthritis is swollen and painful with some restriction of movement. In the younger child, however, a history of pain is often absent. Parents may describe a child who refuses to stand or has a limp first thing in the morning but runs about normally later in the day. In the youngest children, JIA may present as delay in walking or regression of achieved motor milestones (see ➜ Clinical skills p1). Examination may be limited by lack of cooperation and findings may be subtle. It is important to examine all joints even if symptoms are not volunteered and a pGALS assessment is needed as a minimum (see ➜ Clinical skills p. 1). Joint involvement may include joints that are hard to assess clinically (e.g. temporomandibular joints, subtalar joints, hips) and imaging may be required; preferably by US or MRI (with gadolinium) as radiographs are often normal.
  - In the young child, joint involvement is usually asymmetrical and subtle loss of range of movement may be detected in comparison with the normal side.
  - Infection and malignancy are not uncommon and require careful consideration.
  - Consider septic arthritis in an unwell child with a single hot, swollen, painful joint (see ➜ pp. 63–8).
  - Consider malignancy in child with severe joint pain, especially at night (see ➜ pp. 55–8).
  - Consider haematological malignancy in a child presenting with suspected systemic JIA but with low white count and/or platelets and/or low ferritin (see ➜ pp. 55–8).
  - Acute rheumatic fever and Lyme disease are both increasingly seen in the UK and should be remembered in the differential diagnosis (see ➜ pp. 395–9 and pp. 400–4 respectively).

Table 3.4 Summary of ILAR classification of JIA

Subtype	Systemic onset	Oligoarthritis	Polyarthritis RF -ve	Polyarthritis RF +ve	Psoriatic arthritis	Enthesitis-related arthritis	Other
Arthritis	In 1 or more joints with or preceded by daily (quotidian) fever for at least 3 days, accompanied by ≥1 of: • Evanescent erythematous rash • Generalized lymphadenopathy • Hepatomegaly and/or splenomegaly • Serositis	In 1–4 joints during first 6 months of disease Subcategories: • Persistent—affecting no more than 4 joints throughout course • Extended—affecting a total of >4 joints after the first 6 months of disease	In 5 or more joints during the first 6 months of disease RF test negative	In 5 or more joints during the first 6 months of disease RF test positive	Arthritis and psoriasis, or arthritis and at least 2 of: • Dactylitis • Nail pitting or onycholysis • Psoriasis in 1ˢᵗ-degree relative	Arthritis and enthesitis or arthritis with at least 2 of the following • Presence or history of sacroiliac joint tenderness and/or inflammatory lumbosacral pain • Presence of HLA B27 antigen • Onset in ♂ >6yr • Acute anterior uveitis • Ankylosing spondylitis, enthesitis-related arthritis • Sacroiliitis with inflammatory bowel disease • Reiter syndrome • Acute uveitis in 1ˢᵗ-degree relative	Undifferentiated with no category or 2 or more categories
Exclusions	A, B, C, D	A, B, C, D, E	A, B, C, D, E	A, B, C, E	B, C, D, E	A, D, E	

A: psoriasis or history of psoriasis in patient or 1ˢᵗ-degree relative, B: arthritis in HLAB27-positive male after 6ᵗʰ birthday, C: ankylosing spondylitis, enthesitis-related arthritis, sacroiliitis with inflammatory bowel disease, Reiter syndrome or acute uveitis, or history of 1 of these in 1ˢᵗ-degree relative. D: presence of IgM RF on at least 2 occasions at least 3 months apart, E: the presence of systemic JIA.

Prognostic indicators in JIA

Despite the recent intensification of early treatment regimes for children with new-onset JIA, and the associated expectation of improved clinical outcomes, it remains difficult to predict the prognosis for an individual child. This is a huge challenge for children and their families.

Outcomes

An ideal outcome for a child or young person with JIA would be lifelong disease remission with no long-term functional or psychological effects. Suboptimal outcomes may result from:

- Poorly controlled joint disease with resultant joint damage.
- Visual loss from JIA-associated uveitis.
- Psychosocial morbidity.
- Delay in diagnosis and starting treatment.

The existing literature on long-term outcomes highlights a poor functional outcome for many young people with JIA. However, these studies reflect historical treatment regimens rather than current best practice. Evidence predicting outcomes from current therapeutic approaches is limited to anecdote and awaits validation from ongoing long-term outcome studies, e.g. the Childhood Arthritis Prospective Study (CAPS, UK) and Research in Arthritis in Canadian Children Emphasizing Outcomes Study (ReACCH-Out, Canada).

Prognosis

In predicting the prognosis for a child with JIA, two main factors require consideration:

- Heterogeneity in the disease and its response to treatment.
- Variability in access to optimal clinical care.

Disease heterogeneity

Indicators of poor outcome related to the disease itself are summarized in Table 3.5 and have traditionally been divided into:

- Risk factors for continuing active disease.
- Risk factors for long-term damage.
- It should be noted that continuing active disease of any disease subtype can lead to long-term damage, and therefore division of indictors of poor outcome in this way may be obsolete.

Access to care

For any child with JIA, regardless of the disease subtype and features, there is increasing consensus that access to appropriate care is an important determinant of outcome. The British Society of Paediatric and Adolescent Rheumatology (BSPAR) Standards of Care for children and young people with JIA (see ➔ BSPAR, pp. 466–8) emphasize the importance of:

- Prompt diagnosis and referral to specialist care.[1]
- Early aggressive treatment to control inflammation.
- Support from a paediatric rheumatology MDT.

[1] Defined as: all children in whom JIA is suspected should be seen by a specialist paediatric rheumatology MDT within 10 weeks from onset of symptoms and 4 weeks from date of referral in order to facilitate early diagnosis, eye screening, and commence appropriate treatment.

Success in achieving a good outcome mandates that the management must remain patient-centred, maximizing both physical and psychosocial wellbeing. Optimal disease control may require challenging drug regimens and compliance may be an issue during adolescence. The support of the MDT is essential for all children, young people and their families. It may be particularly important for lower socioeconomic groups where increased problems with daily activities and lower perception of disease consequences have been reported.

Adverse prognostic factors

Adverse prognostic factors for any child with JIA therefore include:
- Delay in diagnosis.
- Delay in referral to specialist team.
- Late disease control.
- Continued disease activity.

Future advances

Paediatric rheumatology is a rapidly changing specialty. In the near future improvements in our ability to predict prognosis for a child with JIA will likely result from further advances in our understanding of:
- Genetic and molecular mechanisms involved in the immunological and inflammatory processes.
- Genetic predictors of response to drugs.
- Detection of subclinical disease with imaging.
- Availability of new targeted therapeutic approaches.

Myeloid related proteins 8 and 14 (MRP 8/14) are calcium-binding proteins secreted by infiltrating phagocytes in inflamed synovium. MRP 8/14 may be a useful indicator in JIA, aiding prognostication, monitoring of treatment efficacy, and risk stratification for disease relapse on therapy cessation. Future targeted treatment trials will help to establish the role of MRP 8/14 as a prognostic indicator in children with JIA.

Table 3.5 JIA subtypes and risk factors for poor disease outcomes

| | Risk factors for: | |
	Continuing active disease	Long-term damage
Subtype of JIA	Psoriatic	*Polyarticular onset:* both onset and disease course (e.g. extended oligoarticular disease)
		sJIA: ongoing active systemic features at 6 months defined as fever, need for corticosteroids, and thrombocytosis
Age	Young age in oligoarticular and RF−ve polyarticular	
Blood markers	RF+ve	RF+ve
	ANA+ve (↑ risk of uveitis)	Normal inflammatory markers with late diagnosis
	Persistently raised platelet count in sJIA	
Clinical features	Subcutaneous nodules	Symmetrical joint disease
	Late presentation	Hip or ankle involvement
	High CHAQ at presentation	Rapid & early involvement of small joints of hand and feet
	Poor response to treatment at 4 months	Early radiographic changes
		Presentation with uveitis as 1st symptom; or visual loss at 1st eye screen

Further reading

CAPS: ℘ http://www.medicine.manchester.ac.uk/musculoskeletal/research/arc/clinicalepidemi-ology/outcomestudies/caps.

ReACCH-Out: ℘ http://www.icaare.ca/index.php?option=com_content&task=view&id=28&Itemid=46.

Uveitis screening in JIA: the approach to screening and guidelines

Rationale for screening
- JIA is associated with a significant risk of developing asymptomatic chronic anterior uveitis (CAU).
- JIA CAU is the leading cause of visual loss from childhood uveitis, and is associated with a high level of eye complications.
- Early regular eye-screening is a key component in the care of JIA patients because it aims to reduce the incidence of visual impairment by early detection and intervention.

Justification for a screening programme
- Provision of expensive screening is justified because it fulfils many, but not all, of the criteria for an effective screening programme, principally:
  - Slit lamp examination is a safe, effective screening test identifying CAU earlier in the disease course than children can themselves identify the subtle eye symptoms.
  - The incidence of CAU is high, affecting 10% of all JIA patients; the highest-risk subgroup of JIA, extended oligoarthritis, has an incidence of 35–57%.
  - 40% of CAU is present at the first eye screen.
  - The duration of persistent inflammation in the eye is a key poor prognostic factor which can be reduced by screening.
- The outcome of JIA CAU remains poor despite screening, indicated by the following:
  - Bilateral disease in 67–85%; significant eye complications in >40% of cases—cataract, glaucoma, macular oedema, hypotony.
  - Early treatment is a key aim to improve outcomes. There is increasingly effective treatment for CAU available.

Population requiring screening
- Screening should equally be offered to children with JIA (all subgroups), whether they have few or many affected joints, and despite some variation in risk.
  - Evidence of significant risk to warrant screening exists for persistent and extended oligoarthritis, RF−ve polyarthritis, psoriatic arthritis, and also undifferentiated arthritis.
- Performing the first screen as early as possible is a key aim and in reality eye screening is often performed before the diagnosis of JIA is absolutely clear (e.g. in cases which are ultimately are diagnosed as reactive arthritis). Screening should be performed before the subgroup of JIA is confirmed as the classification evolves over time.
- Uveitis is more common in the following:
  - Girls, younger age patients.
  - JIA patients who are ANA+ve (albeit of patients with uveitis, 50% are ANA−ve)—therefore children with JIA and who are ANA−ve also need eye screening).
  - Severe uveitis is associated with younger age and male sex.

- Enthesitis-related arthritis (ERA) is usually associated with acute anterior uveitis (and often patients carry HLA B27) which presents promptly with a painful red eye. However, reports of asymptomatic CAU in ERA, leads to its inclusion in some screening programmes.

Exclusions to screening

- Two subgroups of JIA are not associated with a high level of CAU, and are not offered screening in all programmes. A single eye screen at presentation of JIA is recommended, particularly where the diagnosis is unclear.
  - RF+ve polyarticular JIA (RF+JIA) is not associated with CAU, and as disease onset is usually in later adolescence may not be considered for screening in some programmes.
  - A small number of case reports exist of CAU in sJIA. Other conditions that could mimic sJIA, such as CINCA (amongst many others), do develop CAU, which raises a question about the diagnosis in these older case reports. *As a rule of thumb developing CAU in sJIA should lead to the question: 'Is this really sJIA?'.*

Structure of the screening programme

The core principles of the screening programmes are listed in Table 3.6. Variations in screening programmes between countries often relate to the lack of a clear evidence base to address these statements. Important points to consider are the following:

- Those providing eye screening should be appropriately trained, skilled at examining young children, and should audit the robustness of their screening programme.
- Most uveitis develops early in the disease course:
  - The first eye screen is critical, and should be made immediately after the diagnosis of JIA, or before certain diagnosis if JIA is likely.
  - Screening in the first and early years should be adhered to robustly.
  - Robust mechanisms to identify non-adherence to the screening programme are important.
- Immediate access to advice and assessment should be offered should eye symptoms develop between screening visits or after discharge from the screening programme.
- A revised screening schedule should be offered if the risk of uveitis increases, such as discontinuation of maintenance drugs (e.g. patients on biologics who stop taking methotrexate—*anecdotally there are reports of de novo uveitis or flares occurring with etanercept use*—see ➜ pp. 493–4).
- Children with JIA who are too young or otherwise unable (e.g. learning difficulties) to recognize subtle changes in their vision associated with the development of CAU must be offered eye screening.
  - Rapid access to an examination under anaesthetic (EUA) should be available for all children unable to comply with screening examinations. The children least likely to comply are at the highest risk for undetected disease, i.e. the youngest or those with learning disability.
- Once considered high enough risk to merit inclusion in the screening programme, the screening interval offered should *not* be related to the risk of developing uveitis, but to the natural history of uveitis should it develop.

- The screening intervals should be short enough so that should uveitis develop, no irreversible damage occurs between screening visits.
- There is a poor evidence base for determining the screening interval.
- Eye screening continues until the child is old enough to detect the symptoms of uveitis and this is usually considered 12yrs of age as a minimum.
  - Whilst the risk of developing uveitis falls with time from the date of last active arthritis, date of diagnosis, and with increasing age, children discharged from screening are still at risk of uveitis, and are discharged because they are considered old enough to identify subtle changes in their vision. In children with learning difficulties screening may be required for longer until the risk is low.

Details of the screening assessment

- Screening involves slit lamp examination of anterior, intermediate, and posterior chambers of the eye:
  - A slit lamp examination by a skilled operator is required, i.e. ophthalmologist (or optometrist) skilled and experienced at examining children's eyes.
  - Examination by ophthalmoscope alone is *not* able to detect the presence of uveitis.
- Anterior uveitis is by far the commonest presentation, but the other chambers are also affected.
- Macular involvement, whilst rare, is associated with a poor prognosis and is particularly important to detect.
- Some screening programmes also check visual acuity, and proceed to intraocular pressure measurements as indicated.

Table 3.6 Comparison of screening programmes between different countries

Core principle	Current UK guidance*	Current USA guidance	German variation on USA guidance
Rapid first eye screen	Within 6 weeks of referral to eye clinic	Within 1 month of diagnosis of arthritis	None given
Minimizing delay of symptom onset of JIA to diagnosis of JIA	Seen within 10 weeks of onset of symptoms and 4 weeks of the referral	Not discussed	
Screening intervals	2-monthly for the first 6 months, then 3–4-monthly	3–12-monthly depending on risk category. No discussion of psoriatic arthritis at all	3–12-monthly depending on risk category. Recognizes psoriatic as important risk factor in addition to oligoarthritis and RF−ve JIA
Access to examination under anaesthetic as appropriate	'Urgent' if deemed high risk—no timescale given	Not discussed	

Table 3.6 Contd.

Core principle	Current UK guidance*	Current USA guidance	German variation on USA guidance
Access if symptomatic	Within 1 week	Urgent access, no time interval given	Not discussed
Altered screening with altered risk	Return to 1st-year screening intervals on discontinuation of methotrexate	Complex algorithm dependent on age, ANA status, and disease duration	
Adherence to screening	Priority to rebook (no time given)	Not discussed	
Ages included, and duration of screening	Complex detail, summarized as until 12th birthday	Continue with 12-monthly screening throughout adolescence	Continue with 12-monthly screening throughout adolescence
Exclusions from screening	RF+ve JIA and sJIA offered baseline screen only	Uses 1986 classification, and screens only sJIA, oligoarthritis, and polyarthritis	None, RF positive JIA, ERA and sJIA offered 12-monthly screening

Note: current screening programmes are not fully evidence-based because of lack of adequate study in large enough numbers of patients. There is little or no evidence to support different screening regimens between subgroups of JIA, nor to determine the best screening interval. This lack of evidence leads to some debate about the validity of the use of the term screening, suggest surveillance as a better term, and also discussion about the validity of guidelines which are not fully evidence-based. Nonetheless screening is performed in many countries with consensus that it is effective and worthwhile.

* Current UK guidance is based on the following:

The Royal College of Ophthalmologists 2006 guidelines for screening for uveitis in juvenile idiopathic arthritis. Produced jointly by BSPAR and the RCPOphth (2006) available at
℘ http://www.rcophth.ac.uk/docs/publications.

BSPAR Standards of Care 2010. BSPAR Standards of Care for JIA.
℘ http://www.bspar.org.uk/downloads/clinical_guidelines/Standards_of_Care.pdf.

Further reading

Cassidy J, Kivlin L, Lindsley C, et al. Ophthalmological examination in children with juvenile rheumatoid arthritis Pediatrics 2006;117:1843–5.

Heiligenhaus A, Niewerth M, Ganser G, et al., and the German Uveitis in Childhood Study Group. Prevalence and complications of uveitis in juvenile idiopathic arthritis in a population-based nationwide study in Germany: suggested modification of the current screening guidelines Rheumatology 2007; 46:1015–19.

JIA in the young adult

Background

A significant percentage of patients with JIA will continue with active disease into adulthood. Young adulthood (age group 16–25 years) is a time of profound personal change and development during which patients with JIA have specific needs which must be addressed in order to optimize their care and subsequent long-term health outcomes. The transition from adolescent to adult care can present challenges for the patient, their family and healthcare professionals–recognizing this and tailoring care appropriately offers the best chance of a healthy present and future.

What makes the young adult (YA) different?

Many new experiences and responsibilities are presented to the YA, often at a time of social upheaval. Life events may include moving out of the parental home, starting work or higher education, the desire for independence from their parents, and introduction of new sexual relationships. The YA may start to engage in behaviours such as substance use (legal and illegal).

Physiologically, middle adolescence (ages 14–17) is a period when there is a rapid increase in dopaminergic activity and so an increase in behaviours such as reward-seeking and risky behaviour where concerns about 'the here and now' predominate, (Steinberg, 2010). This is in contra-distinction to the maturation of the pre-frontal cortex, responsible for executive functions such as planning, abstract thought, problem-solving ability, and impulse control/delay of gratification, which is much slower and may not fully mature until the third decade of life. The YA with JIA may lack the executive functions and therefore skills required to manage their disease optimally. In adult services, such patients may be expected to start to attend appointments alone, take responsibility for their medications and drug monitoring, be encouraged to self-manage and take the initiative to report problems themselves and participate in decision-making with regards to treatment. These are skills which may not have been fully developed yet. In this context, it is perhaps not surprising that a high rate of unsuccessful transfer from paediatric to adult rheumatology care can occur. (Hazel et al., 2010). The YA Rheumatology team must tailor their services and the way in which they interact with the YA to engage patients successfully with healthcare and foster their skills and resilience to self-manage disease.

Specific areas to consider

General issues

- **Developmental stage:** as part of an effective patient–professional relationship, assessment should be made of the ability of a YA to use executive functions in their interactions. This capability may vary from attendance to attendance but will shape the way information is presented and discussed.
- **Communication skills:** some YA patients may not respond to reasoning about the health of their joints in 10-years time (remember: 'the here and now') but may respond better to arguments about what the treatment can provide for them in the immediate/short-term. Non-judgmental, honest, and jargon-free communication should be a

cornerstone of the YA consultation and staff need specific training to develop such skills.

- **Knowledge**: assess your patient's knowledge of their disease and its management and fill in knowledge gaps. Provide information in paper and electronic form.
- **Confidentiality**: should be discussed with the patient (and if necessary, explained to parents).
- **Developing self-advocacy**: patients may begin to attend appointments alone. This should be supported but not forced upon the YA before they are ready. On the other hand, some parents/guardians as well as patients themselves may experience difficulty adjusting to this concept. A relationship of trust between the patient, physician, and parents/guardians is key in enabling the gradual shift towards the YA taking the primary role in consultations. The timing of this transition will vary between patients. The YA may also require guidance on developing skills to access rheumatology services independently (use of multimedia/technological resources may aid this) and to be their own advocate (Fig. 3.2).
- **Taking the lead in decision-making**: use an individualized approach—some YAs may need more guidance than others when it comes to making decisions about their own treatment.
- **Attendance**: Non-attendance is a common occurrence—reasons for non-attendance should be explored via a telephone consultation at the earliest opportunity—this will also enable you to make an, albeit limited, disease assessment, 'troubleshoot' and plan future care.

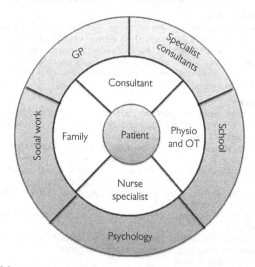

Fig. 3.2 Ideal structure of Rheumatology Services from childhood, through adolescence and into young adulthood and beyond.

- **Adherence**: barriers to adherence include busy social circumstances, long-distance travel, unwillingness to appear different to their peers, and (in the case of methotrexate [MTX]) alcohol use, as well as the usual problems of adverse side-effects. Needle phobia as well as MTX intolerance is common in this population and must be specifically addressed.

Medical issues
- **Medication**
  - Patients may wish to consider a change from subcutaneous to oral MTX if they have not done so already.
  - Patients may wish to start self-injecting MTX/biologics, taking over this role from their parents or guardians.
  - Physicians should continue to use triamcinolone hexacetonide for intra-articular injections.
- **Osteoporosis**: a risk assessment should be performed, risk factors addressed and vitamin D supplementation considered.
- **Recognizing adults with JIA as a separate disease group**: disease phenotypes and treatments differ from adult disease. Re-labelling some sub-types of JIA as 'rheumatoid arthritis' or 'ankylosing spondylitis' may lead to patients being lost to follow-up in registry studies of biologics in JIA which contributes to the relative lack of knowledge of JIA in adulthood.
- **Reproductive health**: an open, non-judgmental dialogue about sexual activity and contraception should be encouraged. Information about how to seek advice on contraception and safe sex should be provided. Patients on MTX should be reminded at regular intervals about teratogenicity.

Psychological issues:
- **Depression and anxiety**: in a cohort study of 246 adults with JIA who had long-term follow-up, 31.6% were anxious, 5.2% were depressed, and 21.1% had previously suffered from depression (Packham et al., 2002). Chronic disease is a risk factor for depression and anxiety—physicians should enquire sensitively about these issues in the consultation—YA may not initiate discussions.

Social issues:
- **Further education and work**: discussion about career aspirations and future work planning should be encouraged. The YA may seek advice on the impact of their arthritis on these issues.
- **Smoking, illicit drug use and alcohol**: sensitive, non-judgmental enquiry is necessary. The impact on their specific disease as well as general health, in the immediate and long-term should be discussed. Excess alcohol is discouraged in the context of MTX and if the patient is unlikely to adhere to treatment for this reason, it may be worthwhile considering an alternative.
- Clinics held in appropriate environments (i.e. dedicated Young Person's Clinic space).
- Clinics held at convenient times for the patient: consider evening clinics or weekend clinics to optimize chances of attendance.
- Telephone consultations.
- Accessibility: email/telephone/SMS contact and a service website/app.

- Higher tolerance of non-attendance and clear plans for chasing non-attenders.
- Built-in psychosocial assessment: consider using the HEADS approach: Home, Education/Employment, Activities outside school and home, Drugs, Sexual Health, Stress/suicidal intent/safety from violence and injury.
- Individualize the consultation (concrete versus abstract) when it comes to communication and shared decision-making.
- Encourage self-advocacy and self-management when developmentally appropriate.

Further reading

Steinberg, L A behavioural scientist looks at the science of adolescent brain development. *Brain Cognit* 2010;72:160–4.

Hazel, E *et al* (2010): High rates of unsuccessful transfer to adult care amongst young adults with juvenile idiopathic arthritis. Paediatr Rheumatol online 2010;11:8:2. doi: 10.1186/1546-0096-8-2.

Packham, JC *et al* Long-term follow-up of 246 adults with juvenile idiopathic arthritis: predictive factors for mood and pain. *Rheumatology* 2002;41(12):1444–9. doi: 10.1093/rheumatology/41.12.14

Transition from children's to adults services for young people using health or social services NICE guidelines NG43 ♒ http://www.nice.org.uk/guidance/ng43

Surgery in the young adult with JIA: practical issues

Introduction

- Surgery has an important but diminishing part in the overall management of JIA.
- Many young adults with JIA in their 20s will have limited physical function and continued disease activity. It should be remembered that current published outcome studies are retrospective and often pre-date the effects of newer treatments such as biologic drugs in combination with MTX. Better treatment has meant that growth has been completed with epiphyseal closure before joints fail and bone density has reached the adult peak.
- Since the advent of these effective drugs, many centres have seen a reduction in need for certain types of surgery such as synovectomy and soft tissue release (tenotomies and capsulotomies), and delay in others such as joint replacement.
- In most centres, surgery for joint failure now occurs into young adulthood, rather than in adolescence when maturation is incomplete.
- There is currently a cohort of young adult patients who have received biologic drugs in their later years after a period of sustained disease activity and who present new problems for those providing services for people with arthritis. It is hoped that newer cohorts of patients who have had optimal control throughout their disease course will need less surgical intervention.
- It is important that the orthopaedic surgeon has skills in this age group and JIA.
- Combined management with a rheumatologist and surgeon is important and should ideally be in a dedicated setting.

Orthopaedic surgery in the young adult

- There is now many years' experience in young people in arthroplasty of the hip, knee, ankle, shoulder, elbow, and wrist. Cervical surgery and arthrodesis of various joints may still be considered.
- The highest requirement for surgery is in RF+ve polyarticular JIA. Other patterns requiring surgery include systemic JIA with polyarticular course, RF−ve polyarticular disease, and extended oligoarticular arthritis, particularly if disease has been active for many years.
- The best results are obtained in fully controlled disease with joints in a good position. If >1 joint needs surgery, the proximal one should be first, and lower limbs should precede upper limbs.

- Intra-articular steroid may reduce synovial activity and fixed flexion deformity although should not be used within 3 months of surgery. Soft tissue release to obtain a good position is equally rarely necessary. Hydrotherapy may be needed to maintain muscle strength.
- There is still a place for synovectomy (usually arthroscopic) if disease remains uncontrolled despite drug treatment.
- Many orthopaedic surgeons are reluctant to operate on young people. However, hip and knee arthroplasty are now the commonest operations in this group with achievement of good 10-yr survival in specialist centres.

The key symptoms requiring surgery are:
- Pain despite control of the other joints with active therapy.
- Reducing exercise tolerance (walking distance in the legs or pain on movement in the arms.
- Night pain or pain at rest.
- Increasing disability and instability (locking or giving way of lower limb joints).

The threshold should be considerably above the level of immobility where the person has to regularly use a wheelchair.

Precautions with surgery in adults with JIA

- Cervical spine: x-rays should be performed prior to surgery; if necessary this should be followed with MRI. PA and lateral views in flexion and extension should be obtained to assess for:
  - Atlanto-axial subluxation (see Fig. 3.3).
  - Cervical spondylolisthesis (slip of one vertebra on another which can be multiple).
  - Cervical fusion with limited range of movement of movement at one level.
- Temporomandibular joint disease: micrognathia and abnormal/restricted jaw opening may cause intubation difficulty.
- Occasionally there may have been previous intubation difficulty due to a small larynx or cricoarytenoid arthritis.

Medications:
- MTX should not be stopped prior to surgery. Infection rates after replacement surgery are less if the drug is continued. Patients who have had MTX as a DMARD have a significantly better prosthesis survival.
- *It is better to be immunosuppressed and have controlled disease than have no immunosuppression and uncontrolled disease.*

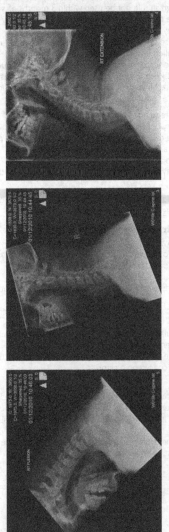

Fig. 3.3 Lateral X rays in flexion, neutral and extension position of 17-year-old man with a 2-yr history, sero+ve polyarticular JIA on MTX and biologic drugs taken prior to hip surgery. The flexion view shows significant atlanto-axial subluxation of 5.0mm not visible in the neutral or extension views. MRI examination did not show significant cord compression. There were no neck symptoms.

- *Biologics*—the current advice is to stop anti-TNF therapy in the peri-operative period—the half-life of etanercept is 100h, adalimumab 15–19 days, infliximab 8–9.5 days, tocilizumab 11-13 days (subcutaneous 5–12 days), and abatacept 13 days.
  - A practical rule is to omit the biologic drug for 14 days before and 14 days after surgery for etanercept, adalimumab, infliximab, tocilizumab, and abatacept, providing the wound is healed and not infected. There is, however, a variation in advice with some studies recommending a 4-week interval for infliximab and tocilizumab. Ideally the timing of surgery should allow for the minimum period without the drug. The American College of Rheumatology recommends that the minimum interval is a week before and a week after surgery.
  - There is a balance between successful wound healing and reduction of infection by stopping anti-TNF therapy or other biologic therapy versus perioperative risk of disease flare.
  - There is some evidence that anti-TNF therapy has a higher incidence of infection and deep vein thrombosis in patients with RA undergoing surgery but the numbers studied were small.

Other considerations
- Small stature—patients should be assessed against standard growth charts and consideration given to a need for greater anaesthetic care for small airways. Special surgical prostheses may be required (small standard prosthesis or a custom-made prosthesis).
- Osteoporosis—bone densitometry is recommended prior to surgery with higher risk in those patients with long disease duration or previous high steroid requirement.
- Down's syndrome—higher risk of atlanto-axial subluxation and also an increased sensitivity to marrow suppression from immunosuppressant and other drugs.
- Corticosteroid usage—steroid dosage may need to be adjusted over the perioperative period depending on the length and dosage of steroid use in the preceding months and years.
- Preoperative assessment—blood counts and liver and renal chemistry should be performed prior to surgery, particularly if the patient is on disease-modifying therapy. Patients with systemic disease may need cardiac assessment with ECG and echocardiogram. Thrombosis risk should be assessed.
- Amyloidosis—it is important not to dehydrate young people with amyloidosis with renal impairment undergoing surgery. An IV line will be needed prior to surgery to maintain hydration.

Perioperative care
- Anaesthetists should be experienced in treating young people with JIA. They should be aware of potential intubation difficulties and the need for nasal intubation using a fibreoptic laryngoscope.
- Pressure-reducing measures may be required to avoid skin ischaemia in vulnerable patients.

- Early mobilization is important and hydrotherapy should be considered once the skin wounds have healed.
- Preoperative physiotherapy assessments should alert the need for temporary or permanent aids and adaptations.
- Written antibiotic advice needs to be given for future surgical and dental procedures.

Advice concerning pregnancy

Young women who have had arthroplasty are often unaware of issues related to pregnancy. All young people should be under consultant care. The physician and obstetrician will need to assess:

- Pelvic size.
- Stability of any hip or other joint prosthesis.
- Neck issues as outlined on ➔ pp. 157–9.
- Drug therapy in pregnancy and risk of postpartum disease flares.
- Physical issues around breastfeeding and child care.
- Timing of reintroduction of drug therapy in relation to delivery and breastfeeding.

Even if the mother has not had an arthroplasty, long labour should be avoided and the mother should be aware of the potential need for assisted delivery and Caesarean section.

Drugs in pregnancy, breastfeeding and paternal exposure

The reader is referred to the guideline reference below for detailed advice.

- Prednisolone is compatible with each trimester of pregnancy, breastfeeding, and paternal exposure.
- MTX should be avoided in pregnancy and stopped 3 months in advance of conception. It is not recommended with breastfeeding. Based on limited evidence it may be compatible with paternal exposure.
- Anti TNF drugs. Infliximab may be continued until 16 weeks. Etanercept, adalimumab may be continued until the end of the second trimester. Women should not be discouraged from breastfeeding on anti-TNF but caution is recommended pending further information. Infliximab, etanercept, and adalimumab are compatible with paternal exposure.
- Tocilizumab should be stopped at least 3 months prior to conception but unintentional exposure early in the first trimester is unlikely to be harmful. There is no data for breastfeeding. While there is no data regarding paternal exposure, it is unlikely to be harmful.
- Abatacept. There is insufficient data to recommend this drug in pregnancy, breastfeeding, or paternal exposure. Unintentional exposure in the first trimester is unlikely to be harmful. Paternal exposure is unlikely to be harmful

Further reading

Ding T, Ledingham J, Luqmani R, et al. BSR and BHPR rheumatoid arthritis guidelines on the safety on anti-TNF therapies. London: BSR, 2010. Available at: http://www.rheumatology.org.uk/includes/documents/cm_docs/2010/d/draft_anti_tnf_safety_guideline_april_2010.pdf. (due for revision 2016)

Flint J, Panchal S, Hurrell A, van den Venne, M et al. BSR and BHPR Guideline on prescribing drugs in pregnancy and breast feeding. Part I: standard and biologic disease modifying anti-rheumatic drugs and corticosteroids. Rheumatology (Oxford). 2016;55(9):1693–7.

Hall MA, Surgical interventions. In Szer IS, Kimura Y, Malleson PN, et al. (eds) Arthritis in Children and Adults. Oxford: Oxford University Press, 2006; 403–14

Treatment approaches in JIA

- JIA is a complex and chronic condition and is therefore optimally managed by an experienced MDT as part of a managed clinical network as outlined in the BSPAR Standards of Care (see ➔ pp. 466–8).
- The MDT is integral to the management with the patient and family at the centre (Fig. 3.4), with input from specialist consultant, specialist nurse, paediatric physiotherapist, and paediatric occupational therapist (with interests in musculoskeletal conditions if possible).
- Access to ophthalmology for monitoring and treatment of JIA-associated eye disease is vital, with other services such as orthopaedic surgeons, radiology, social work, and psychology services able to be accessed readily as required; these disciplines all have to interlink efficiently to achieve the best possible outcome. See ➔ pp. 418–19 and related chapters for more information on MDT members and their specific roles.
- The general treatment approach is to achieve early diagnosis and rapid control of the inflammatory process, whilst minimizing adverse effects of treatment and supporting general physical and mental health (Fig. 3.5).
- Early and adequate treatment aims to prevent long-term joint damage and the need for joint replacement therapy.
- Each member of the team contributes to the holistic management of the patient and family, with medical treatment forming only one strand of the overall picture.
- Education and information form one of the most important features of management throughout the duration of disease and should be undertaken by all members of the team, although the nurse specialist often takes an ongoing role in this area.
- Physiotherapy and occupational therapy have important roles in maintaining maximum function—the aim of treatment is as near to functional normality as possible. It is important to maintain muscle strength despite inflammatory processes within joints and these disciplines aim to achieve this by teaching specific exercises, pain management, and joint protection techniques as necessary.
- A healthy balanced diet with particular emphasis on calcium and vitamin D intake for bone health are recommended in JIA but there is no evidence for dietary modification affecting the inflammatory process in this disease.

Specific medical management in subtypes of JIA

- Table 3.7 illustrates some of the similarities and differences in the specific management of the different subtypes but should only be regarded as a guide to management.
- There is a lack of good evidence for many aspects of JIA management, therefore variability in practice between specialists exists.
- Particular management controversies remain around joint injection; dose, timing, number, and duration of treatment whilst in remission; and the use of specific disease-modifying drugs in particular disease types.
- In future, the possibility of genetic and phenotypic subtyping may determine prognosis and more predictable response to particular drugs.
- Further information is available (See ➔ Treatments used in paediatric rheumatism, p. 472; ➔ Share guidance, pp. 519–21; ➔ CARRA guidance, pp. 515–18; ➔ Corticosteroids joint injections, pp. 438–47)

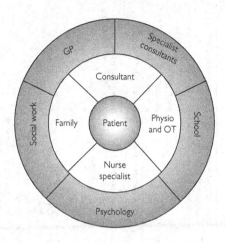

Fig. 3.4 Patient-centred MDT management of JIA.

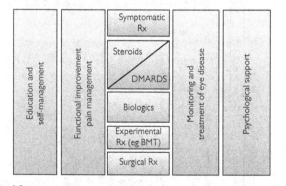

Fig. 3.5 General treatment approach in JIA.

Rx=Treatment; DMARDS=Disease modifying anti-rheumatic drugs; BMT=Bone marrow transplant.

Table 3.7 Specific management of subtypes of JIA

	Systemic onset JIA	Oligoarthritis Psoriatic arthritis	Polyarthritis	Established polyarthritis/ oligoarthritis	Enthesitis related arthritis
Early/mild disease	Medium-dose corticosteroids	Intra-articular steroids NSAIDs	MTX Steroids (intra-articular or systemic)		NSAID IVMP/high-dose corticosteroids followed by 2–4 weeks of low dose
Established/ severe disease	Pulsed IV methyl prednisolone (IVMP)* Methotrexate (MTX) (usually given by subcutaneous (SC) route) Consider ciclosporin, and biologics (e.g. anakinra or tocilizumab)	See next column		MTX (ensure maximum dose, SC route) May need to add etanercept ± corticosteroids + joint injections	Disease >2–4 months' duration Sulphasalazine (may work better than other DMARDS) MTX/anti-TNF
Remission	Wean prednisolone slowly Reduce other treatment with extreme caution—high risk of relapse	Ongoing monitoring	Wean off Steroid first DMARD continues longer then consider reduction or discontinuation	Continue treatment for several months Wean and discontinue steroids first Wait 1 year before weaning off DMARDs—off MTX last	Continue sulfasalazine 6 months–1yr

Relapse	Repeat high-dose corticosteroids Consider other biologic agents	If previous IACs effect >4 months repeat injection If lasted <4 months add NSAID, repeat IAC consider DMARD	Reintroduce all drugs on which remission was achieved.	Reintroduce all drugs that induced remission Often requires step up in treatment to reinduce remission	Generally episodic course Short courses of NSAID and sulphasalazine sufficient to obtain remission in recurrences
Persistent disease	Anti IL-6 and IL-1 directed treatments Tocilizumab (anti-IL-6) canakinumab (anti-IL-1B), anakinra (IL1ra)		IAC targeted joints	Consider alternate biologic agents In severe cases consider bone marrow transplant (see ⊕ pp. 461–4)	

* If macrophage activation syndrome develops (see ⊕ pp. 321–4).

MTX, methotrexate; IAC, intra-articular corticosteroid; DMARD, disease-modifying anti-rheumatic drug; NSAID, non-steroidal anti-inflammatory drug.

Disease activity scores in JIA

The purpose of disease activity scores is to guide and assess treatment strategies, whether pharmaceutical or other. These are formal, valid, typically composite measures that in adult rheumatology have been shown to be more effective than subjective assessment in routine practice to inform treat to target strategies. These validated tools include patient preferred outcomes, joint counts, visual analogue scales, and quality of life assessment.

The prime aim of disease management in juvenile arthritis has to be inactive disease or remission. With more aggressive use of DMARDS and access to biologics this has become a reality and is similar to adult experience.

Outcome measures in JIA

There are several measures for inactive disease in JIA and include core, or conventional, outcome variables (such as active joint count (AJC), ESR, and global assessments – see below) plus, importantly, features of systemic disease, uveitis, and morning stiffness (see ⊃ Outcome measures in paediatric rheumatology, pp. 43–9).

Once inactive disease ('minimal disease activity') has been achieved then the burden of chronic disease on quality of life (pain, anxiety, disability, sleep, loss of schooling and impact on family life) can be better understood. These parameters are currently measured in JIA by health related quality of life (HRQoL) tools (see ⊃ Outcome measures in paediatric rheumatology, pp. 43–9)

Where there is persistent disease activity, further tools have been developed for use in clinical trials, to determine what meaningful improvement is and also what defines a flare. The principle tool for polyarticular course JIA is the American College of Rheumatology (ACR) Core Outcome Variables (COV) which compares a baseline disease activity to subsequent assessments in the form of a percentage improvement; e.g ACR-30 being 30% improvement in 3 of 6 variables. The ACR is based upon:

- Active joint count (71-joints).
- Restrictive joint count (71-joints).
- CHAQ (see ⊃ Chapter 1, p. 1).
- Parent (or patient) global evaluation (visual analogue scale of 0 to 10)—ParGE.
- Physician global assessment (VAS of 0 to 10)—PhysGA.
- ESR.

Core outcome variables are the gold standard for use in research trials although have limited use in clinical practice. They are not a measure of individual disease severity or status, have less responsiveness in oligoarticular disease, and are hampered by the use of CHAQ, which is often completed incorrectly (especially as a proxy measure completed by parents), and is influenced by comorbid conditions such as chronic pain. However, the CHAQ is useful in early disease assessment and has prognostic value in determining poor long term outcome.

The DAS28

In adults, DAS-28 has become the routine measure of disease activity using a complex formula that combines swollen joint count, tender joint count,

Table 3.8 EULAR response criteria to compare DAS at two different points in time

DAS28 improvement → Present DAS28 ↓	> 1.2	> 0.6 and ≤ 1.2	≤ 0.6
≤ 3.2	Good response	Moderate response	No response
> 3.2 and ≤ 5.1	Moderate response	Moderate response	No response
> 5.1	Moderate response	No response	No response

ESR, or CRP, and a patient global assessment (VAS 1 to 100). A score of >5.1 after intensive therapy with a combination of conventional DMARDs, permits the use of a biologic and a moderate EULAR response (Table 3.8) after 6 months will allow drug continuation.

In clinical practice the DAS-28 is now used to provide other targets whereby monthly assessment of RA disease activity is followed by a change in treatment (higher doses or new drugs) until disease activity is brought into remission (DAS<2.6) or low disease activity (DAS< 3.2) or to low CRP or ESR. Persistently high scores are associated with an increased likelihood of progressive joint damage, even in patients seemingly doing well.

A misleadingly low DAS-28 score may occur when the feet are predominantly involved or when neither the ESR nor the CRP have been ever high; these scenarios are both common in JIA. In addition, tenderness is not specific to active disease and it can be difficult to decide whether an individual joint is swollen or tender (leading to inter and intra observer error). The Simple Disease Activity Index (SDAI) has been developed to simplify the complex formulae required to calculate the DAS whilst maintaining sensitivity.

The JADAS

The problems with scoring systems are amplified in paediatric practice and the reliance of scores based on blood tests can be particularly problematic in JIA assessment. Nonetheless the Juvenile Arthritis Disease Activity Score (JADAS) has been developed and comprises PhysGE, ParGA, AJC, and ESR. The ESR is normalized (ESR (mm/hr)-20)/10) to give a score between 0–10.

The three versions of JADAS depend on the number of joints assessed:
- JADAS-71 (all joints).
- JADAS-27 (cervical spine, elbows, wrists, 1st–3rd MCPJs, PIPJs, hips, knees and ankles).
- JADAS-10 (any joints up to a maximum of 10).

Defining active disease presents a challenge when in children joint restriction indicates activity rather than damage and there may be little swelling. JADAS-3 has proposed omitting the ESR to further improve clinical feasibility of the tool. This is equivalent to the Clinical Disease activity Index (CDAI) in adults.

The JADAS has good responsiveness to change and correlates well with ACR-Pedi 30, 50, and 70 in studies of polyarticular JIA. To accommodate the limitations in some forms of JIA, the JADAS scores have been defined as:
- Inactive disease score of <1 in both oligo-JIA and poly-JIA.
- Minimally active disease score of 1–2 in oligo-JIA and score of 1–3.2 in poly-JIA.

There is low correlation between JADAS and DAS-28 and CDAI.

Patient and parent reported measures

More recently, tools have included patient or parent reported outcome measures (PROMs) and in adults these multidimensional tools include the MDHAQ and the simpler form (called RAPID-3). There is good correlation between PROMs and AJC, ESR, and radiographic scores, and they are reproducible and informative to encompass impact of disease on the patient. Comparison of RAPID 3 and DAS-28 shows that they correlate well and in particular in defining disease states of remission, low, moderate, and high activity. Furthermore there is evidence that PROMs minimize the placebo effect of physician assessed AJC seen in trials.

In paediatrics, these tools have to accommodate development, growth and a disagreement between parent (or proxy) and child assessment of activity and PROMs. There is currently the Juvenile Arthritis Multidimensional Assessment Report (JAMAR) and Juvenile Arthritis Parent Assessment Index (JAPAI).

Disease activity in enthesitis-related arthritis

Currently there are no validated tools to measure disease activity in enthesitis-related arthritis or juvenile-onset spondyloarthritis. Although axial involvement is uncommon at presentation the adult tools such as Bath Ankylosing Spondylitis Disease Activity index (BASDAI) and Bath Ankylosing Spondylitis Functional Index (BASFI) show early promise with some degree of responsiveness and good correlation with CHAQ and PhysGA.

Imaging as a disease activity measure in JIA

Ultrasonography (US) is an important real-time diagnostic tool in diagnosis of joint swelling and synovitis. A number of studies suggest grey scale and power Doppler US are more sensitive to detect swelling and subclinical inflammation compared to clinical examination. MRI bone marrow oedema (as a precursor to erosive bone disease), is a good predictor of disease activity although due to the cost, availability and practical challenges in young children, routine use of MRI in clinical practice is limited. A number of scoring systems have been formulated using radiography of specific joints to evaluate joint activity in adult RA; however, measuring joint space narrowing, the number of erosions and cartilage loss in children is challenging due to changes of bone morphology and musculoskeletal maturation.

Further reading

Consolaro, A, Giancane G, Schiappapietra B, et al. Clinical outcome measures in juvenile idiopathic arthritis. *Pediatr Rheumatol* 2016;**14**:23 DOI 10.1186/s12969-016-0085-5

Ringold S et al. Performance of rheumatoid arthritis disease activity measures and juvenile arthritis disease activity scores in polyarticular-course juvenile idiopathic arthritis: analysis of their ability to classify the American College of Rheumatology pediatric measures of response and the preliminary criteria for flare and inactive disease. *Arthritis Care Res* 2010;**62**:1095–1102

McErlane F et al. Validity of a three-variable Juvenile Arthritis Disease Activity Score in children with new-onset juvenile idiopathic arthritis. *Ann Rheum Dis* 2013;**72**:1983–8.

Colebatch-Bourn et al. EULAR-PReS Points to consider for the use of imaging in the diagnosis and management if JIA in clinical practice *Ann Rheum Dis* 2015;**74**:1946–57.

Cardiovascular disease and JIA

Introduction

Individuals with rheumatoid arthritis, psoriatic arthritis and ankylosing spondylitis have an increased risk of cardiovascular disease (CVD). The increased risk is due to a combination of:

1. high prevalence of traditional risk factors for CVD, such as hypertension and smoking
2. accelerated atherosclerosis and plaque instability caused by systemic inflammation
3. treatment, particularly long-term corticosteroids

Registry data and studies using surrogate cardiovascular outcome measures (examples are given in Table 3.9) suggest improved cardiovascular outcomes in adult-onset inflammatory arthritis with adequate disease control and the use of biologics.

EULAR recommends annual cardiovascular risk factor screening for adults with rheumatoid arthritis. The recommendations are summarized in Box 3.2.

Table 3.9 Examples of commonly used surrogate cardiovascular outcome measures[a]

Outcome measure	Component of cardiovascular risk assessed
Pulse wave velocity	Arterial stiffness
Flow mediated dilatation	Endothelial dysfunction
Carotid intima-media thickness	Carotid atherosclerosis
Coronary computed tomography	Coronary artery calcium/ atherosclerotic burden

[a]A surrogate outcome measure is a substitute for a clinical endpoint. It is a predictor for clinical outcome based on scientific evidence.

Box 3.2 EULAR recommendations for cardiovascular (CV) risk management in rheumatoid arthritis (RA), psoriatic arthritis (PsA) and ankylosing spondylitis (AS)

- RA should be regarded as a condition with higher CV risk. This may apply to AS and PsA
- Adequate control of the disease is necessary to lower CV risk
- CV risk assessment using national guidelines is recommended for all patients with RA (and considered in PsA and AS)
- CV risk score models should be adapted for patients with RA by introducing a 1.5 multiplication factor
- TC/HDL cholesterol ratio should be used when SCORE model is used
- Intervention should be carried out according to national guidelines
- Statins, ACE inhibitors and angiotensin II blockers are preferred treatment options
- Caution should be used when prescribing NSAIDs and coxibs
- Use the lowest possible corticosteroid dose
- Recommend smoking cessation

Evidence for cardiovascular risk in JIA

There is a paucity of data on cardiovascular risk either in children or adults with JIA. Preliminary evidence, however, suggests a higher prevalence of some traditional cardiovascular risk factors:

- Children with JIA have higher systolic and diastolic blood pressure (although values remain within normal range).
- Hypertension may be more prevalent in adults with JIA.
- Some studies found ↓ HDL and ↑ triglycerides in JIA. The lipid profile is difficult to interpret in JIA: variability occurs with disease activity and medications (e.g. steroids, anti-TNFa and anti-IL6 agents).
- Children with JIA may be less physically active.
- Individuals with JIA may have higher total body fat for a given BMI.
- Medications used frequently in JIA are known to increase cardiovascular risk in adults (eg steroids, NSAIDs).
- There is insufficient evidence to comment on the prevalence of smoking, diabetes or family history of CVD in JIA.

Different subtypes may have different cardiovascular risk profiles: the JuMBO registry (see Further reading) found a high prevalence of CVD in systemic onset JIA but not in other subtypes. High disease activity is likely to be associated with increased cardiovascular risk, as observed in adult-onset inflammatory arthritides. Long-term cohort studies spanning several decades would be needed to determine the cardiovascular event risk in JIA. Surrogate cardiovascular outcomes (Table 3.10) have potential for assessing cardiovascular risk in JIA prior to such studies being available.

Guidelines for cardiovascular risk assessment in JIA

In the absence of clear increased cardiovascular risk in JIA, no evidence-based guidelines for managing risk are available. Atherosclerosis begins in childhood hence there is potential to improve cardiovascular outcomes from a young age. Extrapolated from the evidence in adult-onset inflammatory arthritides and other childhood conditions associated with increased cardiovascular risk (e.g. diabetes mellitus, familial hypercholesterolaemia, obesity), the following are pragmatic suggestions:

- Determine relevant family history: cardiovascular event <55 years (male) or <60 years (female) in first-degree relatives.
- Review family history for obesity, hyperlipidaemia, diabetes mellitus, and hypertension.
- Commence active anti-smoking advice at an early age and advise against passive smoking including a smoke-free home environment.
- Growth/diet—monitor height/weight/BMI and promote healthy nutrition.
- Measure blood pressure annually for all children and young people.
- Physical activity promotion—recommend >1hr moderate-to-vigorous physical activity per day.
- Cardiovascular health assessment and promotion should be a routine part of transitional care, including serum lipid and glucose measurement.
- Health care professionals involved in the care of children and young adults with JIA should be aware of the potential for increased cardiovascular risk.

Further reading

Coulson EJ, Ng WF, Goff, I, Foster HE. Cardiovascular risk in juvenile idiopathic arthritis. *Rheumatology (Oxford)* 2013;52(7):1163–71.

Bohr, AH, Fuhlbrigge RC, Pedersen FK, de Ferranti SD, Mu¨ller K. Premature subclinical atherosclerosis in children and young adults with juvenile idiopathic arthritis. A review considering preventive measures. *Pediatric Rheumatol* 2016;14:3 DOI 10.1186/s12969-015-0061-5.

Kerekes G, Soltész P, Nurmohamed,MT, et al. Validated methods for assessment of subclinical atherosclerosis in rheumatology. *Nature Rev Rheumatol* 2012;8(4):224–34.

Minden K, Klotsche J, Nieworth M, et al. Biologics register JuMBO. Long-term safety of biologic therapy of juvenile idiopathic arthritis. *Z Rheumatol*. 2013;72(4):339–46. doi: 10.1007/s00393-012-1063-z.

Expert Panel on Integrated Guidelines for Cardiovascular Health and Risk Reduction in Children and Adolescents. Expert Panel on Integrated Guidelines for Cardiovascular Health and Risk Reduction in Children and Adolescents: summary report. *Pediatrics* 2011;128(suppl 5):S213–S256.

Peters, MJ, Symmons DP, McCarey D, et al. EULAR evidence-based recommendations for cardiovascular risk management in patients with rheumatoid arthritis and other forms of inflammatory arthritis. *Ann Rheum Dis* 2010;69:325–31.

Systemic diseases

The classification of paediatric vasculitis

Background to classification criteria

- Classification criteria are often described for diseases where the pathogenesis and/or molecular mechanisms are poorly understood.
- They are used to facilitate clinical trials and improve epidemiological descriptions by providing a set of agreed criteria that can be used by investigators anywhere in the world.
- Classification criteria for vasculitis are designed to differentiate one form of vasculitis from another once the diagnosis of vasculitis has been secured. They are not the same as diagnostic criteria (such as those described for Kawasaki disease), but are often *misused* as such.
- Thus, *classification criteria aim to:*
  - Identify a set of clinical findings (criteria) that recognize a high proportion of patients with the particular disease (sensitivity), and
  - Exclude a high proportion of patients with other diseases (specificity).
- Classification criteria typically include manifestations that are characteristics of the disease in question that occur with less frequency or are absent in other conditions.
- Symptoms or findings that might be typical or common but may also be present in other diseases tend to be excluded.
- An important limitation to these criteria is that they are not based on a robust understanding of the pathogenesis and as such are relatively crude tools that are likely to be modified as scientific understanding of these diseases progresses.

Paediatric vasculitis classification 2010

- New paediatric classification criteria are described, and validated on >1300 cases worldwide (Table 4.1).
- These criteria do not include Kawasaki disease (see → Kawasaki disease, pp. 190–5); nor do they include definitions for microscopic polyangiitis (too few cases included in dataset).
- For Takayasu arteritis, care must be taken to exclude fibromuscular dysplasia (or other cause of non-inflammatory large- and medium-vessel arteriopathy) since undoubtedly there could be scope for overlap in the clinical presentation between these 2 entities, although the pathogenesis and treatment for these are clearly distinct.

General scheme for the classification of paediatric vasculitides

- This is based on the size of the vessel *predominantly* involved in the vasculitic syndrome and is summarized below.
- It should be noted, however, that most vasculitides exhibit a significant degree of 'polyangiitis overlap': e.g. Granulomatosis with polyangiitis can affect the aorta and its major branches; and small vessel vasculitis can occur in polyarteritis nodosa.

Table 4.1 Classification criteria for specific vasculitic syndromes

Vasculitis	Classification criteria	Sensitivity[1]	Specificity*
HSP	Purpura, predominantly lower limb *or* diffuse* (mandatory) *plus* 1 out of 4 of: • Abdo pain • IgA on biopsy • Haematuria/proteinuria • Arthritis/arthralgia *If diffuse (i.e. atypical distribution) then IgA deposition on biopsy required	100%	87%
GPA	At least 3 out of 6 of the following criteria: • Histopathology • Upper airway involvement • Laryngo-tracheobronchial stenoses • Pulmonary involvement • ANCA positivity • Renal involvement	93%	99%
PAN	Histopathology or angiographic abnormalities (mandatory) plus 1 of the following 5 criteria: • Skin involvement • Myalgia/muscle tenderness • Hypertension • Peripheral neuropathy • Renal involvement	89%	99%
TA	Angiographic abnormalities of the aorta or its main branches (also pulmonary arteries) showing aneurysm/dilatation (mandatory criterion), plus 1 of the following criteria: • Pulse deficit or claudication • 4 limb BP discrepancy • Bruits • Hypertension • Acute phase response	100%	99%

[1]Based on 13,47 children with miscellaneous vasculitides.

Source: data from Ruperto N, Ozen S, Pistorio A, et al.; for the Paediatric Rheumatology International Trials Organisation (PRINTO). EULAR/PRINTO/PRES criteria for Henoch–Schönlein purpura, childhood polyarteritis nodosa, childhood Wegener granulomatosis and childhood Takayasu arteritis: Ankara 2008. Part I: Overall methodology and clinical characterisation. *Annals of the Rheumatic Diseases*, Volume 69, Issue 5, pp. 790–7, Copyright © 2010 BMJ Publishing Group Ltd.; Ozen S, Pistorio A, Iusan SM, et al. Paediatric Rheumatology International Trials Organisation (PRINTO). EULAR/PRINTO/PRES criteria for Henoch–Schönlein purpura, childhood polyarteritis nodosa, childhood Wegener granulomatosis and childhood Takayasu arteritis: Ankara 2008. Part II: Final classification criteria. *Annals of the Rheumatic Diseases*, Volume 69, Issue 5, pp. 798–806, Copyright © 2010 BMJ Publishing Group Ltd.

1. Predominantly large-vessel vasculitis
- Takayasu arteritis.

2. Predominantly medium-sized vessel vasculitis
- Childhood polyarteritis nodosa.
- Cutaneous polyarteritis.
- Kawasaki disease.

3. Predominantly small-vessel vasculitis
- Granulomatous:
  • Granulomatosis with polyangiitis (GPA).
  • Eosinophilic granulomatosis with polyangiitis (EGPA; formerly known as Churg–Strauss syndrome).
- Non-granulomatous:
  • Microscopic polyangiitis.
  • Henoch–Schönlein purpura.
  • Isolated cutaneous leucocytoclastic vasculitis.
  • Hypocomplementemic urticarial vasculitis.

4. Other vasculitides
- Behçet's disease.
- Vasculitis secondary to known cause: infection (including hepatitis B-associated PAN), malignancies and drugs, including hypersensitivity vasculitis; an emerging group of monogenic vasculitis syndromes also fall into this category, e.g. DADA2 or SAVI.
- Vasculitis associated with other connective tissue diseases.
- Isolated vasculitis of the CNS (childhood primary angiitis of the central nervous system: cPACNS).
- Cogan's syndrome.
- Unclassified.

The epidemiology of paediatric vasculitis

- Childhood vasculitis is rare and the incidence and prevalence are not accurately described.
- Henoch–Schönlein purpura (HSP) and Kawasaki disease (KD) are the 2 commonest childhood vasculitides and as such those with the most epidemiological information.
  - There is undoubtedly some ethnic variation for these diseases (see ➜ individual sections).
- In paediatric populations other systemic vasculitides including polyarteritis nodosa (PAN), granulomatosis with polyangiitis (and other ANCA-associated vasculitides), Behçet's disease, and Takayasu arteritis are rare and epidemiology difficult to assess.
  - Some ethnic variation has been noted: Takayasu arteritis being more common in Asians than North Americans and Europeans.

Henoch–Schönlein purpura

The estimated annual incidence varies (9–86/100,000 children) and is influenced by ethnicity, age, socioeconomic status, and seasonality:
- In one study, incidence was highest in Hispanic children (86/100,000); and children from lower socioeconomic groups (69/100,000).
- In the West Midlands, UK incidence has been reported as 20.4 per 100,000 children, but was much higher in the 4–6yr age group (70.3/ 100,000 children in this age group).
- Incidence in the Czech Republic was 10.2/100,000; and Taiwan 12.9/ 100,000 children.
- Striking seasonal variations are observed, most cases occurring in winter, often (30–50%) preceded by an upper respiratory tract infection.

Kawasaki disease

- KD has the highest incidence and prevalence in Asian populations, particularly Japan (Fig. 4.1).
  - Nationwide surveys conducted in Japan show the incidence of KD in children under 5years continues to rise with a current incidence of 265/100,000 children under 5.
- This compares to an incidence of 8.39/100,000 (0–5yr) in the UK
- Other incidences per country are provided in Fig. 4.1.
- There are limitations to these studies, as they were all done by survey or questionnaire reporting with <100% response rates; it should also be remembered that KD occurs in children >5 years old.

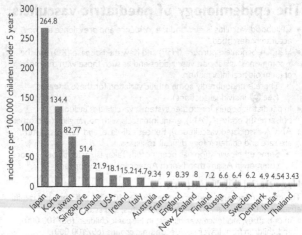

* Incidence per 100,000 children under 15 years

Fig. 4.1 Incidence of Kawasaki disease per 100,000 children aged less than 5 years across the globe.

Reproduced with permission from Singh S et al. The epidemiology of Kawasaki disease: a global update. *Archives of Disease in Childhood*, Volume 100, Issue 11, pp. 1084–1088, Copyright © 2015 BMJ Publishing Ltd.

Further reading

Chapter 33: Leukocytoclastic Vasculitis. In *Textbook of Pediatric Rheumatology* seventh edition. Eds Petty, Laxer, Lindsley, Wedderburn. 2016. Elsevier, Philadelphia.

Singh S et al. The epidemiology of Kawasaki disease: a global update. *Arch Dis Child* 2015:100:1084–88.

The investigation of primary systemic vasculitis

Background
Clinical features that suggest a vasculitic syndrome:
- Pyrexia of unknown origin.
- Palpable purpura, urticaria, dermal necrosis.
- Mononeuritis multiplex.
- Unexplained arthritis, myositis, serositis.
- Unexplained pulmonary, cardiovascular, or renal disease.
- *Plus* 1 or more of:
  - Leucocytosis, eosinophilia.
  - Hypocomplementaemia, cryoglobulinaemia.
  - Circulating immune complexes.
  - Raised ESR or CRP, thrombocytosis.

Level 1 investigations—to be performed in all
- Haematology and acute phase reactants:
  - FBC, ESR, CRP, clotting, prothrombotic screen (if patchy ischaemia of digits or skin), blood film.
- Basic biochemistry:
  - Renal and liver function, CPK, thyroid function, LDH, amylase/lipase, urine dip and UA:UC (spot urine albumin:creatinine ratio).
- Infectious disease screen:
  - Blood cultures.
  - Urine MC&S.
  - ASOT and anti-DNase b.
  - *Mycoplasma pneumoniae* serology.
- Immunological tests:
  - ANA, dsDNA Abs, ENAs, ANCA, RF.
  - Anti-GBM antibodies.
  - TTG (tissue transglutaminase) antibodies (coeliac disease screen).
  - Immunoglobulins: IgG, IgA, IgM, and IgE.
  - Anticardiolipin antibodies, lupus anticoagulant.
  - C3/C4, and functional complement assay (for the classical and alternate pathways) if available.
  - VZV antibody status (prior to starting immunosuppressive therapy).
  - Serum ACE.
- Radiological: CXR, abdominal and renal USS.
- Other: ECG, echocardiography, digital clinical photography of lesions.

Level 2 investigations—to be considered on an individual basis
- Infection screen:
  - Mantoux 1:1000, and/or quantiferon.
  - PCR for CMV, EBV, enterovirus, adenovirus, VZV, HBV, HCV.
  - Serology for HIV, Rickettsiae, *Borrelia burgdorferi*.
  - Viral serology for: hepatitis B & C, parvovirus B19.

- Imaging:
  - Radiograph of bones and joints.
  - Selective contrast visceral angiography.
  - DMSA scan.
  - MRI/MRA of brain (for suspected cerebral vasculitis).
  - CT abdomen, thorax, brain, sinus X ray (for GPA).
  - Cerebral catheter contrast angiography (for suspected cerebral vasculitis).
  - PET-CT (or PET-MRI if available): for differential of malignancy or Castleman's disease.
  - DEXA scan.
  - V/Q scan.
  - USS Doppler of peripheral arteries (if available: seek expert advice).
  - Thermography and nailfold capillaroscopy.
- Tissue biopsy: skin, nasal or sinus, kidney, sural nerve, lung, liver, gut, temporal artery, brain, other.
- Bone marrow analysis and/or lymph node excision biopsy (for suspected malignancy).
- Biochemistry, immunology, and immunogenetics:
  - Serum amyloid A.
  - Formal GFR.
  - Organ-specific autoantibodies (see ➔ Chapter 1, Autoantibodies, pp. 33–6).
  - β2 Glycoprotein 1 antibodies.
  - Urinary catecholamines (consider plasma catecholamines as well), and urine VMA, HVA (for phaeochromocytoma, or neuroblastoma).
  - Cryoglobulins (if there is a history of cold sensitivity/vasculitis mainly present in exposed areas of the body).
  - Basic lymphocyte panel and CD19 count if monitoring post rituximab.
  - Mitochondrial DNA mutations.
  - DNA analysis for *MEFV* (familial Mediterranean fever gene), TNFRSF1A (TNF alpha receptor associated periodic fever syndrome, TRAPS), MVK (mevalonate kinase deficiency; previously referred to as hyper IgD syndrome HIDS), NLRP3 (cryopyrin associated periodic syndrome, CAPS), NOD2 (Crohn's/Blau's/juvenile sarcoid mutations), CECR1 (deficiency of ADA2), genetic screening for SAVI (TMEM173) and CANDLE (PSMB8, 4 and 9; if available).
  - Nitroblue tertrazolium test if granulomatous inflammation found on biopsy.
- Nerve conduction studies (PAN, AAV, Behçet's [before starting thalidomide]).
- Ophthalmology screen.
- Ambulatory 24h BP/4-limb BP.

The standard treatment of childhood vasculitis

Guidelines for the use and monitoring of cytotoxic drugs in non-malignant disease are shown in Table 4.2. Standard vasculitis therapy (*excluding* crescentic glomerulonephritis) is described in Fig. 4.2. Prior to using this approach, remember there should be:

• A well-established diagnosis.
• Severe, potentially life-threatening disease.
• Inadequate response to less toxic therapy—milder cases of vasculitis (e.g. isolated cutaneous forms) may respond to less toxic agents such as colchicine. Therapy should always be tailored for each individual.
• No known infection or neoplasm.
• No pregnancy or possibility thereof.
• Informed consent obtained and documented in notes.

Other points of note

• IV cyclophosphamide is favoured over the oral route in children and adults because of reduced side-effects and lower cumulative dose associated with IV regimens, with comparable efficacy as suggested by a number of studies in adults with ANCA vasculitis (e.g. the 'CYCLOPS' trial).
• IV cyclophosphamide has the added advantage of ensuring adherence to therapy, of particular relevance in adolescents with vasculitis.

Use of biologic therapy in systemic vasculitis of the young

• Whilst the therapeutic approach and drugs used as suggested in Fig. 4.2 and Fig 4.3 undoubtedly have improved survival and long-term outlook for children with severe vasculitis, concerns relating to toxicity particularly with cyclophosphamide, and relapses despite this conventional therapeutic approach have led to the increasing use of biologic therapy such as rituximab, anti-TNF alpha, or other biologic therapy.
• Evidence to support the use of rituximab as an induction agent in place of cyclophosphamide for the treatment of ANCA-associated vasculitis is now available for adults with this group of diseases (RITUXIVAS, and RAVE trials).
• The PEPRS clinical trial is currently assessing the efficacy of Rituximab in treatment of newly diagnosed or relapsing AAV in children; undoubtedly rituximab is being increasingly used for children with ANCA vasculitis that is not adequately controlled using the conventional cyclophosphamide followed by azathioprine therapeutic regimen outlined in Fig 4.2.
• Evidence for the use of anti-TNFα remains anecdotal for children and adults with vasculitis (KD, PAN, and TA; not recommended routinely for AAV).
• Tocilizumab may be effective in large vessel vasculitis.
• Whilst there is not enough evidence to recommend specific biologic therapy for specific vasculitic syndromes, a general approach favoured by the authors is given in Table 4.3.

Table 4.2 Doses, side-effects, and clinical monitoring of commonly used immunosuppressant and cytotoxic immunosuppressant drugs used for the treatment of vasculitis (see also Fig. 4.2 and Fig. 4.3)

	Cyclophosphamide (CYC)	Azathioprine	Mycophenolate mofetil (MMF)	Methotrexate
Dose	0.5–1.0g/m² [max 1.2g] IV every 3–4 weeks with mesna to prevent cystitis (see ❍ pp. 485–9 for mesna dose and IV CYC administration protocol)	0.5–2.5mg/kg once a day PO for 1yr or more	600 mg/m² twice a day, max 1g twice a day	10–15mg/m²/week PO or SC (single dose)
Side effects	Leucopenia; haemorrhagic cystitis; reversible alopecia; infertility; leukaemia, lymphoma, transitional cell carcinoma of bladder	GI toxicity; hepatotoxicity; rash; leucopenia; teratogenicity; ↑ increase in malignancy in adults with RA; no conclusive data for cancer risk in children	Bone marrow suppression; severe diarrhoea; pulmonary fibrosis; increased risk of skin cancer	Bone marrow suppression and interstitial pneumonitis (decreased risk with folic acid); reversible elevation of transaminases; hepatic fibrosis
Cumulative toxic dose	Not described for malignancy; 500mg/kg for azoospermia	Not described	Not described	Not described
Clinical monitoring	Baseline and monthly renal and liver function. Temporarily discontinue and/or reduce dose if neutropenia <1.5 × 10⁹/L, platelets <150 × 10⁹/L, or haematuria. Day 10 FBC post IV dose. Reduce dose if renal or hepatic failure e.g. to 250–300mg/m².	Weekly FBC for 1 month, then 3-monthly. Temporarily discontinue and/or reduce dose if neutropenia <1.5 × 10⁹/L, platelets <150 × 10⁹/L, and check TPMT enzyme—patients deficient in TPMT require reduced doses or may not tolerate) azathioprine because of ↑ marrow toxicity	Fortnightly FBC for 2 months, then monthly for 2/12. 3-monthly when stable. Baseline monthly renal and liver function until stable. Discontinue temporarily and/or reduce dose if neutropenia <1.5 × 10⁹/L, platelets <15⁰ × 10⁹/L, or significant GI side-effects	Baseline CXR, FBC, and LFTs, then FBC and LFTs fortnightly until dose stable, then monthly to every 6 weeks (after 6 months). Reduce or discontinue if hepatic enzymes >3× upper limit of normal, neutropenia <1.5 × 10⁹/L, new or worsening cough, severe nausea, vomiting, or diarrhoea, platelets <150 × 10⁹/L or falling rapidly

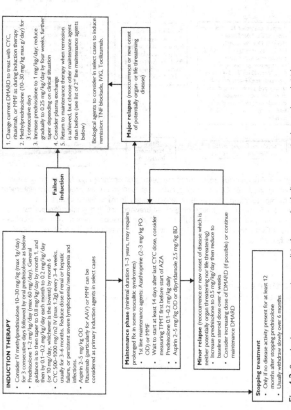

INDUCTION THERAPY
- Consider IV methylprednisolone 10–30 mg/kg (max 1g/day) for 3 consecutive days followed by oral prednisolone as below
- Prednisolone 1–2 mg/kg/day (max 60 mg/day). General guidance is to then taper to 0.8 mg/kg/day by month 1, and then by 0.1–0.2 mg/kg/day each month to 0.2 mg/kg/day (or 10 mg/day, whichever is the lowest) by month 6
- CYC 500–1000 mg/m2 IV (max 1.2g) every 3–4 weeks, usually for 3–6 months. Reduce dose if renal or hepatic failure, or persistent severe lymphopenia/neutropenia and infections.
- Aspirin 2–5 mg/kg OD
- Rituximab (particularly for AAV) or MMF can be considered as primary induction agents in select cases

Failed induction

1. Change current DMARD to treat with CYC, rituximab, or MMF as during induction therapy
2. Methylprednisolone (10–30 mg/kg max g/day) for 3 consecutive days
3. Increase prednisolone to 1 mg/kg/day, reduce gradually to 0.25 mg/kg/day by four weeks, further taper depending on clinical situation
4. Consider plasma exchange
5. Return to maintenance therapy when remission is achieved, but choose other maintenance agent than before (see list of 2nd line maintenance agents below)

Biological agents to consider in select cases to induce remission: TNF blockade, IVIG, Tocilizumab.

Maintenance phase (minimal duration 1–3 years, may require prolonged Rx in some vasculitic syndromes)
- 1st line maintenance agents: Azathioprine (2–3 mg/kg PO OD) or MMF
- Wait to start at least 14 days after last CYC dose, consider measuring TPMT first before start of AZA
- Prednisolone 0.1–0.2 mg/kg daily
- Aspirin 2–5 mg/kg OD or dipyridamole 2.5 mg/kg BD

Major relapse (reoccurrence or new onset of potentially organ- or life threatening disease)

Minor relapse (reoccurrence or new onset of disease which is neither potentially organ threatening nor life threatening)
- Increase prednisolone to 0.5 mg/kg/day then reduce to baseline steroid dose over 4 weeks
- Consider increasing dose of DMARD (if possible) or continue maintenance DMARD

Stopping treatment
- Only if no disease activity present for at least 12 months after stopping prednisolone
- Usually withdraw slowly over 6 months

Fig. 4.2 Standard severe systemic vasculitis therapy (excluding crescentic glomerulonephritis)

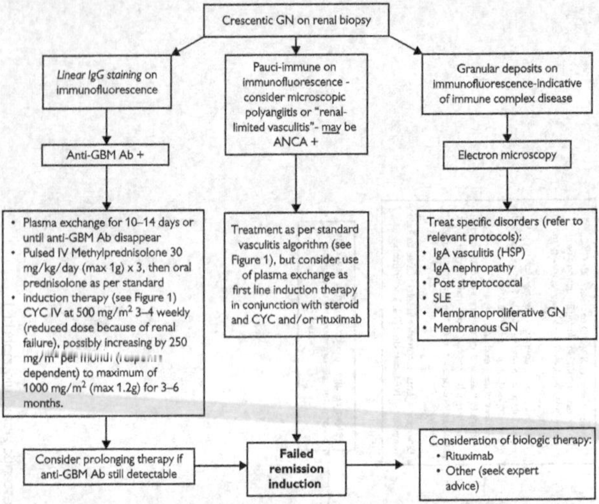

Fig. 4.3 Guideline for treatment of crescentic glomerulonephritis/rapidly progressive glomerulonephritis. Of major importance is early diagnosis and prompt commencement of therapy to maximize chances of renal recovery. Management is always with expertise from paediatric nephrologists. Abbreviations: GN = glomerulonephritis; IgG = Immunoglobulin G; Anti-GBM = Anti-glomerular basement membrane antibody; CYC = Cyclophosphamide; HSP = Henoch Schönlein purpura; SLE = systemic lupus erythematosus.

Further reading

Eleftheriou D, Melo M, Marks SD, *et al*. Biologic therapy in primary systemic vasculitis of the young. *Rheumatology* 2009;48:978–86.

IgA vasculitis (Henoch–Schönlein purpura)

Introduction

- IgA vasculitis is the new term for Henoch-Schönlein purpura (HSP), and is the commonest systemic vasculitis in childhood.
- It is defined in the latest Chapel Hill nomenclature (2012) as:
  - Vasculitis with IgA1-dominant immune deposits affecting small vessels (predominantly capillaries, venules, or arterioles).
  - Often involving skin, gastrointestinal tract and frequently causes arthritis.
  - Associated with glomerulonephritis which is indistinguishable from IgA nephropathy.
- Classification criteria (Ankara 2008) are: palpable purpura in a predominantly lower limb distribution with at least 1 of 4 of:
  - Diffuse abdominal pain.
  - Any biopsy showing IgA deposition (mandatory criterion if rash is atypical).
  - Arthritis and/or arthralgia.
  - Haematuria and/or proteinuria.
- Variable and often relapsing course without specific laboratory findings with 1/3 of children having symptoms up to a fortnight, another 1/3 up to 1 month, and recurrence of symptoms within 4 months of resolution in 1/3.
- Henoch–Schönlein nephritis (HSN) accounts for 1.6–3% of all childhood cases of end-stage renal failure (ESRF) in the UK.

Epidemiology

See also ➔ vasculitis epidemiology pp. 177–8.
- Commoner in Caucasian and Asian populations and boys:
  - ♂:♀ ratio of 1.5–2:1.
  - 50% present before the age of 5yr, 75% present before the age of 10yr.
- Incidence of 10–20.4 (mean of 13.5) per 100,000 children.
  - 22.1 per 100,000 children under 14yr of age.
  - 70.3 per 100,000 children aged 4–7yr.
- Almost 20× rarer in adults.
  - 0.8 cases per 100,000 adults.
  - More severe in adults.
- Seasonal variation (commoner in winter) with infectious triggers.
  - Associations with bacteria (e.g. Group A beta-haemolytic streptococci) and viruses (hepatitis, CMV, HSV, human parvovirus B19, coxsackie, and adenovirus), and some cases after vaccination described.

Immunopathology

- Type III hypersensitivity reaction with IgA1 immune complex formation is central to the pathogenesis.

- Individuals who develop IgA vasculitis have galactose deficient IgA, which contributes to immune complex formation:
  - Galactose-deficient IgA1 is recognized by anti-glycan antibodies, leading to the formation of circulating immune complexes and their mesangial deposition, alternate pathway complement activation, immune-complex-mediated vasculitis of small blood vessels with diffuse angiitis and renal injury in some patients.
  - There may be an associated C2 deficiency.
- Polygenic inheritance with renal involvement associated with HLA-B35, IL-1β (−511) T allele, and IL-8 allele A.
  - Mutations in the familial Mediterranean fever gene (*MEFV*) may be more frequent in patients with IgA vasculitis in Turkey and Israel.
  - The genes controlling IgA1 glycosylation are unknown, but future studies are examining this mechanism as a possible genetic predisposition.
- It is suggested that the 'second hit' in a genetically susceptible individual is the formation of anti-glycan IgG or IgA antibodies (perhaps triggered by infection) that can then go on to form circulating immune complexes containing poorly galactosylated IgA1, which are more prone to deposition.

Systemic involvement

Dermatological

- All patients have purpura but skin involvement may not be present at time of initial presentation.
- Generally symmetrical purpura involving lower limbs and buttocks but can spread to upper limbs (rarely abdomen, chest or face).
- Urticaria and angio-oedema can occur.

Gastrointestinal

- Commonly occurs (68% of patients).
- Abdominal pain precedes rash by 1–14 days in 43% of patients.
- Presents with intermittent colicky abdominal pain, vomiting with or without haematemesis or melaena (faecal occult blood may be positive) as a result of haemorrhage into gut wall.
- Involvement may result in intussusception, appendicitis, cholecystitis, pancreatitis, GI haemorrhage, ulceration, infarction, or perforation.

Rheumatological

60% of patients will have joint involvement with arthritis and/or arthralgia usually affecting the knees and ankles resulting in pain, swelling, and ↓ range of movement.

Renal

- 25–60% of patients will have renal involvement with HSN:
  - 76% will develop within 4 weeks of disease onset.
  - 97% will develop within 3 months of disease onset.
- Most cases are usually asymptomatic which necessitates screening up to 6 months after last recrudescence of rash or HSP symptoms with <10% having significant involvement requiring referral for consideration of renal biopsy (Fig. 4.3).
  - Microscopic haematuria without proteinuria is benign.
  - 82% have normal renal function after 23yr.

- Good prognosis with isolated haematuria and mild proteinuria with mild histological changes as less than 5% will develop chronic kidney disease (CKD) within 10–25yr.
  - Improved renal prognosis in children <7yr.
- Severe disease indicated by increasing proteinuria, development of nephrotic syndrome and/or renal failure.
  - 20% of patients with acute mixed nephritic and nephrotic syndrome progress to ESRF.
  - 44–50% develop hypertension or CKD.
  - Histological pattern is identical to IgA nephropathy and includes focal segmental proliferative glomerulonephritis and rapidly progressive crescentic glomerulonephritis (Table 4.3).

Other

Patients may present with orchitis, severe pulmonary haemorrhage, and/or cerebral vasculitis (which may respond to immunosuppression combined with plasmapheresis).

Management of IgA vasculitis including glomerulonephritis

- No role for antibiotics unless suspected or proven infection.
- Prophylactic corticosteroid therapy at commencement of HSP does not prevent renal or GI involvement.
- However, corticosteroids do seem to be effective in treating these complications and severe facial and/or scrotal haemorrhagic oedema.
- Patients with severe renal involvement may require other immunosuppressive agents, antiproteinuric and antihypertensive agents.

Definitions of nephritis severity

- Mild HSP nephritis: normal GFR[1] and mild[2] or moderate[3] proteinuria.
- Moderate HSP nephritis: <50% crescents on renal biopsy and impaired GFR[4] or marked proteinuria.[5]
- Severe HSP nephritis: >50% crescents on renal biopsy and impaired GFR[4] or marked proteinuria.[5]

Table 4.3 ISKDC classification of Henoch–Schönlein nephritis

ISKDC grade	Pathoanatomical findings
I	Minimal alterations
II	Mesangial proliferation
III A	Focal proliferation or sclerosis with <50% crescents
III B	Diffuse proliferation or sclerosis with <50% crescents
IV A	Focal proliferation or sclerosis with 50–75% crescents
IV B	Diffuse proliferation or sclerosis with 50–75% crescents
V A	Focal proliferation or sclerosis with >75% crescents
V B	Diffuse proliferation or sclerosis with >75% crescents
VI	Membranoproliferative glomerulonephritis

ISKDC=International Study of Kidney Diseases in Children.

- Persistent proteinuria:
  - UP:UC ratio (early morning urine protein : creatinine ratio) > 250mg/mmol for four weeks.
  - UP:UC ratio > 100mg/mmol for three months
  - UP:UC ratio > 50mg/mmol for six months
- Normal GFR: >80ml/min/1.73m².
- Impaired GFR: <80 ml/min/1.73m².
- Mild proteinuria: UP:UC ratio < 100 mg/mmol (in an early morning urine sample).
- Moderate proteinuria: UP:UC ratio 100–250mg/mmol (in an early morning urine sample).
- Marked proteinuria: UP:UC ratio > 250mg/mmol (in an early morning urine sample).

Investigation

Biopsy

- A skin biopsy including specific staining for IgA should be performed in case of atypical rash and/or to exclude alternative diagnoses
- Absence of IgA staining on biopsy does not exclude the diagnosis of IgA vasculitis (HSP).

Renal work-up

- Renal involvement should be investigated using eGFR and urinalysis (hematuria and UP:UC ratio).
- A paediatric nephrologist should be consulted if an IgA vasculitis patient has moderate proteinuria* and/or impaired GFR**
- A renal biopsy should be performed if an IgA vasculitis (HSP) patient has marked proteinuria* or impaired GFR**

Imaging

- In severe abdominal pain, an ultrasound should be performed by an ultrasonographer with paediatric expertise to exclude intussusception.

Treatment

Analgesia

- Adequate analgesia should be prescribed for IgA vasculitis associated arthropathy.
- NSAIDS are not contraindicated if renal function is normal in IgA vasculitis.
- Adequate analgesia should be prescribed for IgA vasculitis associated abdominal pain.

Corticosteroids

- Corticosteroid treatment is indicated in cases of:
  - Orchitis/
  - Cerebral vasculitis/
  - Pulmonary haemorrhage/
  - Other severe organ or life-threatening vasculitis manifestations.
- In patients with severe abdominal pain and/or rectal bleeding (in whom intussusception has been excluded), corticosteroid treatment could be considered

- The dose of oral corticosteroids should be 1–2 mg/kg/day
- If corticosteroids are indicated, pulsed IV methylprednisolone (e.g. 10–30 mg/kg with a maximum of 1 gram per day on 3 consecutive days) may be considered for severe cases.
- Prophylactic corticosteroid treatment to *prevent* the development of IgA vasculitis (HSP) nephritis is not indicated.

IgA vasculitis (HSP) nephritis

- When starting treatment of IgA vasculitis (HSP) nephritis, a paediatric nephrologist should be consulted.
- In the absence of robust data for evidence supporting the treatment of nephritis, a randomised controlled trial for the treatment of IgA vasculitis (HSP) nephritis is urgently needed.
- One treatment approach for IgA vasculitis (HSP) nephritis is:
  - Microscopic haematuria without renal dysfunction or proteinuria is usually benign and does not need to paediatric nephrology follow-up.
  - Similarly, non-persistent mild or moderate proteinuria may not require paediatric nephrology review but does require follow-up to ensure this settles.
  - Always consult a paediatric nephrologist if marked proteinuria, impaired GFR, or persistent proteinuria.
  - Mild HSP nephritis: 1st line treatment oral prednisolone; 2nd line treatment AZA, MMF, pulsed MP.
  - Moderate HSP nephritis: 1st line treatment oral prednisolone and/or pulsed MP; 1st or 2nd line treatment: AZA, MMF, IV CYC.
  - Severe HSP nephritis: 1st line treatment: IV CYC with pulsed MP and oral prednisolone; 2nd line AZA/MMF and oral prednisolone.
  - For all forms of nephritis consider ACE inhibitors if there is persistent proteinuria.
  - Oral CYC and ciclosporin are not routinely indicated for HSP nephritis.
  - For IgA crescentic glomerulonephritis, see ➜ pp. 181–4.

Kawasaki disease

Kawasaki disease (KD) is a self-limiting vasculitic syndrome that predominantly affects medium- and small-sized arteries. It is the 2nd commonest vasculitic illness of childhood (the commonest being HSP) and it is the leading cause of childhood acquired heart disease in developed countries.

Pathogenesis and epidemiology

- Pronounced seasonality and clustering of KD cases have led to the hunt for infectious agents as a cause. However, so far no single agent has been identified.
- The aetiology of KD remains unknown but it is currently believed that one or more widely distributed infectious agents evoke an abnormal immunological response in genetically susceptible individuals, leading to the characteristic clinical presentation of the disease.
- KD has a worldwide distribution with a male preponderance, an ethnic bias towards Asian and in particular Japanese or Chinese children, some seasonality, and occasional epidemics.
- The incidence of KD is rising worldwide, including the UK. The current reported incidence in the UK is 8.39/100,000 children aged <5yr. This may reflect a truly rising incidence or increased clinician awareness. See also → pp. 177–8 for a full description of the epidemiology of KD worldwide.

Clinical features

See Box 4.1.
- The cardiovascular features are the most important manifestations of the condition with widespread vasculitis affecting predominantly medium-size muscular arteries, especially the coronary arteries. Coronary artery involvement occurs in 15–25% of untreated cases with additional cardiac features in a significant proportion of these including pericardial effusion, electrocardiographic abnormalities, pericarditis, myocarditis, valvular incompetence, cardiac failure, and myocardial infarction.
- Of note, irritability is an important sign, which is virtually universally present although not included in the diagnostic criteria.

Box 4.1 Principal clinical features of KD

The principal clinical features of KD are:
- Fever persisting for 5 days or more.
- Peripheral extremity changes (reddening of the palms and soles, indurative oedema, and subsequent desquamation).
- A polymorphous exanthema.
- Bilateral conjunctival injection/congestion.
- Lips and oral cavity changes (reddening/cracking of lips, strawberry tongue, oral and pharyngeal injection), and
- Acute non-purulent cervical lymphadenopathy.

- Another clinical sign that may be relatively specific to KD is the development of erythema and induration at sites of BCG inoculations. The mechanism of this sign is thought to be cross-reactivity of T cells in KD patients between specific epitopes of mycobacterial and human heat shock proteins.
- An important point worthy of emphasis is that the principal symptoms and signs may present sequentially such that the full set of criteria may not be present at any one time. Awareness of other non-principal signs (such as BCG scar reactivation) may improve the diagnostic pick-up rate of KD.
- Other clinical features include: arthritis, aseptic meningitis, pneumonitis, uveitis, gastroenteritis, meatitis and dysuria, and otitis.
- Relatively uncommon abnormalities include hydrops of the gallbladder, GI ischaemia, jaundice, petechial rash, febrile convulsions, and encephalopathy or ataxia, macrophage activation syndrome, and syndrome of inappropriate anti-diuretic hormone secretion (SIADH).

Making a diagnosis of KD

- For the diagnosis of KD to be established 5 of the 6 clinical features should be present, but:
- The diagnosis of KD should be considered in any child with a febrile exanthematous illness and evidence of inflammation, particularly if it persists longer than 4 days.
- The diagnosis of KD may be considered with fewer than 5 days of fever when typical clinical symptoms are present.
- In particular, KD diagnosis and treatment should also be considered if:
  - 5/6 diagnostic criteria of KD are present before day 5 of fever.
  - Coronary artery aneurysm (CAA) or coronary dilatation is present.
  - There is evidence of persistent elevation (>5 days) of inflammatory markers and/or persistent fever, especially in infants or younger children without other explanation
- In a patient in whom KD is suspected, but all criteria have not yet been fulfilled, the following clinical signs strengthen the suspicion of KD:
  - Disproportionate or marked irritability.
  - New erythema and/or induration at the site of previous BCG immunization.

Incomplete KD

- It is recognized that there are incomplete cases of KD (who do not fulfil the AHA-criteria); however, these patients may still be at risk of CAA, particularly infants.
- In children presenting with <5 out of 6 criteria for KD ('incomplete KD'), with evidence of unexplained systemic inflammation (e.g. elevated CRP, ESR, or WBC), an echocardiogram should be considered.
- Patients with <5 or 6 principal features can be diagnosed with KD when coronary aneurysm or dilatation is recognized by two-dimensional (2D) echocardiography or coronary angiography.

Differential diagnosis

Conditions that can cause similar symptoms to KD and must be considered in the differential diagnosis include:
• Scarlet fever.
• Rheumatic fever.
• Streptococcal or staphylococcal toxic shock syndrome.
• Staphylococcal scalded skin syndrome.
• Systemic JIA.
• Infantile PAN.
• SLE.
• Adenovirus, enterovirus, EBV, CMV, parvovirus, influenza virus infection.
• *Mycoplasma pneumoniae* infection.
• Measles.
• Leptospirosis.
• Rickettsiae infection.
• Adverse drug reaction.
• Mercury toxicity (acrodynia).
• Lymphoma—particularly for IVIg resistant cases.

Investigations

In cases of suspected KD the following investigations should be considered:
• FBC and blood film.
• ESR.
• CRP.
• Blood cultures.
• ASOT and anti-DNase B.
• Nose and throat swab, and stool sample for culture (superantigen toxin typing if *Staphylococcus aureus* and/or beta-haemolytic streptococci detected).
• Renal and liver function tests.
• Coagulation screen.
• Autoantibody profile (ANA, ENA, RF, ANCA).
• Serology (IgG and IgM) for *Mycoplasma pneumoniae*, enterovirus, adenovirus, measles, parvovirus, EBV, CMV.
• Urine MC&S.
• Dip test of urine for blood and protein.
• Consider serology for rickettsiae and leptospirosis if history suggestive.
• Consider CXR.
• ECG.
• 2D echocardiography to identify coronary artery involvement acutely and monitoring changes long term.
• Coronary arteriography has an important role for delineating detailed anatomical injury, particularly for children with giant CAAs (>8mm, or internal artery diameter Z score ≥10), where stenoses adjacent to the inlet/outlet of the aneurysms are a concern. Note that the procedure may need to be delayed until at least 6 months after disease onset since there could be a risk of myocardial infarction if performed in children with ongoing severe coronary artery inflammation.

Treatment

See Fig. 4.5.

The treatment of KD comprises of:

- IVIg at a dose of 2g/kg as a single infusion over 12h (consider splitting the dose over 2–4 days in infants with cardiac failure).
- IVIg should be started early preferably within the first 10 days of the illness. However, clinicians should not hesitate to give IVIg to patients who present after 10 days if there are signs of persisting inflammation.
  - IVIg resistance occurs up to 20% of cases; these patients are at increased risk of CAA.
- Aspirin 30–50mg/kg/day in 4 divided doses. The dose of aspirin can be reduced to 2–5mg/kg/day when the fever settles (disease defervescence). Aspirin at antiplatelet doses is continued for a minimum of 6 weeks.
- Corticosteroids (see Fig. 4.4 for suggested doses) should be considered for:
  1. Patients who have already declared themselves as IVIg resistant.
  2. Patients with features of the most severe disease (and therefore the greatest likelihood of developing CAA). In the absence of validated risk scores outside of Japan, we suggest that such patients include:
     - the very young (<12 months).
     - those with markers of severe inflammation, including: persistently elevated C reactive protein despite IVIg, liver dysfunction, hypoalbuminaemia, and anaemia.
     - and the small group who develop features of haemophagocytic lymphohistiocytosis (HLH) and/or shock.
  3. Patients who already have evolving coronary and/or peripheral aneurysms with ongoing inflammation at presentation.
- In patients who have shown some but not complete response to IVIg, we suggest that a second dose of IVIg is given at the same time as commencing steroids if they have not already been commenced for signs of severe disease.
- In refractory cases infliximab, a human chimeric anti-TNFα monoclonal antibody, given IV at a single dose of 6mg/kg has been reported to be effective, and is increasingly used for IVIg-resistant cases.
- Echocardiography should be repeated at 2 weeks and 6 weeks from initiation of treatment (refer to paediatric cardiology).
  - If the repeat echocardiogram shows no CAAs at 6 weeks, aspirin can be discontinued and lifelong follow-up at least every 2yr should be considered.
- In cases of CAA <8mm with no stenoses present, aspirin should be continued until aneurysms resolve.
- If CAA >8mm (or Z score of internal coronary artery diameter ≥10 in infants) and/or stenoses is present, aspirin at a dose of 2–5mg/kg/day should be continued lifelong. The combination of aspirin and warfarin therapy in these patients with giant aneurysms has been shown to decrease the risk of myocardial infarction.
- In patients who develop CAA, echocardiography and ECG should be repeated at 6-monthly intervals and an exercise stress test considered.

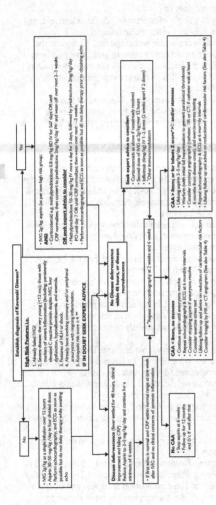

Fig. 4.4 Guideline for the management of Kawasaki disease. Since risk scores for IVIg resistance perform sub-optimally in non-Japanese patients, we cannot recommend their use to define high risk definitively; clinicians may, however, choose to score for the clinical and laboratory parameters listed to identify 'high risk' patients. If the Kobayashi risk score is 'positive' in a non-Japanese patient (e.g. ≥ 4) then IVIg resistance is likely; however a score <4 does not reliably exclude IVIg resistance. The aim of treatment is to switch off the inflammatory process that is damaging the coronary arteries as rapidly as possible. In the absence of a strong evidence base favouring a specific corticosteroid regimen, two suggested corticosteroid regimens for high-risk cases are provided for clinicians to choose from. For those on low dose aspirin, we also recommend avoiding the concomitant use of non-steroidal anti-inflammatory drugs (NSAIDs) as these interfere with the anti-platelet effect of low dose aspirin. *Treatment can be commenced before 5 days of fever if sepsis excluded; treatment should also be given if the presentation is >10 days from fever onset if there are signs of persistent inflammation; **Kobayashi risk score ≥4 points ¶Refer to paediatric cardiologist. ‡ Other specific interventions such as PET scanning, addition of calcium channel blocker therapy, and coronary angioplasty at discretion of paediatric cardiologist. + Other immunomodulators may include ciclosporin. ◆For infants, Z score for internal coronary artery diameter ≥10 based on Montreal normative data: http://parameterz.blogspot.co.uk/2010/11/montreal-coronary-artery-z-scores.html.

Adapted with permission from D Eleftheriou, M Levin, D Shingadia, R Tulloh, NJ Klein, PA Brogan. Management of Kawasaki Disease, *Archives of Childhood Disease*, Copyright © 2013 BMJ Publishing Ltd.

- Other specific interventions such as positron emission tomography (PET) scanning, addition of calcium channel blocker therapy, and coronary angioplasty should be organized at the discretion of a paediatric cardiologist.

Outcome

- Treatment with IVIg and aspirin reduces CAA from 25% for untreated cases to 4–9%.
- IVIg resistance occurs in approximately 20%, and is associated with a higher risk of CAA.
- The overall outlook of children with KD is good, with the acute mortality rate due to myocardial infarction having been reduced to <1% by increased alertness of the clinicians to the diagnosis and prompt treatment.
- Nonetheless the disease may contribute to the burden of adult cardiovascular disease and be associated with late KD vasculopathy of the coronaries and/or contribute to premature atherosclerosis, an area of active ongoing research.

Further reading

Eleftheriou D, Levin M, Shingadia D, Tulloh R, Klein NJ, Brogan P. Management of Kawasaki disease. Arch Dis Child 2014;99:74–83.

The anti-neutrophil cytoplasmic antibody (ANCA)-associated vasculitides

Background

- The ANCA-associated vasculitides (AAV) are:
  - Granulomatosis with polyangiitis (GPA; formerly known as Wegener's granulomatosis).
  - Microscopic polyangiitis (MPA).
  - Eosinophilic granulomatosis with polyangiitis (EGPA) and
  - Renal limited vasculitis (previously referred to as idiopathic crescentic glomerulonephritis).
- Although rare, the AAV do occur in childhood.

Definitions of AAV

Definitions for each of the AAV describing the salient major clinical and laboratory features are given here. These are not the same as classification criteria, which (for GPA) are provided in a separate section on classification.

- *GPA:* granulomatous inflammation involving the respiratory tract and necrotizing vasculitis affecting small- to medium-size vessels.
- *MPA:* necrotizing vasculitis, with few or no immune deposits, affecting small vessels; necrotizing arteritis involving small- and medium-sized arteries may be present; pulmonary capillaritis often occurs. Clinically, it often presents with rapidly progressive pauci-immune glomerulonephritis, in association with perinuclear ANCA (pANCA, MPO-ANCA) positivity.
- *EGPA:* an eosinophil-rich and granulomatous inflammation involving the respiratory tract and necrotizing vasculitis affecting small- to medium-sized vessels; there is an association with asthma and eosinophilia.
- *Renal limited:* rapidly progressive glomerulonephritis, often with ANCA positivity (usually MPO-ANCA) but without other organ involvement.

Pathogenesis

- It is not known why patients develop ANCA in the first instance.
- When ANCA are present, the most accepted current model of pathogenesis proposes that ANCA activate cytokine-primed neutrophils, leading to bystander damage of endothelial cells and an escalation of inflammation with recruitment of mononuclear cells.
- However, other concomitant exogenous factors and genetic susceptibility appear to be necessary for disease expression.

Clinical features of GPA

From a clinical perspective GPA may be broadly considered as having 2 forms:

- Predominantly granulomatous form with mainly localized disease, and
- Florid, acute, small vessel vasculitic form characterized by severe pulmonary haemorrhage and/or rapidly progressive vasculitis or other severe vasculitic manifestation.

These 2 broad presentations may coexist or present sequentially in individual patients.

Organ specific involvement includes:
- Upper respiratory tract:
  - Epistaxis.
  - Otalgia, and hearing loss (conductive and/or sensorineural); chronic otitis media; mastoiditis.
  - Nasal septal involvement with cartilaginous collapse results in the characteristic saddle nose deformity (Fig. 4.5).
  - Chronic sinusitis.
  - Glottic and subglottic polyps and/or large- and medium-sized airway stenosis.
- Lower respiratory tract manifestations include (singly or in combination):
  - Granulomatous pulmonary nodules with or without central cavitation.
  - Pulmonary haemorrhage with respiratory distress, frank haemoptysis, and/or evanescent pulmonary shadows (CXR).
  - Interstitial pneumonitis.
- Renal involvement: typically a focal segmental necrotizing glomerulonephritis, with pauci-immune crescentic glomerular changes. The clinical manifestations associated with this lesion are:
  - Hypertension.
  - Significant proteinuria.
  - Nephritic and nephrotic syndrome.
  - Other protean manifestations of renal failure.

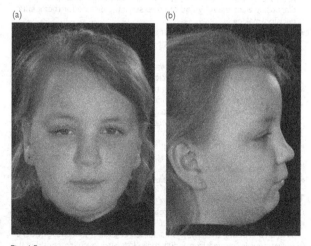

(a)　　　　　　　　　　(b)

Fig. 4.5 Right orbital and characteristic saddle nose deformity in granulomatosis with polyangiitis (GPA).

- Ophthalmological disease: retinal vasculitis, conjunctivitis, episcleritis, uveitis, optic neuritis. Unilateral or bilateral proptosis may be caused by granulomatous inflammation affecting the orbit (pseudotumour) (Fig. 4.6).
- Malaise, fever, weight loss or growth failure, arthralgia, and arthritis.
- Other manifestations include: peripheral gangrene with tissue loss, and vasculitis of the skin, gut (including appendicitis), heart, central nervous system and/or peripheral nerves (mononeuritis multiplex), salivary glands, gonads, and breast.

Investigations

(also see ➔ Vasculitis investigation, pp. 179–180)

- GPA is commonly associated with a cytoplasmic staining pattern of ANCA by IIF, and ELISA reveals specificity against PR3 (PR3-ANCA), although MPO-ANCA are occasionally observed in GPA.
- MPA and renal limited AAV are typically associated with pANCA by IIF and with MPO-ANCA specificity on ELISA, although PR3-ANCA can be observed.
- ANCA-negative forms of GPA, MPA, renal limited vasculitis, and EGPA are well described in children, but care should be exercised before diagnosing AAV in an ANCA-negative child since the differential diagnosis is broad.
- While the diagnostic value of ANCA is without question important, the value of ANCA for the longitudinal monitoring of disease activity is probably unreliable in many patients with GPA.
- Tissue diagnosis, in particular renal biopsy but also biopsy of skin, nasal septum, or other tissue, can be important diagnostically for diagnosing all of the AAV and can help stage the disease for therapeutic decision-making.
- Other commonly observed non-specific findings include:
  - Mild normochromic normocytic anaemia together with a leucocytosis and thrombocytosis.
  - Elevated ESR and CRP.
  - Raised immunoglobulins (polyclonal IgG).
- Laboratory manifestations relating to renal involvement include:
  - Dipstick haematuria and proteinuria positive.
  - Raised urinary spot protein creatinine ratio.
  - Raised serum creatinine and other associated laboratory features of renal failure.
- Chest radiography may be abnormal but high resolution CT chest has better sensitivity for demonstrating pulmonary infiltrates or discrete nodular and/or cavitating lesions.
- Plain x-ray or CT sinuses for sinusitis.

Treatment of AAV

(See also ➔ BSPAR guidelines for treatments used in paediatric rheumatology, p. 472.)

When considering therapy, it is useful to remember that most evidence for treatment is derived from adult trials. It is also useful to consider the different phases of the therapeutic journey for AAV:

- The pre-diagnostic phase: occasionally lasting years. Significant organ damage can accrue in this phase, or even death.
- Induction of remission phase: typically 3–6 months.
- Maintenance of remission phase: usually 18–24 months.
- Therapy withdrawal phase: not all patients achieve this.

The following general points are worthy of note:
- The key to successful treatment is early diagnosis to limit organ damage.
- Treatment for paediatric AAV is broadly similar to the approach used in adults and involves corticosteroids, cyclophosphamide, and in some individuals plasma exchange (particularly for pulmonary capillaritis and/or rapidly progressive glomerulonephritis—'pulmonary-renal syndrome') to induce remission; followed by low-dose corticosteroids and azathioprine to maintain remission.
- Increasingly, rituximab or MMF are also used for induction of remission (see ➲ pp. 181–184).
- Antiplatelet doses of aspirin can also be considered empirically on the basis of the increased risk of thrombosis associated with the disease process.
- MTX in combination with corticosteroids may have a role for inducing remission in patients with limited GPA.
- Co-trimoxazole is commonly added to therapeutic regimens for the treatment of GPA, particularly in those with upper respiratory tract involvement, serving both as prophylaxis against opportunistic infection and as a possible disease-modifying agent.
- Newer immunosuppressive agents and immunomodulatory strategies such as MMF and rituximab have been reported to be effective at inducing or maintaining remission in adults with AAV and are increasingly used in children for recalcitrant disease. PEPRS (the Pediatric Polyangiitis Rituximab Study) is an ongoing open label trial exploring the efficacy and safety of Rituximab in children with newly diagnosed or relapsing AAV.
- Anti-TNF therapy is less effective for the treatment of AAV, although has been used anecdotally in this context with some success in select patients, but is usually not recommended.
- More recently, an adult trial has demonstrated superiority of 6-monthly rituximab to maintain remission of AAV compared with azathioprine. This approach requires further study in children, since hypogammaglobulinemia may be more of a concern in paediatric patients.

Outcome of AAV

- The AAV still carry considerable disease-related morbidity and mortality, particularly due to progressive renal failure or aggressive respiratory involvement, and therapy-related complications, such as sepsis.
- The mortality for GPA from one recent paediatric series was 12% over a 17yr period of study inclusion. The largest paediatric series of patients with GPA reported 40% of cases with chronic renal impairment at 33 months of follow-up despite therapy.

- Mortality in paediatric patients with MPA during follow-up has been reported to be 0–14%.
- For EGPA in children, the most recent series quotes a related mortality of 15%

Further reading

Brogan P, Eleftheriou D, Dillon M. Small vessel vasculitis. *Pediatr Nephrol* 2010;25:1025–35.
Eleftheriou D, Batu ED, Ozen S, Brogan PA. Vasculitis in children. *Nephrol Dial Transplant*. 2015;30 Suppl 1:i94–103.

Polyarteritis nodosa (PAN)

Background

- PAN is a necrotizing vasculitis associated with aneurysmal nodules along the walls of medium-sized muscular arteries.
- Despite some overlap with smaller-vessel disease, PAN appears to be a distinct entity and, in adults in Europe and the USA, has an estimated annual incidence of 2.0–9.0/million.
- Although comparatively rare in childhood, it is the most common form of systemic vasculitis after HSP and KD.
- Peak age of onset in childhood is 7–11yr, often with a ♂ preponderance.
- Classification criteria for PAN are not diagnostic criteria, and meeting classification criteria is not equivalent to making a diagnosis in an individual patient—see rest of section and ➔ Vasculitis classification, p. 175.
- A recent discovery is that of a monogenic form of PAN: deficiency of adenosine deaminase Type 2 (DADA2)
  - consider this diagnosis for early-onset PAN (< 5yr) and/or familial PAN.

Aetiology

- Unknown: possible interaction between infection and aberrant host response.
- There may be genetic factors that make individuals vulnerable to PAN and other vasculitides, but with the exception of DADA2 caused by recessive mutation in *CECR1*, these are not yet fully defined.
  - There is a well-recognized association of PAN and familial Mediterranean fever in parts of the world where this is common.
- There are data to support roles for hepatitis B and reports of a higher frequency of exposure to parvovirus B19 and CMV in PAN patients compared with control populations.
- HIV has also been implicated, and PAN-like illnesses have been reported in association with cancers and haematological malignancies. However, in childhood, associations between PAN and these infections or other conditions are rare.
- Bacterial superantigens may play a role in some cases.
- Occasional reports suggest immunization as a cause, but this is not proven.
- A relatively common infectious trigger may be infection with *Streptococcus*.

Clinical features of PAN

A diagnosis is made by considering all clinical features in a patient, only some of which may be classification criteria. Clinical manifestations (and investigation findings) can be very confusing, especially in the early phase of the disease with absence of conclusive diagnostic evidence.

- The main *systemic clinical features* of PAN are malaise, fever, weight loss, skin rash, myalgia, abdominal pain, and arthropathy.

- *Skin lesions* are variable, and may masquerade as those of HSP or erythema multiforma. The cutaneous features described in a recent international classification exercise for PAN in children occurred commonly and were defined as follows:
  - *Livedo reticularis*—purplish reticular pattern usually irregularly distributed around subcutaneous fat lobules, often more prominent with cooling.
  - *Skin nodules*—tender subcutaneous nodules.
  - *Superficial skin infarctions*—superficial skin ulcers (involving skin and superficial subcutaneous tissue) or other minor ischaemic changes (nailbed infarctions, splinter haemorrhages, digital pulp necrosis).
  - *Deep skin infarctions*—deep skin ulcers (involving deep subcutaneous tissue and underlying structures), digital phalanx or other peripheral tissue (nose and ear tips) necrosis/gangrene.
- *Renal manifestations* such as haematuria, proteinuria, and hypertension.
- *GI features* and abdominal pain are relatively common and include:
  - Indeterminate intestinal inflammation: intestinal inflammation without characteristic histological features of either ulcerative colitis or Crohn's disease. NB: routine mucosal gut biopsies rarely detect overt vasculitis since the small- and medium-sized arteries lie below the mucosa.
  - GI haemorrhage (upper and lower).
  - Intestinal perforation.
  - Pancreatitis.
- *Neurological features* such as focal defects, hemiplegia, visual loss, mononeuritis multiplex; and organic psychosis may be present.
- *Other important clinical features* include: ischaemic heart and testicular pain. Rupture of arterial aneurysms can cause retroperitoneal and peritoneal bleeding, with perirenal haematomata being a recognized manifestation of this phenomenon, although this is rare.

Differential diagnosis

- Other primary vasculitides: HSP, EGPA, MPA, KD. See ➜ relevant chapters, HSP p. 177, EGPA pp. 196–200, MPA pp. 196–200, KD pp. 190–5.
- Autoimmune or autoinflammatory diseases:
  - JIA—particularly the systemic form.
  - JDM.
  - SLE.
  - Undifferentiated connective tissue disease.
  - Sarcoidosis.
  - Behçet's disease.
- Infections:
  - Bacterial, particularly streptococcal infections, and sub-acute bacterial endocarditis.
  - Viral—many: specifically look for hepatitis B/C, CMV, EBV, parvovirus B19 and consider HIV.
- Malignancy: lymphoma, leukaemia, and other malignancies can mimic PAN.
- DADA2; cardinal clinical features are livedo racemosa, lacunar stroke, and systemic inflammation.

Diagnostic laboratory and radiological investigation

Blood tests
- Anaemia, polymorphonuclear leucocytosis, thrombocytosis, increased ESR and CRP.
- Platelets are hyper-aggregable.
- Circulating immune complexes or cryoglobulins may be present.
- Positive hepatitis B serology in children is unusual in association with PAN but can occur.
- ANCA are not thought to play a major part in the causality of PAN, but there are reports demonstrating their presence in some adults and children with PAN.
  - The presence of cytoplasmic ANCA (C-ANCA) with antibodies to proteinase 3 in a patient suspected of having PAN makes it mandatory to consider GPA as a diagnosis.
  - Likewise, a significant titre of perinuclear ANCA (P-ANCA) with antibodies to myeloperoxidase would necessitate steps to consider microscopic polyangiitis (MPA) as the diagnosis.
  - Genetic testing for DADA2 if early onset disease, familial cases and patients with disease refractory to treatment.

Tissue biopsy
- Biopsy material is diagnostically important, especially skin or muscle, although tissue biopsy has overall low diagnostic sensitivity since the disease is patchy and vasculitis can be easily missed.
- The characteristic histopathological changes of PAN are fibrinoid necrosis of the walls of medium or small arteries, with a marked inflammatory response within or surrounding the vessel (Fig. 4.6).

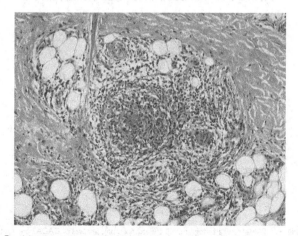

Fig. 4.6 PAN—skin biopsy (also see color plate).

- However, absence of such changes would not exclude the diagnosis, as the vasculitic features are variable and affected tissue may not have been sampled.
- Renal biopsy is usually not helpful and carries a greater risk than usual of bleeding and the formation of arteriovenous fistulae.

Radiological tests
- The most valuable investigative procedure is catheter-selective visceral digital subtraction arteriography to include flush aortogram and selective renal, hepatic, and mesenteric arteriography. This should be performed and interpreted only by those with expertise in this test in paediatric patients.
  - Arteriography findings include aneurysms, segmental narrowing, and variations in the calibre of arteries, together with pruning of the peripheral renal vascular tree (Fig. 4.7).
  - Treatment with prior corticosteroids will alter the arteriography and can result in false negatives.
  - Non-invasive arteriography such as CT or MR angiography (CTA/MRA) are *not* as sensitive as catheter arteriography for the detection of medium-sized vessel vasculitis such as PAN (discussed later in this list).
  - Consider formal cerebral arteriography if clinical and MRI features suggest cerebral vasculitis (see ➔ Cerebral vasculitis, pp. 220–4).
- Indirect evidence of the presence of medium-size artery vasculitis affecting renal arteries may be obtained by demonstrating patchy areas within the renal parenchyma of ↓ isotope uptake on Tc-99m dimercaptosuccinic acid (DMSA) scanning of the kidneys.
- Magnetic resonance angiography (MRA) usually fails to detect aneurysms of small- and medium-sized muscular arteries, although it

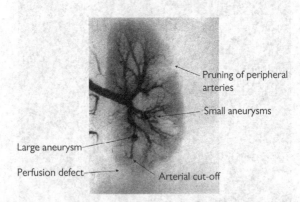

Pruning of peripheral arteries

Small aneurysms

Large aneurysm

Perfusion defect

Arterial cut-off

Fig. 4.7 PAN—renal arteriogram; NB the arteriographic features of DADA2 are identical thus arteriography cannot differentiate sporadic PAN from DADA2.

may demonstrate large intra- and extrarenal aneurysms and stenoses/occlusions of the main renal arteries, and areas of ischaemia and infarction.

- A caveat is that MRA may overestimate vascular stenotic lesions—CTA may also reveal larger aneurysms and arterial occlusive lesions and demonstrate areas of renal cortical ischaemia and infarction, but at the expense of high ionizing radiation exposure with less sensitivity than catheter arteriography.
- Echocardiography can be useful for the identification of pericarditis, valve insufficiency, myocarditis, or coronary artery abnormalities.

Treatment

(See ➔ The standard treatment of childhood vasculitis, pp. 181–4, for specific drug doses and protocols, and ➔ BSPAR guidelines for treatments used in paediatric rheumatology, p. 472.)

- In most patients, it is appropriate to treat aggressively to induce remission (typically 3–6 months), followed by less aggressive therapy to maintain remission (typically 18–24 months).
- In those presenting with mild predominantly cutaneous disease (see ➔ Cutaneous PAN, p. 207), corticosteroid alone may be appropriate, with careful monitoring of clinical and laboratory parameters as this is weaned.
- *Induction therapy*: high-dose corticosteroid with an additional cytotoxic agent such as cyclophosphamide:
  - Cyclophosphamide is usually given as pulsed monthly IV injections for up to 6 months or for shorter periods in children if remission is achieved.
  - Oral cyclophosphamide is no longer recommended since the IV regimen has been shown to have a more favourable therapeutic index.
  - An ongoing clinical trial is comparing cyclophosphamide versus MMF for induction of remission in children with PAN (www.mypan.org).
- Aspirin 1–5mg/kg/day as an antiplatelet agent may be considered.
- *Maintenance therapy*: once remission is achieved, therapy with daily low-dose prednisolone and oral azathioprine is frequently used for up to 18–24 months.
  - Other maintenance agents include MTX, MMF, and ciclosporin.
  - Some advocate alternate day low-dose prednisolone in the maintenance phase with the intention of limiting steroid toxicity such as growth impairment although data to support this approach are limited.
- Adjunctive plasma exchange can be used in life-threatening situations (see ➔ Vasculitis treatment, pp. 181–4).
- Biologic agents such as anti-TNFα or rituximab have been used for those unresponsive to conventional therapy.
- Anti-TNFα is particularly effective for DADA2. The role of HSCT in this condition remains to be established.
- Treatment response can be assessed using the PVAS: paediatric vasculitis activity score; and by monitoring of conventional acute phase reactants, urinary sediment, BP, and growth.

Outcome

- PAN, unlike some other vasculitides, such as GPA, appears to be a condition in which permanent remission can be achieved. Relapses can occur, but despite these, a real possibility of cure can be anticipated.
- However, if treatment is delayed or inadequate, life-threatening complications can occur due to the vasculitic process.
- Severe complications, especially infections, can occur from immunosuppressive treatment.
- In comparison with the almost 100% mortality rate in the pre-steroid era, mortality rates as low as 1.1% were reported in a recent retrospective multicentre analysis. However, this may not truly reflect mortality in circumstances of severe disease because 30% of patients in that series were considered to have predominantly cutaneous PAN.
- A major tertiary referral centre seeing predominantly children with aggressive advanced disease; reported the following outcomes:
  - Relapse rate 35%.
  - Mortality rate 4%.
- Severe GI involvement was associated with increased risk of relapse; longer time to induce remission and increased cumulative dose of cyclophosphamide were associated with lower relapse risk.
- Late morbidity can occur years after childhood PAN from chronic vascular injury, possibly resulting in premature atherosclerosis. This remains a cause for concern and an area of ongoing research.

Further reading

Ozen S, Anton J, Arisoy N, et al. Juvenile polyarteritis: results of a multicenter survey of 110 children. J Pediatr 2004;145:517–22.

Navon Elkan P, Pierce SB et al. Mutant adenosine deaminase 2 in a polyarteritis nodosa vasculopathy. N Engl J Med. 2014;370:921–31.

Zhou Q, Yang D. Early-onset stroke and vasculopathy associated with mutations in ADA2. N Engl J Med. 2014; 6:370(10):911–20.

Eleftheriou D, Dillon MJ, Tullus K, et al. Systemic polyarteritis nodosa in the young: a single-center experience over thirty-two years. Arthritis Rheum. 2013;65:2476–85.

Cutaneous polyarteritis nodosa (cPAN)

Background and clinical features

- Cutaneous PAN (cPAN) is a form of vasculitis affecting small- and medium-sized vessels limited to the skin.
- It is characterized by the presence of fever; subcutaneous nodular, painful, non-purpuric lesions with or without livedo reticularis occurring predominantly in the lower extremities; with no systemic involvement (except for myalgia, arthralgia, and non-erosive arthritis).
- In an international survey of childhood vasculitis, approximately 1/3 of children identified as having PAN were categorized as cutaneous PAN.
- The clinical course is characterized by periodic exacerbations and remissions that may persist for many years.
- Skin biopsy shows features identical to systemic PAN.
- ANCA are usually negative and the condition is often associated with serological or microbiological evidence of streptococcal infection.
- There is debate as to whether the condition should be classed as a separate entity or as a part of the spectrum of PAN since a proportion of cases appear to evolve into full-blown PAN.

Treatment of cutaneous PAN

- NSAIDs may suffice.
- Some require moderate doses of oral steroids.
- When streptococcal infection is implicated, penicillin may be effective.
  - Some recommend continuing prophylactic penicillin throughout childhood, as relapses are common and occur in up to 25% of cases in association with further streptococcal infections.
- When there is a lack of response to the above, or concerns about possible steroid toxicity, other agents may be considered:
  - IVIg has been successfully used.
  - Alternatives with anecdotal success for cutaneous PAN therapy include colchicine, hydroxychloroquine, azathioprine, MTX, dapsone (beware haemolytic anaemia as a relatively common and severe side-effect of this agent), cyclophosphamide, and pentoxifylline.

Outcome of cutaneous PAN

- A minority of patients experience a persistence of cutaneous lesions through childhood.
- Overall it is uncommon for the condition to progress to PAN.
- However, it is mandatory for such patients to remain under surveillance to detect any evidence of developing systemic disease that would be an indication for intensification of treatment as per that of PAN.
- Cutaneous PAN patients who develop neurological complications should be considered for screening for deficiency of adenosine deaminase Type 2 (DADA2) by genetic testing for mutations *CECR1*.

Further reading

Dillon MJ, Eleftheriou D, Brogan PA. Medium-size-vessel vasculitis. *Pediatr Nephrol* 2010; 25(9):1641–52.

Ozen S, Anton J, Arisoy N, et al. Juvenile polyarteritis: results of a multicenter survey of 110 children. *J Pediatr* 2004;145:517–22.

Takayasu arteritis

Background

- Takayasu arteritis (TA) is an idiopathic, chronic inflammation of the large vessels, affecting the aorta and its major branches.
- The disease is named after Mikito Takayasu, a Japanese ophthalmologist, who first described an association between retinal peri-papillary arterio-venous anastomoses and absent radial pulses.
- Other names include 'pulseless disease', aortic arch syndrome, or idiopathic aortoarteritis.
- Classification criteria are provided in the ➋ Vasculitis classification, p. 175.

Epidemiology

- TA is more prevalent in Asian and African populations, and is rarer in Europe and North America. Most studies report an incidence of 1–3 per million/year in Caucasian populations—in Japan the estimated incidence is up to 100 times higher: 1 per 3000/year.
- In adult studies there is a 9:1 F:M predominance. In children however gender ratios vary amongst different studies. A recent study from Southeast Asia and Africa report a F:M ratio of 2:1.
- TA is a rare vasculitis in children. Age of onset may range from infancy to middle age. The peak period of onset is in the 3rd decade of life.

Aetiopathogenesis

- The cause remains unknown.
- Genetic factors may play a role, and there are several reports of familial TA including in identical twins.
  - HLA associations include: HLA-A10, HLA-B5, HLA-Bw52, HLA-DR2, and HLADR4 in Japan and Korea; HLA B22 association has been described in the US population.
  - The presence of HLA Bw52 has been associated with coronary artery and myocardial involvement and worse prognosis.
- TA is described in association with RA, ulcerative colitis, and other auto-immune diseases suggesting an autoimmune mechanism for the pathogenesis of the disease.
- Circulating anti-aortic endothelial cell antibodies in patients with TA have been reported; their exact role however is yet to be determined.

Histopathology

- TA is characterized by granulomatous inflammation of all layers of the arterial vessels (panarteritis).
  - Inflammation of the tunica intima is followed by intimal hyperplasia leading to stenoses or occlusions.
  - Destruction of tunica elastica and muscularis cause dilatation and aneurysms.
  - Endothelial cell damage leads to a prothrombotic tendency.
  - The lesions have a patchy distribution.

- The initial finding is neutrophil infiltration of the adventitia and cuffing of the vasa vasorum with proliferation and penetration of the latter within the tunica intima.
- Various mixed chronic inflammatory cells including T cells contribute to granuloma formation in the tunica media and adventitia mediated by the release of interferon-γ and TNFα.
- Later, the adventitia and media are replaced by fibrous sclerotic tissue and the intima undergoes acellular thickening, thus narrowing the vessel's lumen and contributing to ischaemia.
- In paediatric series:
  - Occlusions and stenoses were present in 98% of the patients while aneurysms were only seen in 15.6% of the patients.
  - Post-stenotic dilatations were present in 34% of cases.
  - Lesions are most commonly seen in the subclavian arteries (90%), the common carotids (60%), the abdominal aorta (45%), the aortic arch (35%), and the renal arteries (35%); pulmonary arteries are involved in 25% of the cases.

Clinical features

Acute phase

Non-specific features of systemic inflammation (systemic, pre-stenotic phase). In children, up to 65% of TA present abruptly with systemic features:
- Pyrexia, malaise, weight loss, headache, arthralgias, and/or myalgias.
- Rash (erythema nodosum, pyoderma gangrenosum).
- Arthritis.
- Myocarditis causing congestive heart failure (± hypertension) or valvular involvement (aortic valve most commonly affected followed by mitral valve).
- Myocardial infarction.
- Hypertension.
- Hypercoagulable state: thrombotic tendency.

Chronic phase

Features and signs 2° to vessel occlusion and ischaemia (stenotic phase):
- Asymmetric or absent pulses; a measured difference of >10mmHg on 4-limb BP monitoring is likely to indicate arterial occlusion.
- Systemic hypertension: commonest finding.
- Arterial bruits.
- Congestive heart failure 2° to hypertension and/or aortic regurgitation when the valve is affected.
- Angiodynia: localized tenderness on palpation of the affected arteries.
- Claudication.
- Coronary angina.
- Mesenteric angina presenting with abdominal pain and diarrhoea from malabsorption.
- Recurrent chest pain from chronic dissection of the thoracic aorta or pulmonary arteritis.
- Pulmonary hypertension.

CNS involvement

May be attributed to ischaemia ± hypertension: dizziness, or headache; seizures; transient ischaemic attacks, stroke.

Eye involvement

- Diplopia, blurry vision, amaurosis, visual field defect. Fundoscopy findings include:
  - Retinal haemorrhage.
  - Micro aneurysms of the peripheral retina.
  - Optic atrophy.

Renal involvement

- Renal hypertension 2° to renal artery stenosis with secondary glomerular damage.
- Chronic renal failure.
- Amyloidosis.
- Glomerulonephritis (GN) has been described in association with TA: IgA nephropathy; membranoproliferative GN; crescentic GN; mesangioproliferative GN.

Differential diagnoses

- Other vasculitides including medium- and small-vessel vasculitis: Kawasaki disease; PAN; GPA is also a recognized cause of aortitis.
- Infections:
  - Bacterial endocarditis.
  - Septicaemia without true endocarditis.
  - TB.
  - Syphilis.
  - HIV.
  - Borelliosis (Lyme disease).
  - Brucellosis (very rare).
- Other autoimmune or autoinflammatory diseases: SLE; rheumatic fever; sarcoidosis; Blau's syndrome.
- Non-inflammatory large vessel vasculopathy of congenital cause. *Treatment with immunosuppression will be ineffective and could be harmful:*
  - Fibromuscular dysplasia.
  - William's syndrome; and autosomal dominant (non-Williams syndrome) elastin mutations.
  - Congenital coartctation of the aorta.
  - Congenital mid-aortic syndrome.
  - Ehler–Danlos type IV.
  - Marfan syndrome.
  - Neurofibromatosis type I.
  - ACTA-2 arteriopathy.
  - An ever increasing number of recently discovered monogenic aortopathies.
- Other: post radiation therapy.

Laboratory investigations

(also see ➔ Vasculitis investigation, pp. 179–80)

- Normochromic normocytic anaemia, leucocytosis, thrombocytosis; raised ESR, raised CRP—may not be present in chronic (stenotic) phase of illness.
- Elevated transaminases and hypoalbuminaemia.
- Deranged renal function tests in cases of renal involvement.
- Polyclonal hyperglobulinaemia.

Further tests required to exclude other causes mimicking TA or for disease monitoring

- Regular 4-limb BP measurement (preferably with a manual sphygmomanometer).
- In cases of significant peripheral artery stenosis, central BP measurements may be required.
- Renal function tests, urinalysis.
- Auto-immune screen.
- Baseline immunology tests including lymphocyte subsets, nitroblue tetrazolium (NBT) test.
- Blood cultures (acute phase).
- Mantoux test or interferon gamma releasing assays (IGRA).
- Syphilis serology.
- Tissue biopsy, rarely performed but should include microbiological culture, 16S and 18S ribosomal PCR if available to exclude bacterial and fungal infection respectively.
- Consider genetic screening for monogenic aortopathy/vasculopathy, e.g. using conventional Sanger sequencing of candidate genes, or next generation sequencing with a targeted gene panel if available.

Imaging

- An echocardiogram (and ECG) and a CXR are simple 1st-line imaging tests and should be performed in all cases where TA is suspected.
- Conventional digital subtraction catheter arteriography is the method used routinely for obtaining a generalized arterial survey when TA is suspected, but essentially only provides 'lumenography' with no imaging of arterial wall pathology.
- MRI and MRA, and CTA, or a combination of these may help accurately diagnose TA and monitor disease activity, and (for MRA and CTA) provide cross-sectional aortic wall images allowing detection of arterial wall thickness and intramural inflammation.
  - MRI and MRA are gradually replacing conventional angiography in most centres and are useful for diagnosis and follow-up.
  - However, MR lacks sensitivity in evaluation of the distal aortic branches, and may overestimate the degree of arterial stenosis, especially in small children.
  - Cardiac MRI is increasingly employed to look for valvular involvement and/or myocarditis.

- Angiographic findings form the basis of one classification for TA (Takayasu Conference, 1994):
  - Type I. Classic pulseless type that affects blood vessels of aortic arch; involving the brachiocephalic trunk, carotid, and subclavian arteries.
  - Type II. Affects middle aorta (thoracic and abdominal aorta).
  - Type III. Affects aortic arch and abdominal aorta.
  - Type IV. Affects pulmonary artery in addition to any of the above types.
  - Type V. Includes patients with involvement of the coronary arteries.

Source: data from Moriwaki R, Noda M, Yajima M, *et al*. Clinical manifestations of Takayasu arteritis in India and Japan—new classification of angiographic findings. *Angiology*, Volume 48, Issue 5, pp. 369-379, Copyright © 1997 SAGE.

- Doppler USS:
  - High resolution duplex US technology is a valuable tool in evaluation and follow-up of TA.
  - This modality offers high-resolution imaging of the vascular wall and can be useful for the detection of ↑ wall thickness.
- ^{18}F-FDG-PET co-registered with CTA can be a powerful technique combining information relating to the metabolic activity of the arterial wall (^{18}F-FDG uptake detected using PET) with detailed lumenography (CTA) thus providing information on disease activity and anatomy. This technique is not available in all centres, and carries a high radiation exposure limiting its use for routine follow-up of disease activity. A newer approach is PET-MRI/MRA (less radiation), which is available in select centres.
- An overall approach to imaging in TA is provided in Fig. 4.8.

Diagnosis

The diagnosis of TA is based on clinical and laboratory findings of systemic inflammation and/or of large-vessel ischaemia, raised and angiographic demonstration of lesions in the aorta or its major branches, with exclusion of other causes listed in the differential diagnosis.

Treatment

(also see ➔ Vasculitis treatment, pp. 181–4)

- Early diagnosis and aggressive treatment is fundamental for the outcome of the disease, although new lesions can continue to develop even in the presence of clinical remission in 60% of cases.
- Vascular damage already established in some patients will usually not respond to medical treatment.
- Medical management of TA includes: high-dose corticosteroids, usually in combination with MTX or cyclophosphamide for induction of remission. Maintenance agents include MTX, azathioprine, and increasingly anti-TNFα or anti-IL6.

Hypertension

- At least 40% of TA patients are hypertensive.
- Optimal control of hypertension is essential in the longer term since it is a major contributor to long-term morbidity.

Imaging algorithm in paediatric large vessel vasculitis (TA)

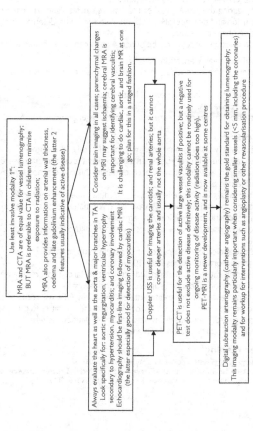

Use least invasive modality 1st:
MRA and CTA are of equal value for vessel lumenography;
BUT MRA is preferable to CTA in children to minimise exposure to radiation;
MRA also provides information on arterial wall thickness, oedema and late gadolinium enhancement (the latter 2 features usually indicative of active disease)

Always evaluate the heart as well as the aorta & major branches in TA
Look specifically for: aortic regurgitation; ventricular hypertrophy secondary to hypertension; myocarditis; and coronary involvement
Echocardiography should be first-line imaging followed by cardiac MRI (the latter especially good for detection of myocarditis)

Consider brain imaging in all cases; parenchymal changes on MRI may suggest ischaemia; cerebral MRA is important for identifying cerebral vasculitis;
It is challenging to do cardiac, aortic, and brain MR at one go; plan for this in a staged fashion.

Doppler USS is useful for imaging the carotids; and renal arteries; but it cannot cover deeper arteries and usually not the whole aorta

PET-CT is useful for the detection of active large vessel vasculitis if positive; but a negative test does not exclude active disease definitively; this modality cannot be routinely used for ongoing monitoring of disease activity (radiation does too high).
PET-MRI is a newer development, and is now available at some centres

Digital subtraction arteriography (catheter angiography) remains the gold standard for obtaining lumenography;
This imaging modality remains particularly important when considering smaller vessels (<5 mm, including the coronaries) and for workup for interventions such as angioplasty or other revascularisation procedure

Fig. 4.8 Suggested imaging algorithm in large vessel vasculitis.

- Medical treatment of hypertension in TA may be challenging since renovascular hypertension may not respond to medical therapy alone. *Seek specialist advice from a paediatric nephrologist.*
- Revascularization procedures may be required.

Revascularization and other surgical procedures

Techniques include:
- Angioplasty (including percutaneous transluminal angioplasty; or patch angioplasty), arterial bypass procedures, endarterectomy, arterial stenting, cardiac valve repair/replacement.
- Surgery during the acute phase of the disease carries significant risk of re-occlusion and procedural complication, so should be deferred until the acute phase is treated.
- These techniques should only be undertaken in centres with expertise.

Indications for revascularization include:
- Hypertension from stenotic coarctation of the aorta or renovascular disease.
- End-organ ischaemia or peripheral limb ischaemia.
- Cerebral ischaemia.
- Aortic or other arterial aneurysms, or aortic regurgitation.

Prognosis

- There is usually a significant time lag (approximately 18 months, occasionally much longer) between initial presentation and diagnosis of TA in children. Arterial damage accrues during this pre-diagnostic phase, and influences prognosis.
- The course of the disease is variable, but most patients experience new lesions over time. Typically vascular inflammation persists even in patients thought to be clinically in remission.
- Aortic valve insufficiency and congestive heart failure are reported in 25%.
- Vascular claudication limiting activities occurs in up to 40%.
- Long-term mortality ranges from 10–30%:
  - The main causes of death include congestive cardiac failure, myocardial infarction, aneurysm rupture, or renal failure.
- After commencement of treatment approximately 60% will respond to corticosteroids while 40% will relapse when these are tapered off.
- Poor prognostic factors are severe aortic regurgitation, severe hypertension, cardiac failure, and aneurysms.

Further reading

Gulati A, Bagga A. Large vessel vasculitis. *Paed Nephrol* 2010 25:1037–48
Eleftheriou D, Varnier G, Dolezalova P, et al. Takayasu arteritis in childhood: retrospective experience from a tertiary referral centre in the United Kingdom. *Arthritis Res Ther.* 2015;17:36.

Behçet's disease

Behçet's disease (BD) is a multisystem disease with a classic triad of recurrent oral aphthous ulcers, genital ulcers, and uveitis, which may also affect the skin, joints, GI tract, and CNS. Both small- and large-vessel vasculitis occurs, and in some patients there is a propensity to arterial and venous thromboses. Many now regard BD within the spectrum of autoinflammatory diseases.

Pathophysiology

- Unknown.
- BD has geographical variability, being more commonly found in the Mediterranean, Middle East, and Japan than in the USA and the UK.
- Likely polygenic auto inflammatory condition with possible environmental triggers in genetically susceptible individuals.
- HLA-B51 is significantly associated with BD.
- Genome wide association studies show an association with the IL10 and IL23/IL17 pathways.
- The familial Mediterranean fever gene (*MEFV*) has been implicated as an additional genetic susceptibility factor in some patients.
- Other genetic associations including *MICA* and *TNF* genes are thought to be the result of linkage disequilibrium with the *HLA-B51* gene, and are thus not causally associated.
- *Pathergy*: the skin hyper-reactivity response or pathergy test is not pathognomic of BD but may be an important diagnostic indicator. Early or pathergy-induced cutaneous lesions in BD show a neutrophilic vascular reaction. This may be vascular or perivascular with a diffuse dermal neutrophilic infiltrate. Longstanding lesions may show a lymphocytic vasculitis. A typical pathergy test protocol is described later in this section.

Diagnostic criteria

- There are several sets of criteria for the diagnosis and/or classification of BD.
  - None have been formally validated in children.
- The most widely used for adult onset disease are the International Behçet's Study Group (ISG) criteria; but these are considered to have suboptimal sensitivity for the classification or diagnosis of BD in adults.
- Recently, International Criteria for Behçet's Disease (ICBD) have been validated in adults (Table 4.4) with 94.8% sensitivity and 90.5% specificity for diagnosis.
- A recent study of children in the UK with BD reported 72% diagnostic sensitivity for the ICBD criteria, versus only 26% for the ISG criteria.

Clinical features

Almost any organ can be involved due to the vasculitis affecting both arteries and veins of all sizes:

- Oral ulcers—painful, occur singly or in crops, affect lips, gingivae, buccal mucosa and tongue, last 1–2 weeks.

Table 4.4 International Criteria for Behçet's Disease (ICBD) – score ≥ 4 required for diagnosis

Sign/symptom	Points
Ocular lesions	2
Genital aphthosis	2
Oral aphthosis	2
Skin lesions	1
Neurological manifestation	1
Vascular manifestations	1
Positive pathergy test*	1

Ocular lesion: anterior uveitis, posterior uveitis and retinal vasculitis; skin lesions: pseudofolliculitis (BD pustulosis), erythema nodosum and skin aphthosis; neurological manifestation includes peripheral and/or central symptoms with evidence of association with disease status; vascular manifestations: arterial thrombosis, large vein thrombosis, phlebitis and superficial phlebitis;

* Pathergy test is optional.

Reproduced with permission from Davatchi, F. et al. The International Criteria for Behçet's Disease (ICBD): a collaborative study of 27 countries on the sensitivity and specificity of the new criteria. *Journal of the European Academy of Dermatology and Venereology*, Volume 28, Issue 3, pp. 338-347, Copyright © 2013 John Wiley and Sons Ltd.

- Genital ulcers—affect scrotum in males, vulva in females, may result in scarring.
- Cutaneous lesions may be erythema nodosum-like, papulopustular, vesicular, abscesses, erythema multiforme-like eruptions, folliculitis, thrombophlebitis. Less commonly are pyoderma gangrenosum-type lesions, palpable purpura, purulent bullae, bullous necrotizing vasculitis and Sweet syndrome-like lesions.
- Ocular—iridocyclitis affecting the anterior segment or chorioretinitis, optic papillitis, retinal thrombophlebitis, arteritis.
- Arthralgia and arthritis usually affecting knees and ankles.
- GI—nausea, vomiting, diarrhoea, weight loss. May mimic inflammatory bowel disease. Ulcers may occur anywhere but usually affect ileum and caecum.
- Neurological—headaches, paralysis, hyperparaesthesia, dementia, behavioural disorders, psychiatric problems, cerebellar signs, peripheral nerve palsies. Underlying pathology includes meningoencephalitis, cerebral venous thrombosis and 'benign intracranial hypertension', parenchymal inflammatory brain disease without obvious vasculitis ('neuro-Behçet's'), and true arterial vasculitis.
- Cardiovascular—myocarditis, pericarditis.
- Vascular—arterial or venous occlusions, varices, aneurysms.
  - Pulmonary arterial aneurysms are of particular concern in adults with BD, and can present with haemoptysis mimicking pulmonary embolism, but anticoagulation can be fatal in this situation so beware this diagnostic pitfall.

- Respiratory—pulmonary infiltrates may be associated with pulmonary haemorrhage.
- Nephro-urological—haematuria and proteinuria (which may cause nephrotic syndrome), urethritis, orchitis, and epididymitis.
- Haematological—thrombocytopenia, neutropenia.
- Systemic—malaise, anorexia, weight loss.

Investigations

- FBC, CRP, ESR, routine clinical chemistry, thrombophilia screen (to exclude other causes of thrombosis), urinalysis.
- IgG, A, and M to exclude common variable immunodeficiency or other cause of low immunoglobulins (can present with oral ulcers).
- Consider a NBT test to exclude chronic granulomatous disease (which can mimic BD in the young)
- ANA, ds-DNA antibodies, RF, C3 and C4, ANCA, anticardiolipin antibodies, and antiphospholipid antibody are negative or normal but should be performed to exclude autoimmune disease.
- Consider genetic testing for mevalonate kinase deficiency (hyper IgD syndrome) in atypical cases of suspected BD.
- Skin pathergy test—A 20-gauge needle is inserted obliquely 5mm into the skin of the anterior forearm. The presence of erythema, papules, erythematous papules, or pustules at 24–48h indicate a positive test result.
- MRI of the brain including MR arteriography and venography should be considered early for those with headaches to exclude neuro-BD or cerebral venous thrombosis.

Treatment

Evidence in children is limited. EULAR recommendations for treatment in adults are based on limited evidence and were not designed with children in mind, but provide a framework for the management of children. See Table 4.5.

General principles of treatment of BD in the young:
- Tailored to the individual and reflecting organ involvement and severity.
- Least toxic therapies should be tried first.
- Oral ulcers should be treated with topical agents before considering systemic drugs.
- Anti-TNFα agents (etanercept, infliximab, and adalimumab) are increasingly used before thalidomide in children.
- Thalidomide is still used on a named-patient basis for children and adolescents with BD, typically for severe and resistant oral and/or genital ulceration, although it may also benefit other systemic symptoms of BD. Peripheral neuropathy and teratogenicity limit its use.
  - Suggested dosing regimen: 0.5–1mg/kg (maximum 100mg) orally once a week at nighttime (to avoid daytime drowsiness). Increase dose by adding another daily dose every week until symptoms controlled or until dose of 1mg/kg daily (whichever achieved first).
  - Exclude pregnancy, and check peripheral nerve conduction studies prior to starting, thereafter repeating nerve conduction 3–6-monthly

Table 4.5 EULAR 2008 recommendations for the treatment of Behçet's disease

Recommendation	Category of evidence
1. Eye involvement: any patient with BD and inflammatory eye disease affecting the posterior segment should be on a treatment regimen that includes azathioprine and systemic corticosteroids	Ib
2. Refractory eye involvement: if the patient has severe eye disease defined as >2 lines of drop in visual acuity on a 10/10 scale and/or retinal disease it is recommended that either ciclosporin or infliximab be used in combination with azathioprine and corticosteroids; alternatively interferon-α with or without corticosteroids could be used instead	Ib/IIb
3. Major vessel disease: there is no firm evidence to guide the management of major vessel disease in BD. For the management of acute deep vein thrombosis immunosuppressive agents such as corticosteroids, azathioprine, cyclophosphamide, or ciclosporin are recommended. For the management of pulmonary and peripheral arterial aneurysms, cyclophosphamide and corticosteroids are recommended	III
4. Anticoagulation: there are no controlled data on, or evidence of benefit from uncontrolled experience with anticoagulants, antiplatelet, or anti-fibrinolytic agents and management of deep vein thrombosis or for the use of anticoagulation for the arterial lesions of BD	IV
5. Gastrointestinal involvement: there is no evidence-based treatment that can be recommended for the management of GI involvement of BD. Agents such as sulfasalazine, corticosteroids, azathioprine, TNFα antagonists and thalidomide should be tried first before surgery, except in emergencies	III
6. Joint involvement: in most patients with BD, arthritis can be managed with colchicine	Ib
7. Neurological involvement: there are no controlled data to guide the management of CNS involvement in BD. For parenchymal involvement agents to be tried may include corticosteroids, interferon-α, azathioprine, cyclophosphamide, MTX, and TNFα antagonists. For dural sinus thrombosis corticosteroids are recommended	III
8. Ciclosporin neurotoxicity: ciclosporin should not be used in BD patients with CNS involvement unless necessary for intra ocular inflammation	III

Table 4.5 *Contd.*

Recommendation	Category of evidence
9. Mucocutaneous involvement: the decision to treat skin and mucosal involvement will depend on the perceived severity by the doctor and patient. Mucocutaneous involvement should be treated according to the dominant or codominant lesions present.	Ib
Topical measures (i.e. topical corticosteroids) should be the 1st-line treatment for isolated oral and genital ulcers	
Acne-like lesions are usually of cosmetic concern only. Thus, topical measures as used in acne vulgaris are sufficient	
Colchicine should be preferred when the dominant lesion is erythema nodosum	
Leg ulcers in BD might have different causes. Treatment should be planned accordingly	
Azathioprine, IFNα and TNFα antagonists may be considered in resistant cases	

CNS, central nervous system; IFN, interferon; TNF, tumour necrosis factor.

Categories of evidence: Ia: meta-analysis of randomized controlled trials; Ib: randomized controlled trial; IIa: controlled study without randomization; IIb: quasi-experimental study; III: non-experimental descriptive studies such as comparative, correlation and case-control studies; IV: expert committee reports or opinion or clinical experience of respected authorities or both.

Adapted with permission from Hatemi G, Silman A, Bang D, Bodaghi B, Chamberlain AM, Gul A, et al. EULAR recommendations for the management of Behcet disease. *Annals of the Rheumatic Diseases*, Volume 67, Issue 12, pp. 1656–62, Copyright © 2008 BMJ Publishing Group Ltd

(or after every 10g of total accumulative dose). Stop immediately if symptoms of neuropathy (e.g. numbness, tingling) develop.
• Remember that teratogenic risk also applies to mothers/female carers who handle the drug–full precautions always must be advised.
• The L-isomer lenalidomide may be less toxic but have greater (or comparable) efficacy, but experience in paediatric BD is limited.
• Use of other biologics, such as anti-IL6, anti-IL1 agents, and interferon-α has been increasingly reported in adults with variable success, but there is limited evidence for their use in children.

Prognosis—variable
• Eye disease can result in long-term visual impairment.
• Course may be worse in children than adults.
• Males tend to be more severely affected.
• Reported mortality of 3%, usually due to vascular complications.

Patient and parental support, including information sheets for children and adults can be found at: ℘ http://www.behcets.org.uk.

Central nervous system vasculitis in children

Background

- Central nervous system (CNS) vasculitis in children is an increasingly recognized inflammatory brain disease that continues to pose great diagnostic and therapeutic challenges. CNS vasculitis may occur as a primary disease that is isolated to the CNS (primary angiitis of the CNS, PACNS) or as a secondary manifestation of an underlying systemic condition.
- The most common systemic inflammatory diseases and infections that may cause secondary CNS vasculitis are summarized in Box 4.2.

Diagnostic criteria

Diagnostic criteria for PACNS in adults were proposed by Calabrese et al. in 1992 and they include the following:

- An acquired neurological deficit.
- Angiographic and/or histopathological features of angiitis within the CNS, and
- No evidence of systemic condition associated with these findings.

Although a paediatric case definition of PACNS in children (cPACNS) has not been proposed, most reported cases fit the Calabrese criteria.
cPACNS is broadly subdivided into two forms of the disease:

- Large–medium-vessel vasculitis (further divided into progressive and non-progressive, according to angiographic evidence of disease progression 3 months after diagnosis).
- Small-vessel vasculitis.

Epidemiology

The true incidence of cPACNS is difficult to establish as the condition is rare and there is lack of consensus on diagnostic criteria.

Clinical features

The clinical presentation of cPACNS is heterogeneous, with some children presenting with a rapidly progressive neurogenic deficit, whereas others have a slowly evolving disease course over weeks or months. Most common presenting features (in isolation or in various combinations) include the following:

- Acute severe headache.
- Focal neurological deficit.
- Gross motor deficit, hemiparesis.
- Cranial nerve involvement and optic neuritis.
- Concentration and cognitive deficits, behaviour, and personality changes.
- New onset of seizures.
- Acute loss of consciousness and symptoms of increased intracranial pressure caused by either intracerebral or subarachnoid haemorrhage, or a CNS mass lesion.
- Movement abnormalities.
- Constitutional symptoms (fever, fatigue, weight loss) are uncommon but can present in a minority of patients with small vessel vasculitis.

Box 4.2 Secondary central nervous system vasculitis in children

Inflammatory disorders
- Systemic lupus erythematosus
- Behçet's disease
- Sjögren's syndrome
- Juvenile dermatomyositis
- Scleroderma (both en coup de sabre and systemic sclerosis)
- Inflammatory bowel disease.
- Sarcoidosis
- Deficiency of adenosine deaminase type 2 (DADA2)

Systemic vasculitides
- Polyarteritis nodosa
- Kawasaki disease
- Henoch–Schönlein purpura
- ANCA-associated vasculitides: GPA; microscopic polyangiitis; EGPA

Infectious/post-infectious
- Bacterial:
  - *Streptococcus pneumoniae*
  - *Salmonella* spp.
  - *Mycoplasma pneumonia*
  - *Mycobacterium tuberculosis*
  - *Treponema pallidum*
- Viral:
  - Hepatitis C virus
  - CMV
  - EBV
  - HIV
  - Parvovirus B19
  - VZV
  - Enterovirus
  - Spirochete
  - *Borrelia burgdorferi.*
- Fungal:
  - *Candida albicans*
  - *Aspergillus*

Other
- Malignancy
- Graft-versus-host disease

Differential diagnosis

CNS vasculitis can be mimicked in both its clinical presentation and radiological manifestations by a number of inflammatory and non-inflammatory disorders, summarized in Box 4.3.

Box 4.3 Mimics of CNS vasculitis in children

- Arterial dissection
- Thromboembolic disease (congenital heart disease, inherited thrombophilia)
- Antiphospholipid syndrome
- Sickle cell disease
- Moyamoya disease (cerebral arteriopathy characterized by progressive steno-occlusive changes at the terminal portions of the bilateral internal carotid arteries with arterial collateral vessels at the base of the brain)
- Fibromuscular dysplasia
- Metabolic diseases:
  - Mitochondrial diseases
  - Leucodystrophies
  - Mucopolysaccharidoses
- Multiple sclerosis (including MOG positive demyelinating disease)
- Acute disseminated encephalomyelitis (ADEM)
- Devic's disease/neuromyelitis optica (CNS demyelinating condition affecting predominantly the spinal cord and optic nerves characterized by the presence of aquaporin-4 water channel IgG antibodies)
- Autoimmune encephalopathies (autoantibody mediated: VGKC, NMDAR, GAD)
- Vitamin B12 deficiency
- Rasmussen syndrome (neurological disorder characterized intractable focal seizures, progressive hemiplegia and increasing cognitive impairment)
- Coeliac disease
- 1° and 2° haemophagocytic lymphohistiocytosis (HLH)
- Progressive multifocal leukoencephalopathy (JC virus)
- Lymphoma
- Glioma
- Migraine/vasospasm
- Post radiation therapy for CNS tumour.
- Fabry's disease
- Sneddon's syndrome (morphologically fixed livedo reticularis and cerebrovascular accidents)
- CADASIL (cerebral autosomal dominant arteriopathy with subcortical infarcts and leukoencephalopathy)
- ACTA2 (Actin, Alpha 2, Smooth Muscle, Aorta) and other congenital arteriopathies
- Susac syndrome (acute encephalopathy, branch retinal artery occlusions and sensorineural hearing loss)
- Hypomyelination with brainstem and spinal cord abnormalities and leg spasticity syndrome due to DARS mutations
- Amyloid angiopathy
- Neurofibromatosis type I
- Hyperhomocysteinaemia
- Drug-exposure (cocaine, amphetamine, methylphenidate)

Glutamic acid decarboxylase-Abs=GAD; Voltage-gated potassium channel=VGKC; N-methyl-d-aspartate receptor =NMDAR; myelin oligodendrocyte glycoprotein=MOG

Investigations

The aim of the diagnostic work-up in patients with suspected cPACNS is to exclude causes of secondary CNS vasculitis or other neuro-inflammatory conditions that can present in the same way. In general there are no consistent or reliable laboratory abnormalities in children with cPACNS, and normal inflammatory markers by no means exclude an active vasculitic process in the CNS. The following investigations should be considered:

Laboratory investigations

- FBC and blood film, haemoglobin electrophoresis/sickle cell screen if patient is black or of Mediterranean ethnicity.
- ESR and CRP.
- ANA/dsDNA, ENA.
- ANCA.
  - Brain/neuronal autoantibodies- such as Voltage-gated potassium channel (VGKC); N-methyl-d-aspartate receptor (NMDAR); myelin oligodendrocyte glycoprotein (MOG); Glutamic acid decarboxylase (GAD) antibodies (see ➔ autoantibodies, pp. 33–6).
- C3 and C4 levels.
- IgG, IgA, IgM.
- Clotting screen.
- Full thrombophilia screen including:
  - Lupus anticoagulant and anticardiolipin antibodies.
  - Protein C.
  - Protein S.
  - Antithrombin.
  - APC resistance ratio.
  - Factor V Leiden.
  - Methylenetetrahydrofolate reductase (MTHFR) and prothrombin G20210A gene mutations.
  - Von Willebrand antigen levels may be elevated.
  - CSF studies to establish cell count, protein levels, and exclude infection. CSF opening pressure should also be measured; CSF oligoclonal bands (simultaneous serum testing for total IgG required).
  - Plasma amino-acids and plasma homocysteine.
  - Plasma lactate and ammonia.
  - Alpha galactosidase A (to exclude Fabry's disease).
  - Serology for mycoplasma, *Borrelia burgdorferi*, VZV.
- *Ophthalmology assessment* to look for retinal vasculitis, infection, or other inflammatory disease.
- Echocardiogram and ECG.
- Consider genetic screening (including next generation sequencing if available) if monogenic neuroinflammation is suspected.

Imaging studies:

- MRI brain/spine and MRA.
  - MRI in cPACNS reveals areas of acute ischemia in a vascular distribution when large–medium vessels are affected. In cases of small-vessel disease, the lesions may be multifocal and not necessarily conform to a specific vascular distribution.

- The parenchymal lesions may involve both grey and white matter, and meningeal enhancement has also been described.
- Diffusion weighted imaging (DWI) identifies areas of ischaemia in large-vessel disease.
- MRA provides an assessment of the vasculature and may reveal beading, tortuosity, stenosis, and occlusion of the vessels.
- Conventional catheter arteriography (CA) continues to be the radiological gold-standard for identifying cerebrovascular changes in patients with suspected CNS vasculitis and is more sensitive than MRA at detecting distal lesions that affect small calibre vessels, and for lesions in the posterior part of the brain.
- Brain biopsy for confirmation of vasculitis should be considered in difficult cases, but is rarely performed in children due to the invasiveness of the procedure. It should however be strongly considered in cases of high clinical suspicion but with negative arteriography findings or in cases of poor response to therapy.
  - Biopsy findings characteristically reveal segmental, non-granulomatous, intramural infiltration of arteries, arterioles, capillaries, or venules.
  - Non-lesional biopsy may be considered when lesions identified on imaging are not easily accessible.

Treatment

There are no randomized control trials (RCTs) to guide therapy.
- Current therapeutic recommendations are based on those for systemic vasculitis (see ➋ Vasculitis therapy, pp. 181–4) and include:
  - 6 months' induction therapy with IV cyclophosphamide: 500–1000mg/m² (max 1.2g) every 3–4 weeks (usually 7 doses); corticosteroids and antiplatelet doses of aspirin, followed by
  - 1–2yr maintenance therapy with azathioprine (1.5–3mg/kg/day), low dose daily or alternate day corticosteroid, and continuation of aspirin.
  - MMF has also been reported to be effective in some cases to maintain remission.
- Full anticoagulation may need to be considered on an individual patient basis.
- Treatment of large-vessel non-progressive disease remains controversial. There may be a role for steroids and aspirin without cytotoxic immunosuppression.

Outcome

- A recent study of 62 children with cPACNS suggested a poorer prognosis for patients presenting with: 1) a neurocognitive dysfunction, 2) multifocal parenchymal lesions on MRI, or 3) evidence of distal stenoses on arteriography.
- Further long-term follow-up studies are necessary to accurately define the prognosis of this condition in children.

Further reading

Elbers J, Benseler SM. Central nervous system vasculitis in children. *Curr Opin Rheumatol* 2008;20:47–54.

Other vasculitides

Background
The EULAR/PReS endorsed consensus criteria for the classification of childhood vasculitides include a category of "other vasculitides" for vasculitides where an aetiological process was defined, or in which no other classification category was appropriate (see ➔ pp. 174–6). These include:
- Behçet's disease.
- Vasculitis secondary to infection (including hepatitis B-associated PAN), malignancies, and drugs, including hypersensitivity vasculitis.
- Vasculitis associated with connective tissue diseases.
- Cogan's syndrome.
- cPACNS.
- Unclassified vasculitides.

Isolated cutaneous leucocytoclastic vasculitis, and hypocomplementaemic urticarial vasculitis are also described in this chapter. Behçet's disease and cPACNS are described in their respective chapters.

Vasculitis secondary to infection, malignancies, and drugs, including hypersensitivity vasculitis
Vasculitis secondary to infection
- Many viruses (HIV, parvovirus B19, CMV, VZV, and human T-cell lymphotropic virus [HTLV1]) can be responsible for systemic vasculitis, the most frequent being hepatitis B virus-related polyarteritis nodosa (HBV-PAN), even though its incidence has ↓ over the past few decades.
- Mixed cryoglobulinemia has been shown to be associated with hepatitis C virus (HCV) infection in adults, but has not been reported in children.
- Some bacteria, fungi, or parasites can also cause vasculitis, mainly by direct invasion of blood vessels or septic embolization.
- Effective antimicrobial drugs are mandatory to treat bacterial, parasitic or fungal infections, while the combination of antiviral agents (vidarabine, interferon-α) and plasma exchange has been proven to be effective against HBV-PAN.

Vasculitis secondary to drugs, including hypersensitivity vasculitis
- Therapeutic agents from virtually every pharmacological class have been implicated in the development of drug-induced vasculitis.
- Typically presents with cutaneous vasculitis alone (palpable purpura, macules, plaques, bullae, and ulcers), low grade fever, arthralgia, and micropic haematuria.
- More rarely can present with life-threatening systemic involvement, which may result in a severe and sometimes fatal illness.
- Withdrawal of the offending agent alone is often sufficient to induce prompt resolution of clinical manifestations.
- Steroids may be used for systemic involvement and azathioprine or other immunosuppressants may be appropriate for refractory disease.

Vasculitis secondary to malignancy
- In some patients, vasculitis occurs during the course of or prior to malignancies, most often haematological rather than solid tumours. Evidence of autoantibodies, immune complexes, and complement consumption is typically absent.
- Vasculitis may also occasionally be a complication of chemotherapy, radiation therapy, and bone marrow transplantation.

Vasculitis associated with connective tissue diseases
- Vasculitis secondary to connective tissue disorders in children most commonly arises in the context of pre-existing SLE, primary Sjögren's syndrome, systemic sclerosis, relapsing polychondritis, primary antiphospholipid syndrome, juvenile dermatomyositis, or mixed connective tissue (see ➲ specific chapters on each of these entities, SLE pp. 238–43, Sjögren's syndrome p. 290, systemic sclerosis pp. 274–9, antiphospholipid syndrome pp. 293–6, mixed connective tissue or overlap syndromes pp. 288–92) and sarcoidosis.
- The vasculitis may involve vessels of any size, but small-vessel involvement is predominant.
- Patterns of involvement vary with the associated underlying disorder, and range from isolated cutaneous involvement to life-threatening internal organ involvement.
- When vasculitis occurs in the setting of a pre-existing connective tissue disorder, it often correlates with disease severity and portends a poorer prognosis. Prompt recognition and treatment of vasculitis can dramatically improve the outcome for these patients.

Isolated cutaneous leucocytoclastic vasculitis
- This refers to cutaneous leucocytoclastic vasculitis without systemic vasculitis or glomerulonephritis.
- Histologically leucocytoclastic vasculitis appears as a neutrophil infiltration in and around small vessels, with neutrophil fragmentation (often referred to as 'nuclear dust' or leucocytoclasis), fibrin deposition, and endothelial cell necrosis.
- Treatment may require corticosteroids, colchicine, hydroxychloroquine, azathioprine, MTX or rarely dapsone (beware severe haemolytic anaemia and/or methaemoglobinaemia with dapsone).

Hypocomplementaemic urticarial vasculitis syndrome
- Hypocomplementaemic urticarial vasculitis syndrome (HUVS) is an uncommon immune complex-mediated entity characterized by urticaria with persistent acquired hypocomplementaemia.
- The disease is extremely rare in the paediatric population.
- In patients with HUVS, systemic findings include leucocytoclastic vasculitis, angio-oedema, laryngeal oedema, pulmonary involvement (interstitial lung disease, haemoptysis, pleural effusions), arthritis, arthralgia, glomerulonephritis, and uveitis.
- Laboratory findings include low levels of C1q, C2, C3, and C4. The binding of C1q antibodies to immune complexes is thought to be important in the pathogenesis of renal disease in HUVS.

- Treatment is individualized and is based on disease severity and will typically include corticosteroids and other immunosuppressive agents such as azathioprine or cyclophosphamide.
- Patients may have significant morbidity and mortality, most commonly caused by chronic obstructive pulmonary disease and acute laryngeal oedema.

Cogan's syndrome

- Cogan syndrome is a rare syndrome of:
  - Interstitial keratitis.
  - Vestibuloauditory symptoms (hearing loss and balance problems).
  - Occasionally aortitis.
- The cause is unknown, although autoantibodies and small-vessel vasculitis have been implicated.
- Typical Cogan's is characterized by:
  - Ocular involvement: primarily interstitial keratitis and occasionally conjunctivitis, uveitis, or subconjuctival haemorrhage.
  - Audiovestibular involvement giving a clinical picture similar to Ménière's disease accompanied with progressive hearing loss of hearing, usually ending in deafness within 1–3 months.
  - Other symptoms include fever, loss of weight, cardiac involvement (aortic insufficiency reported to up to 15% of patients), myalgia, arthralgia, mucocutaneous manifestations, GI and neurological involvement.
- The differential diagnosis is:
  - Vogt–Koyanagi–Harada syndrome (audiovestibular involvement with uveitis, vitiligo, alopecia).
  - Susac syndrome (retinocochleocerebral vasculopathy, presenting with acute or subacute encephalopathy, branch retinal artery occlusions and sensorineural hearing loss as a result of small infarcts in the brain, retina, and cochlea).
  - Other vasculitides.
  - Relapsing polychondritis.
  - SLE or Sjögren's may cause similar symptoms.
- During attacks patients may have raised inflammatory markers. Detection of antibodies against corneal or inner ear antigens has been studied in small case series.
- Treatment includes corticosteroid therapy, while other immunosuppressants such as MTX, cyclophosphamide have been used with variable efficacy. Cochlear implantation may ultimately be necessary for hearing loss, and physiotherapy is required for the vestibular symptoms.
- The course of the disease is variable, with some patients experiencing episodes of ocular and audiovestibular symptoms at variable intervals with complete remission in between. In the longer term >90% of patients suffer severe hearing loss while long-term ocular sequelae are rare. Systemic involvement is associated with the worst prognosis and can develop years after the initial onset of symptoms justifying prolonged close monitoring.

Further reading

Jara LJ, Navarro, C, Medina, G, et al, Hypocomplementemic urticarial vasculitis syndrome *Curr Rheumatol Rep* 2009, 11:410–15.

Ozen S. The 'other' vasculitis syndromes and kidney involvement. *Pediatr Nephrol* 2010;25:1633–9.

Grasland A, Pouchot J, Hachulla E, et al, Typical and atypical Cogan's s syndrome: 32 cases and review of the literature, *Rheumatology* 2004;43:1007–15.

Vasculitis mimics: non-inflammatory vasculopathies

Background

There are numerous non-inflammatory vasculopathies that may mimic the clinical, laboratory, radiological, and/or pathological features of the primary vasculitides. Some will have associated musculoskeletal manifestations and will be referred to the paediatric rheumatologist. Awareness of these mimics is essential to avoid the use of unnecessary and potentially harmful immunosuppression and to direct management to the correct underlying cause of disease. The commonest of these vasculitis mimics are discussed in this section. Mimics of CNS vasculitis are covered in ➔ p. 222.

Fibromuscular dysplasia (FMD)

- FMD is a non-inflammatory vasculopathy leading to stenoses of small- and medium-sized arteries, sometimes with poststenotic dilatation resembling aneurysms. It is a major differential diagnosis for Takayasu disease.
- FMD has been detected in almost every vascular bed although the most commonly affected are renal arteries (60–75%) followed by the cervico-cranial arteries (25–30%), non-renal visceral arteries (5%), and arteries in the extremities (5%). Intracranial arterial poststenotic dilatations have been reported in 7% of adult patients, but rarely in children.
- Patients can remain asymptomatic or present with signs of vascular insufficiency such as hypertension, stroke, abdominal pain, or claudication.
- The pathological classification for FMD is based on the arterial layer involved. Medial fibroplasia accounts for 80–90% of all cases and is characterized by a 'string of beads' appearance on angiography due to alternating areas of stenosis and aneurysmal dilatation involving the mid-to-distal portions of the vessel.
- It can be difficult to differentiate diffuse intimal FMD from large-vessel vasculitis, since their angiographic appearance can be similar. Histological examination may be required in these cases.
- Imaging investigations to be considered include:
  - Renal ultrasonography and Doppler studies.
  - CTA and MRA have been increasingly used for non-invasive imaging of the vascular tree.
  - However, selective catheter arteriography continues to be the radiological gold standard for delineating the extent of vascular involvement.
  - Cerebral perfusion scans or other measures to exclude cerebral arterial insufficiency should be carried out before angioplasty or surgical correction of renal artery stenosis to relieve hypertension, since a drop in BP can precipitate stroke in this situation.
- The management of hypertension associated with renal artery FMD involves antihypertensive therapy and revascularization with percutaneous angioplasty or other revascularization procedures for patients with significant renal artery stenosis, severe hypertension with

inadequate response, or intolerance of antihypertensive medication. Management of dissecting carotid artery due to FMD includes antiplatelet therapy and percutaneous angioplasty or surgical repair for patients with signs of cerebral vascular insufficiency.

Vasculopathies involving the TGFβ-signaling pathway

Marfan syndrome

- Incidence of Marfan syndrome is reported to be 1 in 10,000.
- Marfan syndrome results from mutations in the fibrillin-1 gene (*FBN1*) on chromosome 15, which encodes the glycoprotein fibrillin. Recent studies have suggested that abnormalities in the transforming growth factor-beta (TGFβ)-signalling pathway may represent a final common pathway for the development of the Marfan phenotype.
- Affected patients are usually taller and thinner than their family members. Their limbs are disproportionately long compared with the trunk (dolichostenomelia). Arachnodatyly, pectus excavatum, or carinatum are common features (Fig. 4.9).
- Ocular findings include ectopia lentis, flat cornea, cataract, glaucoma, retinal detachment.
- Cardiovascular involvement is the most serious complication associated with Marfan syndrome and comprises aortic root dilatation, aortic dissection involving the ascending aorta, and mitral valve prolapse.

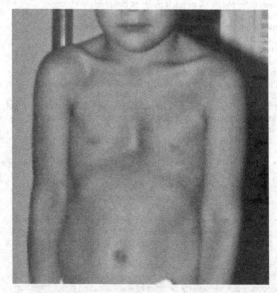

Fig. 4.9 Pectus excavatum of moderate severity.

- Patients can also present with spontaneous pneumothorax, stretch marks (striae atrophicae in the lower back), recurrent or incisional hernia, and dural ectasia (causing peripheral neurological symptoms and signs).

Management: seek expert cardiological advice

The paediatric rheumatologist should be aware that evidence now suggests that the vasculopathy of Marfan syndrome is associated with dysregulation of TGFβ, and that this can be blocked using angiotensin II receptor 1 blockade (AT1 antagonists) such as losartan. Animal and human data have demonstrated that this can significantly slow the progression of aortic root dilatation and prolong life. Thus early referral to a paediatric cardiologist is essential. Other management of the vasculopathy under expert paediatric cardiology supervision may include:

- General measures: moderate restriction of physical activity, endocarditis prophylaxis, echocardiography at annual intervals.
- Beta-blocker therapy (propanolol 2–4mg/kg/day in divided doses) should be considered at any age if the aorta is dilated, but prophylactic treatment may be more effective in those with an aortic diameter of <4cm.
- ACE inhibitors (enalapril 0.08mg/kg/day—up to 5mg) reduce central arterial pressure and conduit arterial stiffness and may be useful.
- Prophylactic aortic root surgery should be considered when the aortic diameter at the sinus of Valsalva is >5cm.

Loeys–Dietz syndrome

- Loeys–Dietz syndrome is considered an autosomal dominant disorder associated with mutations in either of the TGFβ receptors (TGFβ R1/ TGFβ R2).
- 2 subtypes of Loeys–Dietz syndrome have been identified:
  - Loeys–Dietz syndrome type I patients have both craniofacial and vascular disorders. The most characteristic craniofacial findings are hypertelorism and broad or bifid uvula or cleft palate, 2 of the 3 components of the clinical triad that also includes arterial aneurysms and tortuosity.
  - Loeys–Dietz syndrome type II patients may have a bifid uvula but do not have a cleft palate, craniosynostosis, or hypertelorism.
- Additional manifestations include blue sclera, malar hypoplasia, exotropia, and retrognathia. Cervical spine instability, pectus deformity, arachnodactyly, craniosynostosis, scoliosis, and joint laxity are some of the many musculoskeletal manifestations. Patients may also have congenital cardiac anomalies (bicuspid aortic valve).
- Due to the high risk of death from aortic aneurysm rupture, patients should be followed closely to monitor aneurysm formation, which can then be corrected with vascular surgery.
- The role of TGFβ antagonism is currently being explored in this condition too.

Ehler–Danlos syndrome (vasculopathic EDS) type IV

- EDS type IV is an autosomal dominant disorder that results from mutations in the type III pro-collagen gene (*COL3A1*).

- Although joint and skin laxity is not common, patients often have easy bruising, thin skin with visible veins, or characteristic facial features (loss of subcutaneous fat and collagen, referred to as acrogeria).
- Arterial complications may include aortic or other arterial aneurysm, dissection, and carotico-cavernous sinus fistulae. Patients can present acutely with life-threatening rupture of the intestines, the gravid uterus, or other viscera.
- There is currently no preventative treatment for this condition but close follow-up to monitor aneurysm formation is recommended.

ACTA2 arteriopathy

- Heterozygous mutation in the actin alpha-2 smooth muscle aorta gene (ACTA2) cause diffuse and diverse vascular diseases, including thoracic aortic aneurysms, aortic dissections, early onset coronary artery disease, stroke and moyamoya disease.
- Mutation in ACTA2 (p.Arg179His) was also reported in association with a unique syndrome characterized by aortic and cerebrovascular disease, persistent ductus arteriosus, congenital fixed dilated pupils and dysfunction of organs dependent on smooth muscle function, including the bladder and gut.

Susac's syndrome

- Susac's syndrome is a microangiopathy of unclear aetiology that is more frequently reported in young adult ♀.
- Susac's syndrome is characterized by the typical clinical triad of acute or subacute encephalopathy, branch retinal artery occlusions, and sensorineural hearing loss that results from small infarcts in the brain, retina, and cochlea.
- Typical findings on brain MRI are multiple small white-matter hyperintensities; grey matter involvement may also be seen. CSF analysis usually reveals a lymphocytic pleocytosis and elevated protein levels. Histological evidence of microangiopathic infarct is seen, without evidence of vasculitis or thrombosis.

Degos disease (DD)

- DD, also known as malignant atrophic papulosis, is characterized by thrombo-occlusive vasculopathy affecting the skin and various internal organs.
- DD has been described in 2 forms: the limited benign cutaneous and the lethal multiorgan systemic variant.
- In the skin, DD initially manifests with erythematous, pink or red papules that leave scars with pathognomonic, central, porcelain white atrophic centres.
- In the systemic form, GI involvement has been reported in the majority of patients and may manifest as abdominal pain, GI bleeding or bowel perforation. Central and peripheral nervous system, heart, lung, eye, pancreas, adrenal gland, and kidney involvement have been described.
- There has been no proven effective treatment for DD. Antiplatelet agents including aspirin and dipyridamole have been reported to reduce the formation of new skin lesions but there is no evidence in their role

to prevent systemic complications. Immunosuppressants, anticoagulants, and plasma exchange have been shown to be ineffective. Since corticosteroids may worsen other forms of occlusive vasculopathy, they should be used with caution in DD. Prompt surgical intervention is often needed for bowel infarction, perforation, or intracranial haemorrhage.

- The systemic form has a poorer prognosis and is usually fatal within the first 2yr after diagnosis because of major organ involvement.

Livedoid vasculopathy (LV)

- LV is an occlusive vasculopathy characterized by thrombosis and ulceration of the lower extremities.
- While the aetiology of LV remains unclear, it likely has a prothrombotic pathogenesis. Factor V Leiden mutation, heterozygous protein C deficiency, and hyperhomocysteinaemia have been associated with LV. In addition, plasminogen activator inhibitor (PAI)–1 promoter 4G/4G genotype has also been linked to the disease.
- Skin biopsies reveal segmental hyalinizing vascular involvement of thickened dermal blood vessels, endothelial proliferation, and focal thrombosis without nuclear dust. No true vasculitis is evident.
- The initial clinical findings are typically painful purpuric macules or papules on the ankles and the adjacent dorsum of the feet. Patients may have a history of livedo reticularis on their lower legs. The initial lesions, which often appear in clusters or groups, eventually ulcerate over a period of months and years and form irregular patterns of superficial ulcers. When the ulcers finally heal, they leave behind atrophic porcelain-white scars, which are referred to as 'atrophie blanche'.
- Small- and medium-sized vasculitides, such as isolated cutaneous leucocytoclastic vasculitis and PAN occasionally present with ulceration resulting in ivory-white, stellate scarring on the lower limbs and may be difficult to differentiate from LV.
- A number of therapies have been employed with variable effect:
  - Corticosteroids in combination with pentoxifyllin have been used in cases of widespread LV. Pentoxifyllin is believed to enhance the blood flow in the capillaries, making red blood cells more flexible and thereby reducing viscosity effectively. *However, anecdotally some report that corticosteroids can worsen the occlusive vasculopathy associated with LV.*
  - As thrombogenic mechanisms may be involved in the disease pathogenesis, anticoagulant therapy (low-molecular-weight heparin, warfarin) and aspirin are often tried, but with variable efficacy.
  - Hyperbaric oxygen therapy has been used in intractable cases of LV with good effect in some cases.

Pseudoxanthoma elasticum (PXE)

- PXE is a rare, genetic disorder characterized by progressive calcification and fragmentation of elastic fibres in the skin, the retina, and the cardiovascular system, which is termed as elastorrhexia.
- PXE is caused by mutations in the ATP-binding cassette transporter C6 gene (*ABCC6*) also known as multidrug resistance-associated protein 6 gene (*MRP6*).

- Patients present with:
  - Characteristic skin lesions that can appear during childhood. These are small, yellow papules of 1–5mm in diameter in a linear or reticular pattern which may coalesce to form plaques. The skin has a cobblestone-like appearance. These skin changes are first noted on the lateral part of the neck and later can involve any part of the body.
  - Ocular manifestations: angioid streaks of the retina, which are slate grey to reddish brown curvilinear bands radiating from the optic disc.
  - Cardiovascular manifestations include: calcification of the elastica media and intima of the blood vessels leading to a variety of physical findings, mitral valve prolapse.
  - Renal artery involvement leads to hypertension.
  - Mucosal involvement leading to GI haemorrhage.
- There is currently no treatment available for PXE.

Further reading

Molloy ES, Langford CA. Vasculitis mimics. *Curr Opin Rheumatol* 2008;20:29–34.

JSLE: epidemiology and aetiology

Systemic lupus erythematosus (SLE) is a multisystem autoimmune disorder characterized by widespread inflammation and damage to any organ. It is a complex disease with marked heterogeneity, causing mild to life-threatening disease in any combination of organ systems and is remitting and relapsing with an unpredictable natural history.

Approximately 15–20% of patients with lupus present before the age of 18 and form the cohort known as juvenile-onset SLE (JSLE).This group has a higher severity of disease and accrues more organ damage than adults (Box 4.4).

Epidemiology

- The annual incidence of SLE per 100,000 children and young people ranges from 0.36–0.8 although this probably underestimates the actual number as many cases go unrecognized, have mild disease, or do not fulfil diagnostic criteria. The F:M ratio varies with age, being 8:1 after puberty and 4:1 before 10yr of age. JSLE is rare before 5yr of age. The incidence of SLE appears to be higher in non-white children especially Black, Hispanic, and Asian children.
- Outcome has improved over recent years from 5yr survival of 60–90% in the 1980s to nearer 95% now. However, long-term outcome and cardiovascular morbidity from premature atherosclerosis is yet to be determined.
- Male gender, early-onset of disease and non-Caucasian ethnicity are factors associated with worse outcome.

Aetiology

- JSLE is the archetypal paediatric systemic autoimmune disease, illustrated by its complex clinical, molecular, and genetic characteristics. The cause of JSLE remains unknown. The principal underlying disorder in JSLE is impaired cellular and humoral immune response. Hormonal and environmental factors act on genetically susceptible individuals over time resulting in development of autoimmunity, eventually leading to disease progression (Box 4.5 and Fig. 4.10).
- The multitude of presenting and clinical features of lupus reflects the complex pathogenesis of SLE.

Box 4.4 Differences between JSLE and adult-onset SLE

- Children have more severe disease at onset than adults.
- Higher rates of organ involvement and more aggressive clinical course.
- Higher use of corticosteroids and immunosuppressive therapies.
- Accrue more organ damage, related to disease and corticosteroid use.
- Higher mortality rates.
- Increased incidence of renal, neurological, and haematological disease.
- Effects of disease and treatments on growth and physical and psychological development.

Box 4.5 Genetic, immunological, and environmental factors contributing to the development of lupus

Genetic factors
- Siblings of patients with SLE have 10–20-fold increased risk of developing disease.
- Monozygotic twins have 24% concordance rate versus 2% for heterozygote pairs.
- Familial autoimmunity is a risk factor for SLE (odds ratio 4.1 with 1 relative, 11.3 with 2 or more relatives).
- Homozygous deficiency of C1q, C1r, C1s, C4, and C2 are strongest susceptibility factors for SLE in humans (80% prevalence for C1 or C4 molecules). Other monogenic forms of SLE are increasingly described.
- Increased susceptibility to SLE is associated with an increasing number of recognized candidate genes, including HLA haplotypes, ITGAM, IFR5, BLK, STAT4, PTPN22, and Fcγ receptor polymorphisms.

Immune dysfunction
- In JSLE it is proposed that immune tolerance is broken and that defects in apoptosis, T-cells, B-cells, dendritic cells (DCs), neutrophil function and signalling pathways interact, leading to inflammation and clinical disease manifestations.
- B-cells and autoantibodies: loss of B-cell tolerance occurs early in the process of developing JSLE. B-cell activating factor (BAFF) (also known as B-lymphocyte stimulator, BLyS) is a protein that promotes survival of B-cells and has been implicated in the expansion of autoreactive B-cells. Immune complexes containing auto-antibodies against endogenous nucleic antigens activate dendritic cells to produce IFN-α which induces differentiation of B-cells into antibody-secreting plasma cells, perpetuating auto-antibody production.
- DCs: abnormal activation causes selection rather than deletion of T cells that have receptors to self-antigens.
- T cells: hyperactivity, loss of tolerance, and expansion of T helper cells has been shown to correlate with increased auto-antibody levels and disease activity.
- Pro-inflammatory cytokines levels elevated: interferon-α, IL-6, IL-10, IL-12, IL-18.
- Apoptosis: impaired clearance of apoptotic cells may lead to over-presentation of nuclear antigens by DCs to T cells.
- Other: abnormalities in monocytes, NK cells, cytokines, and immunoglobulins also identified.

Environmental
- Ultra-violet (UV) light can induce flares, possibly by altering DNA methylation.
- Viruses.
- Hormones.
- Drugs (e.g. procainamide, hydralazine have been shown to impair T cell DNA methylation leading to ↑ autoreactivity).

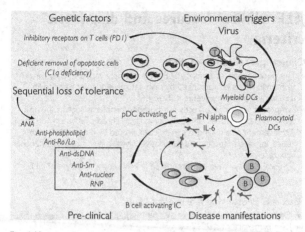

Genetic factors   Environmental triggers
                                        Virus

Inhibitory receptors on T cells (PD1)

*Deficient removal of apoptotic cells
(C1q deficiency)*

Sequential loss of tolerance
                                        Myeloid DCs

                     pDC activating IC   IFN alpha   Plasmacytoid
ANA   IL-6   DCs
   Anti-phospholipid
      Anti-Ro/La
         Anti-dsDNA
           Anti-Sm
             Anti-nuclear
               RNP

              B cell activating IC
        Pre-clinical   Disease manifestations

Fig. 4.10 Roles played by both genetic and environmental factors in the
development of paediatric SLE. Genetic alterations may contribute to a progressive
loss of tolerance to nuclear antigens, which has been shown to precede the
development of clinical disease. IFN-α will also activate monocytes and other
myeloid DC precursors to become immunogenic DCs able to activate T and B cells.
Viruses and other environmental triggers can activate DCs to secrete IFN-α which
amplifies these loops and precipitates the development of clinical disease.

Further reading

Crispin JC, Liossis SN, Kis-Toth K, *et al*. Pathogenesis of human systemic lupus erythematosus: Recent advances. *Trends Mol Med* 2010;**16**:47–57.

Stichweh D, Arce E, Pascual V. Update on pediatric systemic lupus erythematosus. *Curr Opin
Rheumatol* 2004; **16**:577–87.

Midgley A, Watson L, Beresford MW. New insights into the pathogenesis and management of lupus
in children. *Arch Dis Child* 2014;**99**(6):563–7.

JSLE: clinical features and diagnostic criteria

Clinical presentation of JSLE

- The clinical manifestations of JSLE are extremely variable. They range from mild illness characterized by rash, fatigue, and joint pains to life-threatening organ involvement (Box 4.6)
- Symptoms may be incorrectly attributed to problems such as 'being a teenager', exam stress, anorexia nervosa, or chronic fatigue syndrome. Achievement of a diagnosis can be complicated by diagnostic features appearing intermittently and cumulatively over many months rather than in parallel.
- Significant delays have been reported in achieving a diagnosis of JSLE

Box 4.6 Presenting features of JSLE

- Constitutional (fever, malaise, weight loss): 40–74%
- Joint pains/arthritis: 20–74%
- Enlarged liver ± spleen: 15–74%
- Renal involvement: 20–82%
- Malar rash: 44–52%
- Lymphadenopathy: 15–30%

Multisystem presentation of JSLE

There is no single diagnostic test for JSLE, therefore diagnosis relies upon awareness and experience, comprehensive clinical assessment, judicious interpretation of investigations, and exclusion of other conditions. Individual patients can display different combinations of the following clinical features:

- Mucocutaneous—malar rash, vasculitic lesions, photosensitive rashes, nasal/oral ulcers, Raynaud's phenomenon, alopecia, discoid lesions.
- Systemic—fever, lethargy, weight loss, arthralgia.
- Arthritis (non-erosive).
- Renal—proteinuria, glomerulonephritis, hypertension, renal failure.
- GI tract: hepatosplenomegaly, autoimmune hepatitis, pancreatitis, diffuse abdominal pain, serositis, colitis, oesophageal dysmotility.
- Cardiopulmonary—pericarditis, myocarditis, pleuritis, interstitial lung disease, pulmonary haemorrhage.
- Neuropsychiatric—headache, migraine, seizures, depression, cognitive impairment, stroke, chorea, cranial and peripheral neuropathies.
- Haematological—anaemia, Coombs positivity, thrombocytopenia, leucopenia.
- Other—lymphadenopathy, ocular (e.g. uveitis, episcleritis, optic neuritis, retinopathy), antiphospholipid antibodies.

Diagnosis of JSLE

- The diagnosis of JSLE is based on a collection of clinical and laboratory features. The American College of Rheumatology (ACR) revised criteria for classification of SLE (Table 4.6) are frequently used for diagnosis and have been shown to be valid in JSLE:
  - The criteria were introduced for the purpose of clinical trials.
  - A person can be said to have SLE if any 4 or more of the 11 criteria are present, serially or simultaneously, during any interval.
  - The presence of 4 out of 11 gives 96% sensitivity and specificity for (adult-onset) SLE.
  - The criteria alone are not a pre-requisite for diagnosis or commencing treatment in patients where there is a high index of suspicion of JSLE. Many individuals with 1 or 2 features will develop others later on and may eventually fulfil the criteria.
- The ability to diagnose JSLE correctly may be challenging especially in those with an insidious onset of symptoms that are common in childhood such as joint pains and tiredness.
- Early referral to a clinician with experience and expertise of JSLE is important to allow prompt and correct diagnosis and the timely commencement of appropriate therapy to prevent long-term damage.
- The most common ACR criteria found in children are ANA positivity, arthritis, immunological disorder, haematological disorder, malar rash, and photosensitivity although many children present with or develop renal or neurological disease, even if not strictly meeting the ACR definitions outlined here.
- In 2012 the Systemic Lupus International Collaborating Clinics (SLICC) group revised and validated the ACR SLE classification criteria in order to improve clinical relevance.
  - According to the new SLICC criteria, the patient must satisfy at least 4 criteria, including at least one clinical criterion and one immunologic criterion *or* the patient must have biopsy proven lupus nephritis in the presence of antinuclear antibodies or anti–dsDNA antibodies (Table 4.7).
  - Criteria are cumulative and need not be present concurrently.
  - The SLICC classification criteria have also been validated in JSLE, performing better than the ACR criteria in terms of sensitivity and accuracy at the first visit, and within the first year of follow-up.
- The median time to achieving a diagnosis of JSLE has been reported to be 0.4 years (interquartile range 0.2–1.4 years), with some patients taking significantly longer (up to 14 years) highlighting the difficulties faced in achieving a diagnosis and access to care for JSLE patients.

Table 4.6 The ACR revised criteria for classification of SLE

Criteria	Definition
Malar rash	Fixed erythema, flat or raised, over malar eminences, tending to spare nasolabial folds
Discoid lupus	Erythematous raised patches of adherent keratotic scaling and follicular plugging. Atrophic scarring may be seen in older lesions
Photosensitivity	Skin rash as a result of unusual reaction to sunlight
Oral or nasal ulceration	Oral or nasopharyngeal ulcers, usually painless, observed by a physician
Non-erosive arthritis	Non-erosive arthritis involving 2 or more peripheral joints, characterized by tenderness, swelling, or effusion
Serositis	Pleuritis—pleuritic pain, rub heard or pleural effusion, or
	Pericarditis—documented by ECG or rub or pericardial effusion
Nephritis	Persistent proteinuria >0.5g/day or >3+, or:
	Cellular casts: red cell, haemoglobin, granular, tubular or mixed
Neurological	Seizures in the absence of offending drugs or metabolic derangement (e.g. uraemia, ketoacidosis, electrolyte imbalance), or
	Psychosis in the absence of offending drugs or metabolic derangement (e.g. uraemia, ketoacidosis, electrolyte imbalance)
Haematological	Haemolytic anaemia with reticulocytes, or
	Leucopenia <4000 per mm^3 on 2 or more occasions, or
	Lymphopenia <1500 per mm^3 on 2 or more occasions, or
	Thrombocytopenia <100,000 per mm^3 in absence of offending drugs
Immunological	Anti-DNA antibody, or
	Anti-Sm antibody, or
	Anti-phospholipid antibodies:
	(i) Abnormal anticardiolipin antibody IgG or IgM
	(ii) Positive lupus anticoagulant
	(iii) False positive for syphilis for >6 months
Anti-nuclear antibody	Abnormal titre of ANA at any point in absence of drugs known to be associated with drug-induced lupus

Table 4.7 The SLICC criteria for classification of SLE

Clinical criteria	Definition
1. Acute cutaneous lupus	Lupus malar rash (do not count if malar discoid)
	Bullous lupus
	Toxic epidermal necrolysis variant of SLE
	Maculopapular lupus rash
	Photosensitive lupus rash (in the absence of dermatomyositis)
	or
	Subacute cutaneous lupus—non-indurated psoriaform and/or annular polycyclic lesions that resolve without scarring, although occasionally with post-inflammatory dyspigmentation or telangiectasias
2. Chronic cutaneous lupus	Classic discoid rash
	Localized (above the neck)
	Generalized (above and below the neck)
	Hypertrophic (verrucous) lupus
	Lupus panniculitis (profundus)
	Mucosal lupus
	Lupus erythematosus tumidus
	Chillblains lupus
	Discoid lupus/lichen planus overlap
3. Oral ulcers *or* nasal ulcers	Palate, buccal, tongue (in the absence of other causes, such as vasculitis, Behcet's disease, infection (herpes virus), inflammatory bowel disease, reactive arthritis or acidic foods)
4. Non-scarring alopecia	Diffuse thinning or hair fragility with visible broken hairs in the absence of other causes such as alopecia areata, drugs, iron deficiency, or androgenic alopecia
5. Arthritis	Synovitis involving 2 or more joints, characterized by swelling or effusion *or*
	Tenderness in 2 or more joints and at least 30 minutes of morning stiffness
6. Serositis	Typical pleurisy for more than 1 day *or* pleural effusions *or* pleural rub
	Typical pericardial pain (pain with recumbency improved by sitting forward) for more than 1 day *or* pericardial effusion
	or pericardial rub *or* pericarditis by electrocardiography
	(in the absence of other causes such as infection, uremia, or Dressler's pericarditis)

Table 4.7 Contd.

Clinical criteria	Definition
7. Renal	Urine protein-to-creatinine ratio (or 24-hour urine protein) representing 500mg protein/24 hours or red blood cell casts
8. Neurologic	Seizures
	Psychosis
	Mononeuritis multiplex (in the absence of other known causes such as primary vasculitis)
	Myelitis
	Peripheral or cranial neuropathy (in the absence of other known causes such as primary vasculitis, infection or diabetes mellitus)
	Acute confusional state (in the absence of other causes, including toxic/metabolic, uremia, drugs)
9. Haemolytic anemia	
10. Leukopenia	< 4000/mm³ at least once, in the absence of other known causes such as Felty's syndrome, drugs, portal hypertension or
Lymphopenia	<1000/mm³ at least once, in the absence of other known causes such as corticosteroids, drugs, and infection
11. Thrombocytopenia	<100,000/mm3 at least once in the absence of other known causes such as drugs, portal hypertension, and thrombotic thrombocytopenic

Immunological criteria	Definition
1. ANA	Level above laboratory reference range
2. Anti-dsDNA antibody	Level above laboratory reference range (or >2-fold the reference range if tested by ELISA)
3. Anti-Sm	Presence of antibody to Sm nuclear antigen
4. Anti-phospholipid antibody	Positivity as determined by any of the following:
	Positive test result for lupus anticoagulant
	False-positive test result for rapid plasma reagin
	Medium- or high-titre anticardiolipin antibody level (IgA, IgG, or IgM)
	Positive test result for anti–β2-glycoprotein I (IgA, IgG, or IgM)
5. Low complement	Low C3
	Low C4
	Low CH50
6. Direct Coombs test	Positive in the absence of hemolytic anemia

Reproduced with permission from Petri M, Orbai AM, Alarcon GS et al. Derivation and validation of the Systemic Lupus International Collaborating Clinics classification criteria for systemic lupus erythematosus. *Arthritis & Rheumatology*, Volume 64, Issue 8, pp. 2677–2686, Copyright © 2012 John Wiley and Sons Ltd.

Further reading

Hochberg MC. Updating the American College of Rheumatology revised criteria for the classification of systemic lupus erythematosus. *Arth Rheum* 1997;**40**:1725.

Petri M, Orbai AM, Alarcón GS, et al. Derivation and validation of the Systemic Lupus International Collaborating Clinics classification criteria for systemic lupus erythematosus. *Arthritis Rheum* 2012;**64**(8):2677–86.

Sag E, Tartaglione A, Batu ED. Performance of the new SLICC classification criteria in childhood systemic lupus erythematosus: a multicentre study. *Clin Exp Rheumatol* 2014;**32**:440–4.

Fonseca AR, Gaspar-Elsas MI, Land MG et al. Comparison between three systems of classification criteria in juvenile systemic lupus erythematous. *Rheumatology (Oxford)* 2015;**54**:241–7.

Smith EM, Foster HE, Gray WK, et al. Predictors of access to care in juvenile systemic lupus erythematosus: evidence from the UK JSLE Cohort Study. *Rheumatology (Oxford)* 2014;**53**(3):557–61.

Assessment of the child with JSLE and monitoring of disease activity

Assessing disease severity and monitoring outcome

Optimizing disease control depends on assessing disease activity. The complexity and variability of paediatric lupus makes this difficult. There is no single 'gold standard' biological marker that accurately reflects this. In the assessment of the child with JSLE it is important to determine the following aspects of their disease across all organ systems:

- Disease activity—potentially reversible with correct therapy.
- Organ damage—reversible or irreversible.
- Effect of lupus on the patient's quality of life (QoL).
- Concurrent pathology, e.g. infection, drug side-effects, disease complications, concomitant conditions.

Clinical approach to assessment

Careful multisystem assessment must be carried out at each clinical visit:

- *History*—detailed multi-system symptom enquiry including effect of disease on social and psychological functioning. Enquire about fatigue.
- *Examination*—cardiovascular including BP, respiratory, abdominal, mucocutaneous, musculoskeletal, and neurological. Growth, pubertal staging, and development.
- Disease activity score assessment: see Box 4.7.
- SLICC/ACR damage index (at least annually): see Box 4.7.

Investigations

Routinely at each review, e.g. 3-monthly or more frequently if unwell

- *FBC*—decreased Hb (anaemia of chronic disease or autoimmune anaemia), decreased WCC (lymphopenia +/- neutropenia), increased WCC (suggests infection or response to corticosteroids), decreased lymphocytes (due to disease or immunosuppression), decreased platelets (autoimmune, due to peripheral destruction or as a complication of drug therapy).
- *NB*: consider macrophage activation syndrome (see ➋ MAS, pp. 321–4) if increasing pancytopenia in sick patient.
- Increased *ESR* (if sudden drop in ESR in sick patient, consider MAS).
- *Urinalysis*—protein or blood in renal involvement. If protein present need quantitative measure such as spot urinary albumin creatinine ratio (UACR) or protein creatinine ratio (UPCR) on an early morning urine sample (to exclude orthostatic proteinuria).
- *Urine MC&S*—presence of casts, WCC, RBC, organisms.
- *U&Es, LFTs, bone profile, and glucose* (consider amylase and lipase in presence of abdominal pain).
- *CRP*—if increased consider infection. Other causes of raised CRP in the context of SLE include serositis and polyarthritis.
- *Complement*—decreased C3 and C4, levels correlate with disease activity.

Box 4.7 JSLE assessment tools

There are several assessment tools available which can be used serially in the clinical setting or in clinical studies/trials to assess response and outcome and allow comparison of therapies.

Lupus disease activity measures
- BILAG (British Isles Lupus Assessment Group)
- SLEDAI (SLE Disease Activity Index)
- SLAM (Systemic Lupus Activity Measure)
- ECLAM (European Community Lupus Activity Measure)

Most widely used are the BILAG and SLEDAI.

Assessment of damage
- The SLICC/ACR damage index (Systemic Lupus International Cooperating Clinics/American College of Rheumatology).

Function and QoL
- Neither the SLEDAI, BILAG, nor SLICC/ACR measure health-related QoL, degree of disability, or impact of disease.
- The Childhood Health Questionnaire (CHQ) and SF36 can be useful in assessing general health and well-being. Specific JSLE-related QoL tools are also being developed (e.g. LupusQoL).
- The CHAQ (Childhood Health Assessment Questionnaire) measures function and includes a visual analogue scale (VAS) for pain and general evaluation of disease.

- *Immunoglobulins*—increased in acute inflammation.
- *ds-DNA*—possible direct pathogenic role and titres are measure of disease activity. Serial measurements of anti-C1q also marker of disease activity particularly renal disease but test not widely available.

At initial assessment then annually
(*Denotes investigations to perform more frequently in sick patients.)
- *Clotting screen** (prolonged in APLS and MAS), *fibrinogen** (increased in acute inflammation, decreased in MAS).
- *Coombs**—positive in autoimmune haemolytic anaemia.
- *Lupus anticoagulant and anticardiolipin IgG and IgM*—see ➔ APLS, pp. 293–6.
- *TFTs** and thyroid antibodies.
- *Lipid profile** (dyslipidaemia increased risk of cardiovascular events; increased TGs in MAS).
- *Vitamin D levels.*
- *ANA* (positive in 95% of SLE), *dsDNA* (positive in 60%), *ENAs*—most common include anti-Ro, anti-La associated with neonatal lupus syndromes, anti-Sm (anti-'Smith', not 'smooth muscle' as often erroneously assumed) associated with renal involvement.
- *Immunity status*—e.g. measles and varicella IgG.

Further systems investigation should be undertaken when appropriate
for select individuals with any disease flare or annual monitoring of progress
depending on previous involvement.

- Renal biopsy.
- ECG, echocardiogram, visceral angiogram, MRA.
- CXR, pulmonary function tests including transfer factor, CT chest.
- Renal USS, renal biopsy, measurement of GFR.
- MRI brain, MRA brain, EEG, psychometric testing.
- Abdominal USS, upper and lower GI endoscopy.
- Bone mineral density scan (DEXA) for those at risk from osteoporosis.
- Skin biopsy.
- Ophthalmology assessment.
- Infection screen, e.g. viral serology, urine MC&S, blood cultures, lumbar puncture, stool MC&S, and virology.

Further reading

Gutierrez-Suarez R, Ruperto N, Gastaldi R et al. A proposal for a pediatric version of the Systemic Lupus International Collaborating Clinics/American College of Rheumatology Damage Index based on the analysis of 1,015 patients with juvenile-onset systemic lupus erythematosus. *Arthritis Rheum* 2006; 54:2989–96.

Haq I, Isenberg DA. How does one assess and monitor patients with systemic lupus erythematosus in daily clinical practice? *Best Pract Res* 2002;16:181–94.

Morgan T, Watson L, McCann LJ, Beresford MW. Children and adolescents with SLE: not just little adults. *Lupus* S013;22(12):1309–19.

JSLE: approach to management

(Also see ➲ Lupus nephritis, pp. 251–4, and chapter on B-cell depletion.)

General principles

- Management of JSLE requires full MDT engagement by professionals experienced in paediatric rheumatology including prompt liaison with other specialists as dictated by disease manifestations.
- As the survival rates for JSLE improve, the late complications of both disease and therapy should be recognized and addressed, such as premature atherosclerosis (Box 4.8), osteoporosis, neurocognitive impairment, and potentially increased risk of malignancy.
- *Early and aggressive therapy* is key for treatment of JSLE to improve outcome and function and reduce organ damage.
- Management should be individualized taking into account patient preference, tolerance of drugs, and disease presentation. Care should be taken to explore the burden of disease and treatment on QoL, education, physical and emotional development. This should improve patient care and adherence.

Evidence base for management of JSLE

- Paucity of robust epidemiological, clinical cohort studies, and clinical trial data in JSLE hamper evidence-based management of JSLE. To date, no large randomized comparative trials have been published in JSLE, so treatment regimens are based primarily on observational cohort studies and adult data (Box 4.9).
- International organizations (e.g. PRINTO, CARRA) and national, collaborative research groups, such as the UK JSLE Study Group, seek to improve the evidence base.

Box 4.8 Premature atherosclerosis

- Leads to marked morbidity in young adults—risk to women with SLE of myocardial infarction (MI) or stroke 6–9× that of healthy controls and MI rate of 8% observed in 24–43yr-olds who developed SLE in childhood.
- Risk factors relate to JSLE itself and its treatment—obesity, smoking, insulin resistance, increased BP, renal disease, dyslipidaemia, inflammation, APLS, vascular disease, and corticosteroid use. Other as yet undefined non-conventional cardiovascular risk factors arising from SLE and its treatment are areas of ongoing study.
- Prevention in JSLE needs to begin in childhood—importance of modifying risk factors, and potential use of statins in JSLE. Atorvastatin use in JSLE has been shown to significantly reduce cholesterol and LDL levels, with a non-significant trend towards reducing carotid intima medial thickness (CIMT) progression rates.
- Use of *hydroxycholoroquine (HCQ)* has been associated with reductions in cholesterol and apolipoprotein B levels in JSLE, and lower vascular event frequency in adult SLE.

Box 4.9 UK JSLE Cohort Study & Repository

Established by the UK JSLE Study Group (𝓡 http://www.liv.ac.uk/ukjsle/index.htm), the study consists of a comprehensive, prospective clinical data set from patients with JSLE from across the UK. The aims of the UK JSLE Cohort Study & Repository include:

• To determine the demographics of JSLE across the UK and to investigate the clinical characteristics of disease presentation, activity, damage, and response to therapy for a national cohort of JSLE patients.

• To undertake comparative studies with other national lupus cohorts.

• Develop a cohort of patients suitable for recruitment to clinical interventional trials in JSLE.

• Facilitate international collaborative studies and trials in JSLE.

• Multinational collaborative paediatric research is essential to define the efficacy and safety of therapies to improve care for JSLE patients.

• Important data from adult studies can help; they may have larger cohorts including patients developing SLE in childhood; however, determining the efficacy and safety within a paediatric population of new and existing therapies is critical.

General management of JSLE

• UV light—advise sun avoidance and prescribe sun block factor 50–60 to reduce flares and photosensitive rashes.

• Vaccination—increased risk of infection in JSLE due to drug therapies and JSLE-associated immune dysfunction. All routine immunizations advised plus pneumococcal and influenza. NB Live vaccines contraindicated if on significant immunosuppression.

• Bone health—ensure adequate dietary intake of calcium and vitamin D. Discourage inactivity. Assess bone density regularly and treat osteoporosis if present.

Corticosteroids in JSLE

• Corticosteroids are needed initially in all but very mild cases to provide rapid control of inflammation but are associated with numerous side-effects (osteoporosis, growth retardation, obesity, Cushingoid facies, cataracts, impaired glucose tolerance) and are a risk factor for damage.

• Prednisolone used as oral therapy (1–2mg/kg initially then tapered). In control of acute flares and at induction high-dose pulsed IVMP may be required (e.g. 30mg/kg on 3 consecutive days) and repeated as according to response, followed by tapering oral steroids. Weekly pulsed IVMP (e.g. 30mg/kg/day for 4–6 weeks), followed by tapering of oral steroids may also be needed. Oral prednisolone may not be absorbed in gut involvement.

• Steroid-sparing immunosuppressive therapy is started early to allow rapid tapering of steroids as clinical response dictates, with the aim to minimize steroid toxicity. Steroid free DMARD based induction regimens are increasingly being considered and examined in clinical trials.

Disease-modifying drugs in JSLE

(see ➜ JSLE: renal involvement, pp. 251–4 and ➜ BSPAR guidelines for treatments used in paediatric rheumatology, p. 472)

Choice of DMARDs in JSLE varies with clinician as evidence of superiority is lacking. Multiple DMARDs may be required in refractory disease.

HCQ e.g. 5–6.5mg/kg/day once a day can be given (maximum 400mg/day)
- Advised in all patients unless contraindicated. Adult studies indicate disease-modifying role; particularly useful for skin and joint disease; some patients can be managed with HCQ and low-dose corticosteroids only.

Azathioprine (AZA) (e.g. start at 1mg/kg/day, increase in increments up to a maximum of 3mg/kg/day)
- Traditionally the 1st-line steroid-sparing DMARD in moderate disease. Side effects uncommon but include nausea, fatigue, hair loss, and bone marrow suppression.

Mycophenolate mofetil (MMF): (e.g. 10–20mg/kg/day per dose twice daily; or 600mg/m² per dose twice daily)
- Increasingly used as induction and/or maintenance of remission therapy in all but mild disease.
- The adult ALMS trial has shown MMF to be as effective but less toxic than cyclophosphamide in the induction phase of lupus nephritis management (class III/IV, see ➜ Lupus nephritis, p. 472), and superior to AZA as maintenance therapy.
- In contrast, the adult MAINTAIN Lupus nephritis trial showed MMF and AZA to be equivalent maintenance treatments.
- Increasingly, however, many clinicians are using MMF before AZA due to anecdotal evidence of increased efficacy and tolerability of MMF.
- Published data from the JSLE population is limited, although it offers a significant therapeutic opportunity.
- It is steroid-sparing, improves renal function, and reduces disease activity in JSLE.
- Relatively well-tolerated, main side-effect is GI upset which can be minimized by slow introduction.

Cyclophosphamide (CYC) (e.g. monthly pulsed IV CYC of 500–1000mg/m² [maximum dose 1.2g for 3–6 months)
- 'Gold standard' until recently as induction agent for major organ involvement or life-threatening lupus together with pulsed IVMP.
- Marked side-effect profile including bone marrow suppression, gonadal suppression, hair loss, haemorrhagic cystitis, and late malignancy.
- IV CYC considered superior to oral CYC (safer therapeutic index).
- More recently, an alternative approach using lower cumulative doses of IV CYC (300–500mg/m², maximum dose 500mg, given every 2 weeks for 6 doses), the so-called 'Eurolupus protocol' have been proposed for induction of remission of JSLE.

Biologic therapies in JSLE (see chapter on B cell depletion)
- The advent of biological therapies offers a major therapeutic advance in the management of JSLE. To date, rituximab, a B-cell depletor has

demonstrated evidence of efficacy in JSLE in retrospective studies and case series. Two randomized controlled trials assessing rituximab in adult SLE have failed to reach their primary and secondary endpoints.

- Belimumab is a fully humanized monoclonal antibody that binds soluble BAFF and prevents it from binding to its receptors. Two adult SLE trials assessing belimumab alongside standard therapy have demonstrated a significant response to treatment (BLISS-52, BLISS-76). A paediatric trial of belimumab treatment alongside standard therapy is on-going (PLUTO trial).
- Further details on rituximab and belimumab are provided in the separate section on B cell depletion therapy in SLE (➔ pp. 256–61). Both treatments should be given under expert advice only.

Anti-phospholipid syndrome

- If positive anticardiolipin Ab or lupus anticoagulant on 2 occasions 3 months apart commence *low-dose aspirin* to prevent thrombotic events.

Other therapies used in refractory JSLE

- Methotrexate (skin and joint disease), ciclosporin (lupus nephritis, particularly for membranous nephritis, Class V), infliximab, IVIg.

Treatment of severe refractory lupus

- *Plasma-exchange*—anecdotal evidence of efficacy in severe refractory lupus with theoretical benefit associated with removal of immune complexes, autoantibodies and other immune mediators (e.g. cytokines).
- *Haematopoietic stem cell transplantation (autologous and allogeneic stem cell transplant, see ➔ Haematopoietic stem cell transplantation, pp. 461–4)*—successfully used in severe refractory disease. Associated with significant mortality rate so only considered in those with severe disease who have failed conventional therapies.

Further reading

Appel GB, Contreras G, Dooley MA, et al. Mycophenolate mofetil versus cyclophosphamide for induction treatment of lupus nephritis. J Am Soc Nephrol 2009;20:1103–1112.

Dooley MA, Jayne D, Ginzler EM, et al. Mycophenolate versus azathioprine as maintenance therapy for lupus nephritis. N Engl J Med 2011;365:1886–1895.

Houssiau FA, D'Cruz D, Sangle S, et al. Azathioprine versus mycophenolate mofetil for long-term immunosuppression in lupus nephritis: results from the MAINTAIN nephritis trial. Ann Rheum Dis 2010;69:2083–2089.

Morgan T, Watson L, McCann LJ, Beresford MW. Children and adolescents with SLE: not just little adults. Lupus. 2013;22(12):1309–1319

JSLE: renal involvement

Introduction

- Renal disease is a major determinant of the long-term outcome of SLE:
  - Present in 60–80% of JSLE cases.
  - Influences management with immunosuppressive agents.
  - Earlier and more severe presentation in patients with JSLE (compared to adult-onset) SLE.
- Presentation of renal involvement:
  - Proteinuria.
  - Microscopic (and rarely macroscopic) haematuria.
  - Nephrotic syndrome.
  - Hypertension.
  - Evidence of renal dysfunction—elevated plasma creatinine or reduced estimated GFR.
- Histopathology of renal involvement with lupus nephritis (LN) cannot be accurately predicted from clinical and serological markers:
  - Renal biopsy is undertaken if deteriorating renal function, significant proteinuria, haematuria or hypertension, or to delineate thrombotic microangiopathy.

Investigations

All JSLE patients should be monitored at least every 3 months for evidence of LN:
- BP measurement.
- Early morning urinary dipstick test.
- Early morning urine albumin:creatinine ratio (or protein:creatinine ratio).
- Consideration of 24h urine collection in adolescent children.
- Markers of renal function (plasma creatinine, estimated GFR, and serum albumin).
- Routine lupus immunological tests.

Histopathology

Classification of LN facilitates clinical management (in guiding treatment and conducting RCTs of therapeutic agents) as well as communication between pathologists and scientists. It standardizes definitions with uniform and reproducible reporting between centres.

The original World Health Organization classification of LN was developed in 1974–1975, and modified in 1982 and 1995 with the current histopathological classification reported by the International Society of Nephrology/Renal Pathology Society working group in 2003 (Fig. 4.11):
- ISN/RPS Class I LN = minimal mesangial LN.
- ISN/RPS Class II LN = mesangial proliferative LN.
- ISN/RPS Class III LN = focal lupus nephritis, subdivided into:
  - III (A) active focal proliferative LN.
  - III (A/C) active and sclerotic focal proliferative LN.
  - III (C) inactive sclerotic focal lupus nephritis.
- ISN/RPS Class IV LN = diffuse segmental (IV-S) or global (IV-G):
  - See Figs. 4.12 and 4.13.
  - IV (A) active diffuse segmental or global proliferative LN.

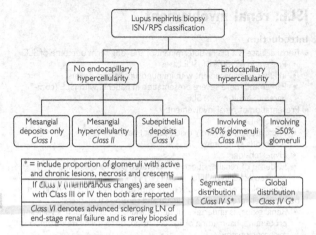

Fig. 4.11 Summary of International Society of Nephrology/Renal Pathology Society classification of lupus nephritis.

- IV (A/C) diffuse segmental or global proliferative and sclerotic.
- IV (C) diffuse segmental or global sclerotic lupus nephritis.
- ISN/RPS Class V LN = diffuse membranous LN:
  - Class III and Class V changes are reported as Class III + V.
  - Class IV and Class V changes are reported as Class IV + V.
- ISN/RPS Class VI LN = advanced sclerotic LN.
- This classification has been validated in JSLE.

Treatment

- The aim of treatment is to induce remission while minimizing side-effects (including infectious complications) and flares of disease activity in order to improve patient morbidity and mortality.
- Once induction of remission to gain control of disease activity is achieved then maintenance therapy is utilized to maintain disease control and minimize therapy related toxicity, including corticosteroid exposure.
- However, due to the increasing use of MMF instead of IV CYC for induction of remission, many clinicians are utilizing MMF for both induction and maintenance phases.
- *ISN Class I and II LN*:
  - The same therapy is employed for those with mild to moderate SLE without LN and may include azathioprine therapy (see ➜ JSLE: non-renal involvement, p. 238).
- *ISN Class III, IV and V LN*:
  - MMF as 1st-line treatment is a safe and efficacious therapy for SLE and LN but can cause more diarrhoea despite less overall side effects than CYC.

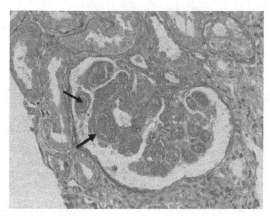

Fig. 4.12 ISN/RPS Class IV LN (PAS stain, original magnification ×250). Wire loop lesion (denoted by lower arrow) and hyaline droplet (upper arrow) change representing massive subendothelial deposits when seen on light microscopy (also see color plate).

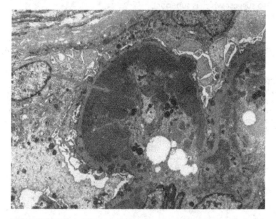

Fig. 4.13 ISN/RPS Class IV LN (electron microscopy). Massive subendothelial deposit corresponding to a wire-loop lesion (see arrow).

- IV CYC may be reserved for patients with severe multisystem disease activity or with poor adherence to oral therapy but is associated with more nausea and vomiting.
- The Aspreva Lupus Management Study (ALMS) showed no difference in response rate in adults with ISN/RPS Class III, IV and V who were randomized to MMF or iv CYC in a 24-week induction study:
  —56% and 53% responded to MMF and IV CYC respectively.
  —No significant differences in rates of adverse events, including infections.
- Plasmapheresis should be considered for children with rapidly progressive crescentic glomerulonephritis (as well as cerebral vasculitis or pulmonary haemorrhage).
- B cell depletion with IV rituximab has been shown to be useful for JSLE patients with severe renal and non-renal disease activity as well as refractory disease, although its use is not yet supported with RCT data (see ❶ B-cell depletion therapy, pp. 256–61).
- *ISN Class VI*
  - The current classification of advanced sclerotic LN implies end-stage renal failure (CKD5) management with renal replacement therapy, although immunosuppressive therapies may be utilized to treat or avoid further non-renal flares of disease activity.
- Maintenance therapy of LN:
  - Oral prednisolone 10–15mg alternate days (where possible; some prefer lower doses of daily prednisolone and there are no hard data to suggest which is superior).
  - Oral hydroxychloroquine 4–6mg/kg/day (maximum dose 400mg/day).
  - Oral AZA 2–3mg/kg once daily, or
  - Oral MMF 300–600mg/m^2/dose twice daily (usual maximum dose of 2g/day although occasionally 3g/day has been used).

Further reading

Appel G, Contreras G, Dooley MA, et al. Mycophenolate mofetil versus cyclophosphamide for induction treatment of lupus nephritis. *J Am Soc Nephrol* 2009; 20:1103–12.

Weening JJ, D'Agati VD, Schwartz MM, et al. The classification of glomerulonephritis in systemic lupus erythematosus revisited. *Kidney Int* 2004; 65:521–30.

Madhok R. Systemic lupus erythematosus: lupus nephritis. *Clinical Evidence* 2015;12:1123 .

Neonatal lupus syndrome

- Autoimmune disease associated with transplacental passage of maternal auto-antibodies (autoAbs) to SSA/Ro and SSB/La antigens from mothers with diseases such as SLE and Sjogren's syndrome.
- Risk of an infant developing NLS in positive mother is 2%
- Risk to subsequent pregnancy is 25%.

Clinical features

Simultaneous involvement of more than two organ systems is uncommon:

- *Skin*—subacute cutaneous lupus-like lesions which can vary including confluent, scaly, periorbital erythema, or erythematous infiltrated plaques with central vesicles and lesions resembling seborrheic eczema or fungal infection and telangiectasia. Skin changes may be present at birth and usually appear within 4–6 weeks of age. Lesions usually appear on sun-exposed areas but can also affect the trunk and extremities.
- *Cardiac*—congenital heart block, cardiomyopathy, prolonged QT interval, sinus bradycardia, cardiac malformations.
- *Hepatobiliary*—elevation in transaminases, cholestasis, fulminant liver failure.
- *Haematological*—thrombocytopenia and less commonly other cytopenias.
- *Neurological*—hydrocephalus and non-specific white matter changes have been reported.

Investigation

- Diagnosis is made by identifying relevant clinical features with positive NLS-associated antibodies in maternal or neonatal serum.
- Skin biopsy may be useful if diagnosis unclear.

Management

- Careful *in utero* and postnatal monitoring of at-risk pregnancies is important to ensure appropriate treatment (serial fetal echo; postnatal ECG).
- Use of maternal fluorinated corticosteroids (dexamethasone or beclamethasone) which cross the placenta may prevent progression of incomplete heart block.
- Infants with cardiac disease may need cardiac pacing.
- Skin lesions can be treated with sun avoidance, sun block, and topical corticosteroids.

Prognosis

- Skin, hepatic, and haematological manifestations tend to resolve spontaneously as maternal autoantibodies disappear from the infant's circulation; complete heart block and cardiomyopathy can be life threatening.
- Affected infants may be at ↑ risk of subsequent autoimmune disease.

Further reading

Lee LA. The clinical spectrum of neonatal lupus. *Arch Dermatol Res* 2009; **301**:107–10.
Pain C, Beresford MW. Neonatal lupus syndrome. *Paediatr Child Health* 2007; **17**:223–7.

B-cell-targeted therapies for systemic lupus erythematosus

Why target B cells in SLE?

- A minority of patients with SLE will not have a sufficient clinical response to the current conventional treatment with MMF, IV CYC, AZA, and corticosteroids.
- In these cases there continues to be clinical and laboratory symptoms and signs of active disease of such a degree that alternative approaches to treatment would be preferable.
- B cells have critical roles in the pathogenesis of SLE, including cytokine production, presentation of self-antigen, T-cell activation, and (indirectly via plasma cells) autoantibody production.
- Several clinical trials have reported different approaches for the induction of remission in adults with SLE by targeting B cells.

Types of B-cell-targeted therapy

- Currently tested B-cell-targeted therapies include rituximab, ocrelizumab, belimumab, epratuzumab, atacicept, blisibimod, and tabalumab. The mechanisms of action of these agents are summarized in Table 4.8.
- Rituximab is currently not licensed for the treatment of SLE. In the UK it is reimbursable by NHS England for treatment of adults if strict criteria are met.
- The vast majority of the paediatric SLE experience to date is only with rituximab, with little or no data on the role of other agents in paediatric patients.
- Rituximab should only be used in conjunction with expert advice and in children with SLE resistant to standard therapy; in rare circumstances, rituximab may be considered for primary induction of remission.
- There is ongoing controversy as to whether rituximab should be given with IV CYC for 'synergistic' B-cell depletion or not, and what immunosuppression to follow rituximab therapy with.
- In 2011, belimumab became the first drug in 50 years to be licensed (by the FDA and EMA) for the treatment of adults with SLE.
  - Belimumab is approved for SLE with the exception of patients with active lupus nephritis or CNS disease.

Clinical trials of B-cell-targeted therapies in adults with SLE

- Several important prospective RCTs of B cell-targeted therapy have been reported in adults (summarized in Table 4.9), with mixed and perhaps (to many) surprising results.
  - Both rituximab trials (EXPLORER and LUNAR) reported negative results.
  - Both belimumab trials reported positive results.

Table 4.8 Different types of B cell-targeted therapy

Drug name	B cell target	Proposed mechanism of efficacy
Rituximab (see ➔ pp. 504–5 guidelines)	Chimeric (mouse-human) monoclonal antibody which binds specifically to the CD20 antigen located on pre-B and mature B lymphocytes, thus mediating B-cell lysis. CD20 is not expressed on plasma cells	Depletion of peripheral blood B cells, with little or no ↓ in serum immunoglobulin because plasma cells are spared Efficacy thought to be the result of autoantibody independent effects of B cell depletion including reduced self-antigen presentation, reduced cytokine production and ↓ T-cell activation
Ocrelizumab	Fully human monoclonal antibody against CD20	Same as rituximab
Belimumab	Fully human monoclonal antibody against BAFF (B-cell activating factor, also referred to as B-lymphocyte stimulator, BLyS). BAFF (and another related molecule called APRIL) are produced mainly by cells of the innate immune system, and promote B cell survival and differentiation	BAFF levels are ↑ in SLE and correlate with disease activity-blocking BAFF therefore reduces pathological B-cell survival and differentiation
Epratuzumab	Fully human monoclonal antibody against CD 22, a B-cell surface antigen involved in the regulation of signalling	B-cell depletion so similar in action to rituximab
Atacicept	Chimeric molecule with a region which binds both BAFF and APRIL, fused to the constant region of human IgG1	Has a dramatic inhibitory effect on plasma cells hence reduces autoantibodies but also reduces immunoglobin—very high rate of infections reported in early trials
Blisibimod	Anti-BAFF monoclonal antibody	Decreases B cell survival by binding to BAFF and inhibiting its binding to BAFF receptors
Tabalumab	Anti-BAFF monoclonal antibody	Same mechanism as blisibimod. Recently, tabalumab failed to meet primary endpoints in two SLE clinical trials

Table 4.9 Summary of RCTs (Phase III) of B-cell-targeted therapy in SLE

Trial name	Description	Design	Primary end point	Result	Adverse events
EXPLORER	The Exploratory Phase II/III SLE Evaluation of Rituximab; Non-renal lupus trial	Double blind RCT; n=257 all receiving PRED, and 1 of AZA, MMF, or MTX. Patients were randomized 2:1 to receive RTX or placebo. Moderate and severe LN or CNS lupus excluded	Pre-defined improvement in BILAG score	No differences between placebo and RTX groups in the 1° endpoint. Serological improvement not observed in RTX group	Safety and tolerability were similar in patients receiving RTX and those receiving placebo
LUNAR	Lupus Nephritis Assessment with Rituximab	Double blind RCT; RTX or placebo was added onto standard therapy with MMF and high-dose corticosteroids; n=144. 1:1 randomization. Active class III or IV LN included; CNS lupus excluded	Proportion of patients who obtained a pre-defined renal response at 52 weeks: either CRR, PRR, or NR	No difference between RTX and placebo groups. Serological improvement not observed in RTX group	More severe neutropenia (3.6% RTX vs 0% placebo); and non-serious herpes virus infections (15% RTX vs 8% placebo); 4 episodes of serum sickness occurred in the RTX group
BLISS-52	Belimumab International SLE study 52 week follow-up	Double blind RCT; n= 865;standard care (corticosteroids and other immunosuppressant) plus either placebo or belimumab 1mg/kg, or 10mg/kg given at days 0, 14, 28, and every 28 days until week 52. Severe LN and active CNS lupus excluded	Improvement at week 52 in SRI, and no worsening of physician global assessment score or BILAG	Reduced disease activity and ↑ time to flare for both the low- and high-dose belimumab groups compared with placebo at week 52	No difference in adverse events between placebo and belimumab groups with the exception of infusion reactions
BLISS-76	Belimumab International SLE study 76 week follow-up	Second phase III RCT of belimumab; identical study design as BLISS-52; only difference is that blinding and follow-up remain for an additional 24 weeks		Reduced disease activity and ↑ time to flare in the high dose belimumab group only, compared with placebo at week 52. Week 76 results not yet reported	As per BLISS-52

AZA: azathioprine; BILAG: British Isles Lupus Assessment Group score; CNS: central nervous system; CRR: complete renal response; LN: lupus nephritis; MTX: methotrexate; PRED: prednisone; PRR: partial renal response; MMF: mycophenolate mofetil; NR: non-response; RCT: randomized controlled trial; RTX: rituximab; SRI: SLE-response index.

- Methodological aspects of the clinical trials of rituximab could explain the 'unexpected' negative results of the EXPLORER and LUNAR trials despite early reported open label success in those with SLE resistant to conventional therapy (including children). Possible reasons include:
  - Improvements in the standard care limb of these trials: MMF in place of IV CYC which may result in a higher than anticipated response rate thus reducing the power of the study.
  - High corticosteroid doses in both the experimental and standard limbs of the trials.
  - Overly optimistic primary endpoints and sensitive cut-offs for non-response.
  - Patient heterogeneity including the fact that some patients with minimal disease activity were included in these trials.
  - The EXPLORER and LUNAR trials do not answer the question relating to efficacy of rituximab for those with SLE resistant to standard induction therapy.
- The RITUXILUP trial of rituximab and mycophenolate mofetil with corticosteroid minimizing regimen is ongoing (and includes children and adults).
- Epratuzumab is currently in a phase III trial of moderate-to-severe SLE (EMBODY).
- Belimumab is currently being studied in a phase II trial for lupus nephritis (BLISS-LN).
- Blisibimod is currently in phase III studies in SLE patients with and without lupus nephritis.

The use of rituximab in paediatric SLE

- Given the negative trial data for rituximab, albeit with positive retrospective clinical experience with this therapy in children with SLE resistant to standard therapy, rituximab should only be given upon expert advice.
- In rare circumstances, rituximab can be considered for primary induction of remission—suggest under expert advice only.
- Adding to the complexity is the still ongoing controversy as to whether rituximab should be given with IV CYC for 'synergistic' B-cell depletion or not, and what immunosuppression to follow rituximab therapy with.
  - Data suggest that B-cell activation in SLE makes these cells more resistant to antibody-mediated cell killing from agents such as rituximab, providing an (unproven) argument for combining rituximab with cyclophosphamide.
  - At the time of writing there are no data to provide firm recommendations on these issues.
  - Treat each case on an individual basis.

Patient selection criteria

- Severe active lupus previously treated with standard lupus treatment either IV CYC or MMF for a minimum of 6 months, or
- As add on to standard induction therapy for those with severe life-threatening disease—little available evidence of its efficacy in this context.
- No known severe reaction to humanized chimeric antibodies.

Exclusion criteria
- Chronic active infection.
- Recent severe infection.
- Pregnancy or planned pregnancy.

Rituximab treatment protocol

Rituximab may be given in addition to cyclophosphamide (see above), except where cumulative cyclophosphamide toxicity, side-effects, or other clinical contraindication preclude this. A suggested protocol is given (also see Guidelines ⊃ pp. 504–5):

Day 1 and day 15
- Rituximab infusion 750mg/m² (rounded up to the nearest 100mg). Max. dose: 1g.
- Pre-medicate with chlorphenamine (5–10mg) and paracetamol (15mg/kg) *1h prior* to the rituximab infusion.
- In addition a dose of methylprednisolone IV 100mg (absolute dose, not per kg) is given *immediately prior* to the rituximab infusion.
- This is followed with oral prednisolone for 3 days after the infusion: 30mg, 20mg, and 10mg (i.e. days 2, 3, & 4 & days 16, 17, & 18), and then with the patient's previous maintenance prednisolone dose.

Day 2 and day 16
- *Cyclophosphamide infusion* 375mg/m² as per infusion protocol (see ⊃ pp. 485–9).

Administration of rituximab: practical aspects
- Dilute the required dose with sodium chloride 0.9% or glucose 5% to a final concentration of 1–4mg/mL.
- The initial infusion rate is 25mg/h, which can be ↑ by increments of 25mg/h every 30min up to a maximum of 200mg/h as tolerated.

Rituximab: side-effects
- Serum sickness: fevers and rigors, which usually present within the first 2h. Other reported symptoms include pruritis and rashes, dyspnoea, bronchospasm, angio-oedema, and transient hypotension.
  - In the event of an infusion-related adverse event, stop the infusion and recommence at half the previous rate once the symptoms have resolved.
  - Premedication with chlorphenamine, paracetamol, and methylprednisolone will reduce the incidence of adverse effects.
- Infections:
  - Herpes zoster infection described in children.
  - Progressive multifocal leucoencephalopathy caused by JC virus (a polyoma virus).
- Rituximab associated neutropenia—occurring usually several months following the administration of rituximab:
  - Usually not clinically significant and is self-limited but should be differentiated with neutropenia from other cause such as active SLE.
  - Mechanism remains largely speculative.

Follow-up post rituximab

Follow-up carefully with:

- Clinical status.
- FBC including diff, ESR, CRP, U&Es, and LFTs; UA:UC (minimum of fortnightly FBC for 6 weeks then monthly).
- ANA, doubled-stranded DNA, C3, C4.
- Screen for B-cell response and hypoagammaglobulinaemia (see Table 4.10). The use of replacement immunoglobulin in deficient patients is not standard practice at this stage, but will be continually monitored. The decision to commence IVIg replacement will be decided on an individual basis and will depend on the findings of hypogammaglobulinaemia and/or the occurrence and nature of infections.

Immune monitoring (Table 4.10) is recommended.

Table 4.10 Monitoring rituximab treatment in patients with SLE

Test	Timing (after 1ˢᵗ dose)	Notes
Lymphocyte subsets	- Days 7–10 - Monthly from 4 months after first dose until B cells normal	Measures T, B (CD19), and NK cells. Must do FBC same day
Immunoglobulins GAM	- Days 7–10 - 2 months after first dose - Monthly from 4 months after first dose until B cells normal	

Note: B cells express CD19 and CD20, and it is routine to measure CD19 as a B-cell marker. Rarely (normally in the context of malignancy) B cells may not express CD20 and will not therefore be eliminated by rituximab. If there is concern that B cells are not eradicated after 7–10 days, routine B cell measurement should be repeated and direct measurement of CD20 may be helpful. This will rarely be required.

Repeat rituximab dosing

- Repeated doses of rituximab are only recommended for those with evidence of return of disease activity after return of peripheral blood lymphocytes.
- Hypersensitivity reactions such as serum sickness and anaphylaxis may be of increasing concern for those re-treated with rituximab.

Further reading

Podolskaya A, Stadermann M, Pilkington C, et al. B cell depletion therapy for 19 patients with refractory systemic lupus erythematosus. Arch Dis Child 2008;93:401–6.
Jordan N et al. Progress with the use of monoclonal antibodies for the treatment of systemic lupus erythematosus. Immunotherapy 2015; 7:255–70.

British Isles Lupus Assessment Group (BILAG) 2004 Index

The BILAG Index is a measure of disease activity developed initially for adult-onset SLE using nominal consensus approach and modified several times to improve its validity and reliability (Table 4.10). It is increasingly used in clinical trials in SLE. Across 9 domains, clinicians indicate whether each parameter is:

• Not present, 0.
• Improving, 1.
• Same, 2.
• Worse, 3 or
• New, 4.

Scoring refers to manifestations present in the last 4 weeks compared to the previous 4 weeks and to features attributable to SLE disease activity and not due to damage, drugs, or infection. For detailed descriptions of definitions of manifestations, see ➋ BILAG 2004 glossary (Table 4.11).

The BILAG rests on the principle of the physicians' intent-to-treat in assigning scores A–E:

• A = Disease necessitating high-dose oral/IV steroids, DMARDs, or biologics.
• B = Low-dose corticosteroids (equivalent to ≤20mg/day prednisolone) and/or HCQ.
• C = Stable mild disease.
• D = Prior involvement of the organ system, no current disease activity.
• E = Organ system never involved.

Several conversion systems have been proposed to translate BILAG A–E ratings into a BILAG disease activity summary score. Newly revised scoring for BILAG 2004 is as follows: A = 12; B = 8; C = 1; D = 0; E = 0.

Use of BILAG in JSLE

The original adult-derived 'Classic' BILAG index has been used in JSLE and shown to be sensitive to change in disease activity. However, it was recognizsed that adaptation of certain parameters of the original BILAG needed to take place for use in children (e.g. age-adjusted BP). In addition, potential scoring problems were noted due to the differences between paediatric and adult management practices (e.g. timing of renal biopsy). Validation of the revised BILAG 2004 in a JSLE cohort is currently underway.

Further reading

Yee CS, Farewell VT, Isenberg DA et al. Numerical scoring for the BILAG 2004 Index. *Rheumatology* 2010;49:1665–9.

Table 4.11 British Isles Lupus Assessment Group (BILAG) 2004 Index

Domain	Manifestations*		Assessment
Constitutional	1. Pyrexia (documented >37.5°C)	A	Pyrexia recorded as 2 (same), 3 (worse), or 4 (new) *and* ≥2 recorded as 2–4: weight loss, lymphadenopathy/splenomegaly, anorexia
	2. Weight loss-unintentional >5%		
	3. Lymphadenopathy/splenomegaly	B	Pyrexia recorded as 2, 3, or 4 *or* ≥2 recorded as 2–4: weight loss, lymphadenopathy/splenomegaly, anorexia *but* do not fulfil criteria for category A
	4. Anorexia		
		C	Pyrexia recorded as 1 (improving) *or* ≥1 recorded as 2 (same), 3 (worse) or 4 (new): weight loss, lymphadenopathy/splenomegaly, anorexia *BUT* does not fulfil criteria for category A or B
		D	Previous involvement
		E	No previous involvement
Mucocutaneous	1. Skin eruption—severe	A	Any of the following recorded as 2 (same), 3 (worse), or 4 (new):
	2. Skin eruption—mild		Skin eruption—severe
	3. Angio-oedema—severe		Angio-oedema—severe
	4. Angio-oedema—mild		Mucosal ulceration—severe
	5. Mucosal ulceration—severe		Panniculitis/bullous lupus—severe
	6. Mucosal ulceration—mild		Major cutaneous vasculitis/thrombosis
	7. Panniculitis/bullous lupus—severe	B	Any category A features recorded as 1 (improving) or any of following recorded as 2 (same), 3 (worse), or 4 (new):
	8. Panniculitis/Bullous lupus—mild		Skin eruption—mild
	9. Major cutaneous vasculitis/thrombosis		Panniculitis/Bullous lupus—mild
	10. Digital infarcts or nodular vasculitis		Digital infarcts or nodular vasculitis
	11. Alopecia—severe		Alopecia—severe

Table 4.11 Contd.

Domain	Manifestations*	Assessment
	12. Alopecia—mild	C Any category B features recorded as 1 (improving) or any of the following
	13. Peri-ungual erythema/chilblains	recorded as ≥1:
	14. Splinter haemorrhages	Angio-oedema—mild
		Mucosal ulceration—mild
		Alopecia—mild
		Periungual erythema/chilblains
		Splinter haemorrhages
		D Previous involvement
		E No previous involvement
Cardiorespiratory	1. Myocarditis—mild	A Any of the following recorded as 2 (same), 3 (worse), or 4 (new):
	2. Myocarditis/endocarditis + cardiac failure	Myocarditis/endocarditis + cardiac failure
	3. Arrhythmia	Arrhythmia
	4. New valvular dysfunction	New valvular dysfunction
	5. Pleurisy/pericarditis	Cardiac tamponade
	6. Cardiac tamponade	Pleural effusion with dyspnoea
	7. Pleural effusion with dyspnoea	Pulmonary haemorrhage/vasculitis
	8. Pulmonary haemorrhage/vasculitis	Interstitial alveolitis/pneumonitis
	9. Interstitial alveolitis/pneumonitis	Shrinking lung syndrome
	10. Shrinking lung syndrome	Aortitis
	11. Aortitis	Coronary vasculitis
	12. Coronary vasculitis	B Any category A features recorded as 1 (improving) **or** pleurisy/pericarditis or mild myocarditis recorded as 2, 3, or 4
		C Any category B features recorded as 1 (improving)

Neuropsychiatric		
1. Aseptic meningitis	D	Previous involvement
2. Cerebral vasculitis	E	No previous involvement
3. Demyelinating syndrome	A	Any of manifestations numbered 1–11 or status epilepticus or cerebellar ataxia recorded as 2 (same), 3 (worse), or 4 (new)
4. Myelopathy	B	Any category A features recorded as 1 (improving) **or** any of the following recorded as 2 (same), 3 (worse), or 4 (new):
5. Acute confusional state		Seizure disorder
6. Psychosis		Cerebrovascular disease (not due to vasculitis)
7. Acute inflammatory demyelinating polyradiculoneuropathy		Cognitive dysfunction
8. Mononeuropathy (single/multiplex)		Movement disorder
9. Cranial neuropathy		Autonomic disorder
10. Plexopathy		Lupus headache—severe unremitting
11. Polyneuropathy		Headache due to raised intracranial hypertension
12. Seizure disorder	C	Any category B features recorded as 1 (improving)
13. Status epilepticus	D	Previous involvement
14. Cerebrovascular disease (not due to vasculitis)	E	No previous involvement
15. Cognitive dysfunction		
16. Movement disorder		
17. Autonomic disorder		
18. Cerebellar ataxia (isolated)		
19. Lupus headache—severe unremitting		
20. Headache from intracranial ↑BP		

Table 4.11 Contd.

Domain	Manifestations*	Assessment
Musculoskeletal	1. Myositis—severe 2. Myositis—mild 3. Arthritis—severe 4. Arthritis(moderate)/tenosynovitis 5. Arthritis (mild)/arthralgia/myalgia	A Severe myositis or severe arthritis recorded as 2 (same), 3 (worse), or 4 (new) B Any category A features recorded as 1 (improving) or mild myositis or moderate arthritis/tendonitis/tenosynovitis recorded as 2–4. C Any category B features recorded ≤1 (improving) or mild arthritis/arthralgia/myalgia scored as ≥1 D Previous involvement E No previous involvement

Gastrointestinal	1. Lupus peritonitis
	2. Abdominal serositis or ascites
	3. Lupus enteritis/colitis
	4. Malabsorption
	5. Protein losing enteropathy
	6. Intestinal pseudo-obstruction
	7. Lupus hepatitis
	8. Acute lupus cholecystitis
	9. Acute lupus pancreatitis
		A Any of the following recorded as 2 (same), 3 (worse), or 4 (new):
		  Peritonitis
		  Lupus enteritis/colitis
		  Intestinal pseudo-obstruction
		  Acute lupus cholecystitis
		  Acute lupus pancreatitis
		B Any category A feature recorded as (improving) or abdominal serositis and/or ascites, malabsorption, protein losing enteropathy, lupus hepatitis recorded as 2 (same), 3 (worse) or 4 (new)
		C Any category B features recorded as (improving)
		D Previous involvement
		E No previous involvement

Ophthalmic
(Usually scored by ophthalmologist)

1. Orbital inflammation/myositis/proptosis
2. Keratitis—severe
3. Keratitis—mild
4. Anterior uveitis
5. Posterior uveitis/retinal vasculitis—severe
6. Post. uveitis/retinal vasculitis—mild
7. Episcleritis
8. Scleritis—severe
9. Scleritis—mild
10. Retinal/choroidal vaso-occlusive disease
11. Isolated cotton-wool spots
12. Optic neuritis
13. Anterior ischaemic optic neuropathy

A Any of the following recorded as 2 (same), 3 (worse), or 4 (new):
Orbital inflammation/myositis/proptosis
Keratitis—severe
Posterior uveitis/retinal vasculitis—severe
Scleritis—severe
Retinal/choroidal vaso-occlusive disease
Optic neuritis
Anterior ischaemic optic neuropathy

B Any category A features recorded as 1 (improving) or any of the following
recorded as 2 (same), 3 (worse), or 4 (new):
Keratitis—mild
Anterior uveitis
Posterior uveitis/retinal vasculitis—mild
Scleritis—mild

C Any category B features recorded as 1 (improving) or episcleritis or isolated
cotton-wool spots (cytoid bodies) recorded as ≥1

D Previous involvement

E No previous involvement

Table 4.11 Contd.

Domain	Manifestations*	Assessment

Renal	1. Systolic BP (mmHg)
	2. Diastolic BP (mmHg)
	3. Accelerated hypertension (Y/N)
	4. Urine dipstick protein (+=1, ++=2, +++=3)
	5. Urine albumin-creatinine ratio (UACR) mg/mmol
	6. Urine protein-creatinine ratio (UPCR) mg/mmol
	7. 24h urine protein (gram)
	8. Nephrotic syndrome (Y/N)
	9. Creatinine (plasma/serum)
	10. GFR (calculated)
	11. Active urinary sediment (Y/N)
	12. Active nephritis
		A Two or more of the following providing 1, 4, or 5 is included:
		  1. Deteriorating proteinuria (severe) defined as:
		    (a) Urine dipstick increased by ≥2 levels or
		    (b) 24h urine protein >1g that has not decreased (improved) by ≥ 25%; or
		    (c) UPCR >100 mg/mmol that has not decreased (improved) by ≥ 25%; or
		    (d) UACR >100 mg/mmol that has not decreased (improved) by ≥ 25%
		  2. Accelerated hypertension
		  3. Deteriorating renal function (severe) defined as
		    (a) plasma creatinine >130μmol/L and having risen to >130% of previous value; or
		    (b) GFR <80mL/min per 1.73m² and having fallen to <67% of previous value; or
		    (c) GFR <50mL/min per 1.73m², and last time was >50mL/min per 1.73 m² or was not measured
		  4. Active urinary sediment
		  5. Histological evidence of active nephritis within last 3 months
		  6. Nephrotic syndrome
		B One of the following:
		  1. One of the category A criteria
		  2. Proteinuria (that has not fulfilled category A criteria):
		    (a) Urine dipstick which has risen to ≥2+ or
		    (b) 24h urine protein ≥0.5 g that has not decreased (improved) by ≥25%; or
		    (c) UPCR or UACR ≥50 mg/mmol that has not decreased (improved) by ≥25%
		  3. Plasma creatinine >130μmol/L and having risen to ≥115% but ≤130% of previous value

C One of the following:
  1. Mild/stable proteinuria defined as that which has not fulfilled criteria for category A & B
  2. Rising BP (>140/90mmHg) which has not fulfilled criteria for category A & B, defined as systolic rise of ≥30 mm Hg; and diastolic rise of ≥15mm Hg
D Previous involvement
E No previous involvement

Haematological	1. Hemoglobin (g/dL)	A	TTP recorded as 2 (same), 3 (worse), or 4 (new) or evidence of haemolysis and Hb <8 g/dL or platelets <25 × 10⁹/L

Haematological
  1. Hemoglobin (g/dL)
  2. Total WBC (×10⁹/L)
  3. Neutrophils (×10⁹/L)
  4. Lymphocytes (×10⁹/L)
  5. Platelets (×10⁹/L)
  6. TTP
  7. Evidence of active haemolysis (Y/N)
  8. Coombs test positive (Y/N)

A TTP recorded as 2 (same), 3 (worse), or 4 (new) or evidence of haemolysis and Hb <8 g/dL or platelets <25 × 10⁹/L

B TTP recorded as 1 (improving) or any of the following:
  1. Evidence of haemolysis and Hb 8–9.9g/dL
  2. Hb <8g/dL (without haemolysis)
  3. WCC <1.0 × 10⁹/L
  4. Neutrophil count <0.5 × 10⁹/L
  5. Platelet count 25–49 × 10⁹/L

C Any 1 of the following:
  1. Evidence of haemolysis and Hb ≥10g/dL
  2. Hb 8–10.9 g/dL (without haemolysis)
  3. WCC 1–3.9 × 10⁹/L
  4. Neutrophil count 0.5–1.9 × 10⁹/L
  5. Lymphocyte count <1.0 × 10⁹/L
  6. Platelet count 50–149 × 10⁹/L
  7. Isolated Coombs' test positive

D Previous involvement
E No previous involvement

Adapted with permission from CheeSeng Yee et al. Numerical scoring for the BILAG 2004 index. Rheumatology, Volume 49, Issue 9, pp. 1665–1669, Copyright © The Author(s) 2010. Published by Oxford University Press on behalf of The British Society for Rheumatology. Form, Scoring and Glossary available from Rheumatology online, https://academic.oup.com/rheumatology

SLEDAI 2000 Disease Activity Index

See Table 4.12.

Table 4.12 SLEDAI 2K—check box: if descriptor is present at time of visit or past 10 days

Weight		Descriptor	Definition
8	☐	Seizure	Recent onset, exclude metabolic, infectious, or drug causes
8	☐	Psychosis	Altered ability to function in normal activity due to severe disturbance in the perception of reality. Include hallucinations, incoherence, marked loose associations, impoverished thought content, marked illogical thinking, bizarre, disorganized, or catatonic behaviour. Exclude uraemia and drug causes
8	☐	Organic brain syndrome	Altered mental function with impaired orientation, memory, or other intellectual function, with rapid onset and fluctuating clinical features, inability to sustain attention to environment, plus at least 2 of the following: perceptual disturbance, incoherent speech, insomnia or daytime drowsiness, or ↑ or ↓ psychomotor activity. Exclude metabolic, infectious, or drug causes
8	☐	Visual disturbance	Retinal changes of SLE. Include cytoid bodies, retinal haemorrhages, serous exudates or haemorrhages in the choroid, or optic neuritis. Exclude hypertension, infection, or drug causes
8	☐	Cranial nerve disorder	New onset of sensory or motor neuropathy involving cranial nerves
8	☐	Lupus headache	Severe, persistent headache, may be migrainous, but must be non-responsive to narcotic analgesia
8	☐	CVA	New onset of cerebrovascular accident(s). Exclude arteriosclerosis
8	☐	Vasculitis	Ulceration, gangrene, tender finger nodules, periungual infarction, splinter haemorrhages, or biopsy or angiogram proof of vasculitis

Table 4.12 Contd.

Weight		Descriptor	Definition
4	☐	Arthritis	≥2 joints with pain and signs of inflammation (i.e. tenderness, swelling or effusion)
4	☐	Myositis	Proximal muscle weakness, associated with elevated creatine phosphokinase/aldolase or electromyogram changes or a biopsy showing myositis
4	☐	Urinary casts	Haem-granular or red blood cell casts
4	☐	Haematuria	>5 red blood cells/high power field, Exclude stone, infection, or other cause
4	☐	Proteinuria	>0.5g/24h
4	☐	Pyuria	>5 white blood cells/high power field. Exclude infection
2	☐	Rash	Inflammatory type rash
2	☐	Alopecia	Abnormal, patchy, or diffuse loss of hair
2	☐	Mucosal ulcers	Oral or nasal ulcerations
2	☐	Pleurisy	Pleuritic chest pain with pleural rub or effusion, or pleural thickening
2	☐	Pericarditis	Pericardial pain with at least 1 of the following: rub, effusion, or electrocardiogram or echocardiogram confirmation
2	☐	Low complement	↓ in CH50, C3, or C4 below the lower limit of normal for testing laboratory
2	☐	Increased DNA binding	↑ DNA binding by Farr assay above normal range for testing laboratory
1	☐	Fever	>38°C. Exclude infectious cause
1	☐	Thrombocytopenia	<100,000 platelets/× 10^9/L, exclude drug causes
1	☐	Leucopenia	<3000 white blood cells/× 10^9/L, exclude drug causes
	☐	TOTAL SCORE (Sum of weights next to descriptors marked present)	

Adapted with permission from Gladman DD, Ibanez D, and Urowitz MB. Systemic lupuserythematosus disease activity index 2000. Journal of Rheumatology, Volume 29, Issue 2, pp. 288–91, Copyright © 2002 by The Journal of Rheumatology Publishing Company Limited.

SLICC/ACR Damage Index (paediatric)

Table 4.13.

Table 4.13 SLICC/ACR Damage Index (paediatric)*

	SCORE (circle)
Ocular (either eye, by clinic assessment)	
• Any cataract ever	0 1
• Retinal change or optic atrophy	0 1
Neuropsychiatric	
• Cognitive impairment or major psychosis	0 1
• Seizures requiring therapy for 6 months	0 1
• Cerebral vascular accident ever (score 2 if >1) or resection not for malignancy	0 1 2
• Cranial or peripheral neuropathy (excluding optic)	0 1
• Transverse myelitis	0 1
Renal	
• Estimated or measured GFR <50%	0 1
• Proteinuria 24h, ≥3.5 g	0 1
• End-stage renal disease (regardless of dialysis or transplantation)	3
Pulmonary	
• Pulmonary hypertension (right ventricular prominence, or loud P2)	0 1
• Pulmonary fibrosis (physical and x-ray)	0 1
• Shrinking lung (x-ray)	0 1
• Pleural fibrosis (x-ray)	0 1
• Pulmonary infarction (x-ray) or resection not for malignancy	0 1
Cardiovascular	
• Angina or coronary artery bypass	0 1
• Myocardial infarction ever (score 2 if >1)	0 1 2
• Cardiomyopathy (ventricular dysfunction)	0 1
• Valvular disease (diastolic murmur, or a systolic murmur >3/6)	0 1
• Pericarditis × 6 months or pericardiectomy	0 1
Peripheral vascular	
• Claudication × 6 months	0 1
• Minor tissue loss (pulp space)	0 1
• Significant tissue loss ever (e.g. loss of digit or limb, resection) (Score 2 if >1)	0 1 2
• Venous thrombosis with swelling, ulceration, or venous stasis	0 1
Gastrointestinal	
• Infarction or resection of bowel (below duodenum), spleen, liver or gall bladder (score 2 if >1)	0 1 2
• Mesenteric insufficiency	0 1
• Chronic peritonitis	0 1
• Stricture or upper GI tract surgery ever	0 1
• Pancreatic insufficiency requiring enzyme replacement or with pseudocyst	0 1

Table 4.13 *Contd.*

	SCORE (circle)
Musculoskeletal	
• Atrophy or weakness	0 1
• Deforming or erosive arthritis (including reducible deformities, excluding avascular necrosis)	0 1
• Osteoporosis with fracture or vertebral collapse (excluding avascular necrosis)	0 1
• Avascular necrosis (score 2 if >1)	0 1 2
• Osteomyelitis	0 1
• Ruptured tendons	0 1
Skin	
• Alopecia	0 1
• Extensive scarring of panniculum other than scalp and pulp space	0 1
• Skin ulceration (not due to thrombosis) >6 months	0 1
Diabetes (regardless of treatment)	0 1
Malignancy (exclude dysplasia) score 2 if >1 site	0 1 2
Premature gonadal failure/secondary amenorrhoea	0 1
Pubertal stage	pre post
Height (cm)	Weight (kg)
Bone age (yr)	
• DEXA scan every 2yr	

Scored by summation of scores for each item in the 12 domains (maximum of 47).

Adapted with permission from Gutierrez- Suarez R et al. A proposal for a pediatric version of the Systemic Lupus International Collaborating Clinics/American College of Rheumatology Damage Index based on the analysis of 1,015 patients with juvenile-onset systemic lupus erythematosus. *Arthritis Rheumatology*, Volume 54, Issue 9, pp. 2989–96, Copyright © 2006 by the American College of Rheumatology.

Scleroderma

The encompassing term scleroderma (literally 'hard skin') is characterized by skin thickening and ↑ collagen and may involve atrophy of subcutaneous fat and/or deeper tissues. Scleroderma has 2 distinct groupings: localized scleroderma (LS) and the much rarer juvenile systemic sclerosis (jSSc)—Table 4.14. Classifications of LS and jSSC are largely clinical and as yet, there is no universal consensus as to their use in clinical practice or clinical trials (Tables 4.15 and 4.16).

Assessment and monitoring

There are currently no validated outcomes of severity or disease activity in LS or jSSc, either of the skin or organ involvement. Current methods of assessment include:

- Clinical examination (skin, joints, muscles, general examination, growth).
  - Need to consider potential multisystem involvement (Table 4.17): check BP, urinalysis, pulmonary function tests/transfer factor, ECHO as baseline and in jSSc, at least annually pending clinical scenario.
- Imaging:
  - Serial photographs and measurement of lesions.
  - Thermography and capillaroscopy.
  - MRI head (especially if facial lesions present).
  - Skin US, Laser Doppler flowmetry (not yet validated).
- Blood tests: autoantibodies (Table 4.16 and see ➋ pp. 33–6). Muscle enzymes (➋ Juvenile dermatomyositis, pp. 280–7).

Approach to management

- Early disease recognition and referral to an experienced paediatric rheumatology MDT.
- There are few placebo-controlled trials in children with scleroderma; therapy decisions are based on reports of clinical cohorts.
- Physiotherapy and occupational therapy optimize physical function to treat and prevent contractures and muscle weakness and facilitate access to make up and cosmetic approaches if there are disfiguring skin lesions. Surgery may be complicated by problems with healing and ischaemia.
- Treatment of skin lesions in LS depends largely on lesion site, size, depth, and potential for growth impairment when the lesions are deep and/or over joints and the presence of extra-cutaneous features. Options include topical treatments (e.g. moisturizers, corticosteroids), UV phototherapy, and systemic immunosuppression are increasingly used (e.g. corticosteroids, MTX, MMF, and anti-TNF treatment—see ➋ p. 472)—case series have demonstrated efficacy in halting progression of skin involvement. Cosmetic procedures in localized scleroderma may be helpful when growth is complete and lesions inactive.
- Use of disease activity and damage measures with the Localized Scleroderma Cutaneous Assessment Tool LoSCAT scores are helpful in monitoring response to treatment.

Table 4.14 Epidemiology and clinical features

	Localized scleroderma (LS)	Juvenile systemic sclerosis (jSSc)
Estimated incidence	3.4 per million	0.27 per million
Survival	Likely normal	Estimated 4yr survival is 95% (cardiac and pulmonary disease)
♀:♂ ratio	Between 1.7:1–2.4:1 (largest cohort 2.4:1)	2.8:1 or greater (largest cohort 3.6:1)
Ethnicity	82–90% Caucasian	
Mean age of onset	Approx 8yr (range: birth–16yr) Delay in diagnosis is common especially in LS as presentation is often insidious	
Clinical features	Articular (19%)— often distant to skin lesions Neurological (4%)— e.g. epilepsy, headaches, behavioural change, learning disabilities Vascular—Raynaud's Ocular—e.g. uveitis, episcleritis, eyelid or eyelash abnormality GI (2%) (reflux oesophagitis) Respiratory, renal & cardiac (<1%)	More generalized skin changes and may include widespread visceral involvement Raynaud's phenomenon (76%), skin induration (66%), sclerodactyly (55%), digital tip ulceration (35%), dysphagia (13%) 3 subtypes recognized: Limited cutaneous systemic sclerosis (lcSSc)—skin change usually confined to distal arm or leg >head and neck. *Previously often termed 'CREST' (calcinosis, Raynaud's, oesophageal involvement, sclerodactyly, telangiectases)* Diffuse cutaneous (dcSSc)—skin involvement extends to proximal limb and/or trunk *Overlap syndromes*—both lcSSc and dcSSc may overlap with other connective tissue diseases (e.g. SLE, Sjögren's syndrome and inflammatory muscle disease)
Differential diagnosis	Amyloidosis, eosinophilic fasciitis, graft-versus-host-disease, juvenile dermatomyositis, juvenile idiopathic arthritis, [lichen sclerosus et atrophicus], lipodystrophy, Lyme disease, lupus erythematosus, mixed connective tissue disease, phenylketonuria, scleredema; PHID syndrome (pigmentary hypertrichosis and non-autoimmune insulin-dependent diabetes mellitus)	

Table 4.15 Localized scleroderma (Mayo Clinic classification).

Localized scleroderma type (relative frequency, %)	Subdivision	Comment
Plaque morphoea (26%)	Plaque morphoea	Most benign subtype (usually on the trunk), lesions may be single or multiple. Often start as localized patch of erythema, induration with erythematous halo or altered skin pigment
	Others—Guttate morphoea, atrophoderma of Pasini and Pierini, keloid morphoea (nodular morphoea), [lichen sclerosus et atrophicus]	Skin lesion patterns are variable and differing patterns may coexist
Generalized morphoea (7%)		No subdivisions. Plaques confluent or affecting >2 separate anatomical sites
Bullous morphoea (<1%)		No subdivisions
Linear morphoea (65%)	Linear morphoea/scleroderma	Commonest subtype usually affecting limbs. May also involve face
	En coup de sabre (Parry-Romberg)	When face is affected, changes are often disfiguring
	Progressive hemifacial atrophy	'En coup de sabre' refers to cranial linear lesion with lack of hair growth in the involved skin; 'Parry–Romberg syndrome' refers to hemifacial atrophy. Intracranial brain lesions are rare (e.g. gadolinium-enhancing lesions, cerebral vasculitis, raised oligoclonal bands, or intracranial calcification)
Deep morphoea (2%)	Various descriptions	Subcutaneous morphoea, eosinophilic fasciitis, morphoea profunda, disabling pansclerotic morphoea of children

Table 4.16 Proposed provisional classification criteria of jSSc

Major criterion (1 required)

Proximal skin sclerosis/induration of the skin

Minor criterion (>2 required)

Cutaneous	Sclerodactyly
Peripheral vascular	Raynaud's phenomenon, nailfold capillary abnormalities, digital tip ulcers
Gastrointestinal	Dysphagia, gastroesophageal reflux
Cardiac	Arrhythmias, heart failure
Renal	Renal crisis, new-onset arterial hypertension
Respiratory	Pulmonary fibrosis (high-resolution CT/radiography) with ↓ transfer factor and restrictive lung disease on pulmonary function tests, pulmonary arterial hypertension
Neurologic	Neuropathy, carpal tunnel syndrome
Musculoskeletal	Tendon friction rubs, arthritis, myositis
Serological	Antinuclear antibodies, jSSc-selective autoantibodies (anticentromere, anti–topoisomerase I [Scl-70], antifibrillarin, anti–PMScl, antifibrillin or anti–RNA polymerase I or III)

These criteria still require validation, particularly with regard to disease subtypes.

Reproduced with permission from Zulian F, Woo P, and Athreya BH. The Pediatric Rheumatology European Society/American College of Rheumatology/European League against Rheumatism provisional classification criteria for juvenile systemic sclerosis. *Arthritis & Rheumatology*, Volume 57, Issue 2, pp. 203–212, Copyright John Wiley and Sons Ltd 2007.

- Raynaud's phenomenon—avoidance of smoking, certain drugs (e.g. beta blockers) and may be helped by gloves, topical GTN, or oral medication (calcium channel blockers) or iloprost (see ➔ Clinical guidelines p. 492, and ➔ Overlap syndromes, pp. 288–92).
- EULAR have proposed evidenced-based treatment recommendations for jSSc (Table 4.17). Treatment of jSSc requires specialist evaluation and treatment (including iloprost (see ➔ Epoprostenol/iloprost, p. 492, and ➔ Overlap syndromes, pp. 288–92) for Raynauds, DMARDs, and cytotoxics for organ involvement and proton pump inhibitors for GI symptoms). There are successful case reports of bone marrow transplantation and autologous haematopoietic stem cell transplantation (see ➔ HSCT, pp. 461–4).
- The UK Scleroderma Study Group (UKSSG) have published a number of consensus-based best practice recommendations with others being prepared. The group includes paediatric representation and current recommendations are available via the group's website.
- Long-term monitoring is imperative and LS often progresses insidiously and frequently relapses following cessation of drug treatment. LS evolving into jSSc is reported, albeit very rarely (and possibly cases were atypical from onset).

Table 4.17 EULAR recommendations for the treatment of SSc (recommendations for adult and paediatric populations)

Organ system	Recommendation	Category of evidence
SSc-related digital vasculopathy (Raynaud's phenomenon (RP), digital ulcers)	Dihydropiridine-type calcium antagonists, usually oral nifedipine, should be considered for first-line therapy for SSc-RP, and IV iloprost, or other available IV prostanoids for severe SSc-RP	A
	IV prostanoids (in particular iloprost) should be considered in the treatment of active digital ulcers in patients with SSc	A
	Bosentan should be considered in diffuse SSc with multiple digital ulcers after failure of calcium antagonists and, usually, prostanoid therapy	A
SSc-related pulmonary arterial hypertension (PAH)	Bosentan should be strongly considered to treat SSc-PAH (pulmonary hypertension)	A/B
	At present, sitaxentan may also be considered to treat SSc-PAH	A/B
	Sildenafil may be considered to treat SSc-PAH	A/B
	Intravenous epoprostenol should be considered for the treatment of patients with severe SSc-PAH	A
SSc-related skin involvement	MTX may be considered for treatment of skin manifestations of early diffuse SSc	A
SSc-related interstitial lung disease (ILD)	In view of the results from 2 high-quality RCTs and despite its known toxicity, cyclophosphamide should be considered for treatment of SSc-ILD (interstitial lung disease)	A
SSc-related renal crisis (SRC)	Despite the lack of RCT, expert consensus is that ACE inhibitors should be used in the treatment of SRC	C
	4 retrospective studies suggest that steroids are associated with a higher risk of SRC. Patients on steroids should be carefully monitored for BP and renal function	C
SSc-related gastrointestinal disease	Despite the lack of specific RCT, experts believe that proton pump inhibitors should be used for the prevention of SSc-related gastro-oesophageal reflux, oesophageal ulcers, and strictures	B
	Despite the lack of specific RCTs, experts believe that prokinetic drugs should be used for the management of SSc-related symptomatic motility disturbances (dysphagia, gastrointestinal reflux disease, early satiety, bloating, pseudo-obstruction)	C
	Despite the lack of specific RCT, experts believe that, when malabsorption is caused by bacterial overgrowth, rotating antibiotics may be useful in SSc patients	D

Further reading

Herrick AL, Ennis H, Bhushan M, et al. Incidence of childhood linear scleroderma and systemic sclerosis in the UK and Ireland. *Arthritis Care Res (Hoboken)* 2010; 62(2):213–18.

Kowal-Bielecka O, Landewé R, Avouac J, et al. EULAR recommendations for the treatment of systemic sclerosis: a report from the EULAR Scleroderma Trials and Research group EUSTAR). *Ann Rheum Dis* 2009; 68(5):620–8.

Zulian F, Athreya BH, Laxer R, et al.; Juvenile Scleroderma Working Group of the Pediatric Rheumatology European Society (PRES). Juvenile localized scleroderma: clinical and epidemiological features in 750 children. An international study. *Rheumatology (Oxford)* 2006; 45(5):614–20.

Zulian F, Woo P, Athreya BH, et al. The Pediatric Rheumatology European Society/American College of Rheumatology/European League against Rheumatism provisional classification criteria for juvenile systemic sclerosis. *Arthritis Rheum* 2007; 57(2):203–12. ℣ http://www.scleroderma-royalfree.org.uk/UKSSG.html accessed 03.12.2015

Juvenile dermatomyosis

Juvenile dermatomyosis (JDM) is a rare autoimmune small-vessel vasculopathy of childhood. It characteristically affects the skin and muscle but can also involve the GI system, heart, joints, and other organs. JDM is the most common of the idiopathic inflammatory myopathies of childhood.

Epidemiology
- The incidence of JDM is between 2 and 3 children per million per year.
- JDM is more commonly seen in girls than boys (2.3:1).
- The mean age of onset is ~7yr; however, 25% of cases present before the age of 4.
- Ethnicity largely reflects that of the population. An analysis of cases from Great Britain and Ireland has shown an over-representation amongst the black population relative to population demographics.
- Seasonality, most notably in birth distribution in certain populations, suggests a role for perinatal environmental factors in the onset of the illness in later childhood.

Clinical features
- Clinical features form the central basis of the diagnosis of all cases of JDM. The typical picture is one of:
  - Heliotrope rash, periorbital oedema.
  - Gottron's papules over the extensor surfaces.
  - Proximal muscle weakness.
- In reality patients can present with any of a number of clinical pictures including:
  - Systemic symptoms (fever, malaise, anorexia, weight loss or irritability).
  - Arthritis, myalgia, contractures.
  - Dysphagia, dyspnoea, dysphonia.
  - Lipoatrophy, calcinosis, skin ulceration, oedema.

Diagnostic criteria
- The diagnostic criteria defined by Bohan and Peter in 1975 remain the most widely used today. These criteria require, for a diagnosis of definite JDM, the presence of 1 of the characteristic rashes in combination with 3 of the following:
  - Symmetric proximal muscle weakness.
  - Raised serum muscle enzymes (creatine kinase, transaminases, lactate dehydrogenase, and aldolase).
  - Abnormal findings on a muscle biopsy (Fig. 4.14) or electromyogram (EMG).
- Probable JDM: 1 of the characteristic rashes plus 2 of the other features; possible JDM: rash +1 feature.
- Over time, changes in clinical practice have made these criteria less reliable as many children with a diagnosis of JDM may not fulfil the criteria as a result of a lack of muscle biopsy or EMG. As such the classification criteria for JDM is under discussion, but may include:
  - Myositis specific autoantibodies.

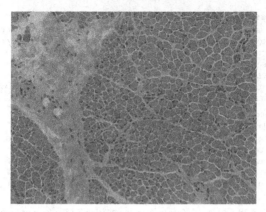

Fig. 4.14 Muscle biopsy in JDM (see plate section).

- Abnormal MRI.
- Abnormal nailfold capillaroscopy.
- Calcinosis.
- Dysphonia.
- Myositis specific autoantibodies: these are essentially still a research tool, but look promising for subcategorizing JDM which may help with prognosis and deciding suitable treatments.

Monitoring during follow-up

Monitoring of disease activity in JDM involves:
- Assessment of muscle disease: muscle strength, contractures, reduced muscle length.
- Assessment of skin disease: rashes, nailbed erythema, and swelling.
- Assessment of other systems: arthritis, lung/liver/heart, calcinosis, cuticular overgrowth, nailbed capillary abnormalities.

Global assessment
- JDM Disease Activity Score—assesses the extent and distribution of cutaneous involvement, muscle weakness, functional status, and vasculopathic manifestations.
- Parent/Patient global assessment of disease activity assessment by Visual Analogue Score (VAS).

Functional ability
Childhood Health Assessment Questionnaire—see ➔ Outcome measures, pp. 43–9.

Health-related quality of life
Child Health Questionnaire—see ➔ Outcome measures, pp. 43–9).

Assessment of muscle disease

The assessment of the extent and severity of muscle involvement is pivotal to the monitoring of JDM. Assessment of muscle disease activity and response to therapy can be subdivided.

- Measures of muscle strength—MMT8 (tests 8 muscle groups).
- Measures of muscle functional ability—CMAS.
- Serological measurement of muscle enzymes (but not always raised with disease activity, especially in long-standing disease).

Childhood Myositis Assessment Scale (CMAS)
(Table 4.18)

- This is an excellent assessment and monitoring tool to assess muscle strength and function, stamina of muscles, task orientated function.
- The CMAS assesses quality of movement as well as whether the task can be completed.
- The maximum score is 52 and this indicates a well, fit, young person.

Table 4.18 Childhood Myositis Assessment Scale (CMAS) scoring sheet

1. Head elevation (neck flexion):	Item
0 = Unable	score ...
1 = 1–9sec	
2 = 10–29sec	
3 = 30–59sec	
4 = 60–119sec	
5 = >2min	
No. of seconds	
2. Leg raise/touch object:	Item
0 = Unable to lift leg off table	score ...
1 = Able to clear table, but cannot touch object	
2 = Able to lift leg high enough to touch object	
3. Straight leg lift/duration:	Item
0 = Unable	score ...
1 = 1–9sec	
2 = 10–29sec	
3 = 30–59sec	
4 = 60–119sec	
5 = >2min	
No. of seconds	
4. Supine to prone:	Item
0 = Unable. Has difficulty even turning onto side; able to pull arms under torso only slightly/not at all	score ...
1 = Turns onto side fairly easily, but cannot fully free arms, but not able to fully assume a prone position	
2 = Easily turns onto side; some difficulty freeing arms, but fully frees them and fully assumes prone position	
3 = Easily turns over, free arms with no difficulty	

(Continued)

Table 4.18 *Contd.*

5. Sit-ups: for each type of sit-up enter either '0' (unable) or '1' (able). Then enter the total subscore. Maximum possible item score 6.	Item score ...
Hands on thighs, with counterbalance	
Hands across chest, with counterbalance	
Hands behind head, with counterbalance	
Hands on thighs, without counterbalance	
Hands across chest, without counterbalance	
Hands behind head, without counterbalance	

6. Supine to sit:	Item score ...
0 = Unable by self	
1 = Much difficulty. Very slow, struggles greatly, barely makes it. Almost unable	
2 = Some difficulty. Able, but is somewhat slow, struggles some	
3 = No difficulty	

7. Arm raise/straighten:	Item score ...
0 = Cannot raise wrists	
1 = Can raise wrists at least up to the level of the acromioclavicular joint, but not above top of head	
2 = Can raise wrists above top of head, but cannot raise arms straight above head so that elbows are in full extension	
3 = Can raise arms straight above head so that elbows are in full extension	

8. Arm raise/duration:	Item score ...
Can maintain wrists above top of head for:	
0 = Unable	
1 = 1–9sec	
2 = 10–29sec	
3 = 30–59sec	
4 > 60sec	
No. of seconds	

9. Floor sit:	Item score ...
Going from a standing position to a sitting position on the floor.	
0 = Unable. Afraid to even try, even if allowed to use a chair for support. Child fears that he/she will collapse, fall into a sit, or harm self.	
1 = Much difficulty. Able, but needs to hold onto a chair for support during descent. (Unable or unwilling to try if not able to use a chair for support.)	
2 = Some difficulty. Can go from stand to sit without using a chair for support, but has at least some difficulty during descent. Descends somewhat slowly and/or apprehensively; may not have full control or balance as maneuvers into a sit.	
3 = No difficulty. Requires no compensatory maneuvering.	

10. All-fours manoeuvre:	Item score ...
0 = Unable to go from a prone to an all-fours position.	
1 = Barely able to assume and maintain an all-fours position.	
2 = Can maintain all-fours position with straight back and head raised (so as to look straight ahead). But, cannot creep (crawl) forward	
3 = Can maintain all fours, look straight ahead, and creep (crawl) forward	
4 = Maintains balance while lifting and extending leg.	

(Continued)

Table 4.18 Contd.

11. Floor rise:	Item
Going from a kneeling position on the floor to a standing position.	score ...
0 = Unable, even if allowed to use a chair for support	
1 = Much difficulty. Able, but needs to use a chair for support. Unable if not allowed to use a chair	
2 = Moderate difficulty. Able to get up without using a chair for support, but needs to place one or both hands on thighs/knees or floor. Unable without using hands	
3 = Mild difficulty. Does not need to place hands on knees, thighs, or floor, but has at least some difficulty during ascent	
4 = No difficulty.	
12. Chair rises:	Item
0 = Unable to rise from chair, even if allowed to place hands on sides of chair seat	score ...
1 = Much difficulty. Able, but needs to place hands on sides of seat. Unable if not allowed to place hands on knees/thighs.	
2 = Moderate difficulty. Able, but needs to place hands on knees/thighs. Does not need to place hands on side of seat.	
3 = Mild difficulty. Able; does not need to use hands at all, but has at least some difficulty;	
4 = No difficulty	
13. Stool step:	Item
0 = Unable	score ...
1 = Much difficulty. Able, but needs to place one hand on exam table or examiner's hand	
2 = Some difficulty. Able; does not need to use exam table for support, but needs to use hand(s) on knee/thigh	
3 = Able. Does not need to use exam table or hand(s) on knee/thigh	
14. Pick up:	Item
0 = Unable to bend over and pick up pencil off floor	score ...
1 = Much difficulty. Able, but relies heavily on support gained by placing hand(s) on knees/thighs	
2 = Some difficulty. Needs to at least minimally and briefly place hand(s) on knees/thighs for support and is somewhat slow	
3 = No difficulty. No compensatory manoeuvre necessary	
TOTAL SCORE (Max = 52)	

Reproduced with permission from Lovell DJ, Lindsley CB, Rennebohm RM, Ballinger SH, Bowyerv SL, Giannini EH, et al. Development of validated disease activity and damage indices for the juvenile idiopathic inflammatory myopathies. II. The Childhood Myositis Assessment Scale (CMAS): a quantitative tool for the evaluation of muscle function. *Arthritis & Rheumatology*, Volume 42, Issue 10, pp. 2213–9, Copyright John Wiley and Sons Ltd 1999.

Manual Muscle Test (MMT8)

JDM affects proximal muscles and in more severe disease, distal muscles. Muscle tests have been validated to provide an outcome tool that measures 8 specific muscle groups, giving an overall score, which can be followed over time. Current Scoring scales include the Oxford MMT and the Kendall MMT (Table 4.19).

Table 4.19 The MMT Standard Scoring systems (Oxford and Kendall) (0–10 scale)

Kendall Manual Muscle Test scoring system		0–10 scale
	Function of the muscle	
No movement		0
Test movement	Movement in horizontal plane	
	Moves through partial range of motion	1
	Moves through complete range of motion	2
	Moves to completion of range against resistance or	3
	Moves to completion of range and holds against pressure or	
	Antigravity position	
	Moves through partial range of motion	
Test position	Gradual release from test position	4
	Holds test position (no added pressure)	5
	Holds test position against slight pressure	6
	Holds test position against slight to moderate pressure	7
	Holds test position against moderate pressure	8
	Holds test position against moderate to strong pressure	9
	Holds test position against strong pressure	10

Oxford MMT:
- 0=no muscle action,
- 1=flicker of muscle action,
- 2=muscle action with gravity counterbalance,
- 3=muscle action against gravity,
- 4=muscle action against gravity with some resistance,
- 5=full muscle strength,
- (9=not done)

The eight muscle groups assessed are:
- Neck flexors (this must be assessed lying flat as this includes gravity)
- Shoulder abductors
- Elbow flexors
- Wrist extensors
- Hip abductors
- Hip extensors
- Ankle dorsiflexors
- Knee extensors

All eight muscle groups are assessed and the score is added up to give a global score (out of 80).

Kendall MMT reproduced with permission from Kendall F et al. Muscles: Testing and Function, with Posture and Pain. Copyright © Wolters Kluwer Health 2005.

Assessment of skin disease
- Cutaneous Assessment Tool—assesses skin activity and damage.
- Disease Activity Score—assesses muscle and skin disease.

Monitoring of extramuscular disease
Myositis Disease Activity Assessment—a combination of a series of organ specific visual analogue scales and a myositis intention to treat activity index.

Assessment of damage
Myositis Damage Index—assesses the extent of damage in many organ systems and includes a visual analogue scale (VAS) to quantify the extent of damage (it includes the assessment of linear growth and pubertal development).

Imaging
MRI is accepted as the most valuable tool in the evaluation of myositis activity and in differentiation between activity and damage (Fig. 4.15).

Capillaroscopy
(see ➔ Nailfold capillaroscopy in rheumatic disease, pp. 39–42)
Nailfold capillary changes correlate strongly with measures of disease activity.

Treatment
- The aims of therapy for JDM are to treat the disease, prevent mortality, and reduce long-term disability and calcinosis.
- The management of JDM continues to vary widely from centre to centre and the evidence base is scant.
- Corticosteroids are the accepted 1st-line therapy;, however, mode of administration, dosage, and duration of therapy still varies.

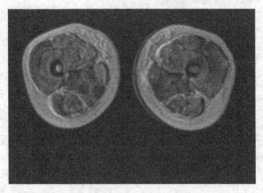

Fig. 4.15 MRI of muscles in JDM.

- The early introduction of agents beyond corticosteroids may shorten disease duration, reduce calcinosis, and help reduce the likelihood of flares later in the disease course.
- Corticosteroid therapy is preferably administered by the parenteral route rather than oral, particularly in patients with vasculopathy as evidenced by periungal nailfold capillary abnormalities.
- *Accepted 1st-line management for a typical case of JDM in the UK*
  - Corticosteroids—IV methylprednisolone 10–30mg/kg/day for 3 days followed by 1–2mg/kg oral prednisolone (weaning course).
  - MTX 15mg/m² preferably by the subcutaneous route.
  - Physical therapy.
  - Photoprotective measures (sunblock, hat, long sleeves).
  - Calcium and vitamin D supplementation.
- *2nd-line agents*
  - Hydroxychloroquine at 3–6mg/kg/day.
  - IVIg.
  - Ciclosporin.
  - AZA.
- *3rd-line agents*
  - Cyclophosphamide.
  - MMF.
  - Tacrolimus.
  - Rituximab.
  - Anti-TNFα agents.

Further reading

Isenberg DA, Allen E, Farewell V, et al. International consensus outcome measures for patients with idiopathic inflammatory myopathies. Development and initial validation of myositis activity and damage indices in patients with adult onset disease. *Rheumatology (Oxford)* 2004; **43**:49–54.

Lowry CA, Pilkington CA. Juvenile dermatomyositis: extramuscular manifestations and their management. *Curr Opin Rheumatol* 2009; 2: 575–80.

Pilkington C. Clinical assessment in juvenile idiopathic inflammatory myopathies and the development of disease activity and damage tools. *Curr Opin Rheumatol* 2004;**16**:673–7.

Overlap syndromes

Background

- Patients of all ages may exhibit features of >1 of the classical autoimmune rheumatic diseases (JIA, SLE, JDM, systemic sclerosis) (Fig. 4.16).
- Patients who do not fully fulfill the diagnostic criteria of any one defined autoimmune rheumatological disease may also fall within this spectrum of disease and are described as having 'undifferentiated' autoimmune rheumatic disease (UAIRD)/connective tissue disease (UCTD).
- Overlap syndromes have been defined as entities satisfying classification criteria of at least two connective tissue diseases occurring at the same or at different times in the same patient.
- Some overlap syndromes may cluster around clinical features and specific autoantibody markers, while others may cluster around clinical features alone. Some have classified these for adults (Table 4.20) with case reports in children.
- Over time, UAIRD and overlap syndromes may 'evolve' so the features of one of the classical autoimmune diseases predominate.
- Sometimes one AIRD, e.g. JDM may 'evolve' into another, e.g. SLE.
- The variability of the clinical manifestations over time in the juvenile population is thought to be more common than in adult patients and thought to be reflective of a more plastic immune system.
- One needs to remain vigilant for features of SLE, myositis, systemic sclerosis, inflammatory arthritis, and vasculitis in any child with an overlap syndrome, and should rigorously avoid a rigid diagnostic label.

Mixed connective tissue disease (MCTD)

- This is the best described of the overlap syndromes, and characterized by:

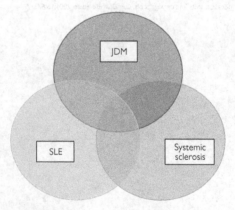

Fig. 4.16 Overlap syndromes.

Table 4.20 The spectrum of overlap syndromes

Associated with a specific autoantibody	• Mixed connective tissue disease (U1RNP) • Anti-synthetase syndrome (anti tRNA synthetase) • Polymyositis and scleroderma (anti-PM/Scl) • SLE and Sjögren's (anti La/SSB)
Not associated with a specific autoantibody	• Rhupus syndrome • Systemic sclerosis and Sjögren's syndrome • Systemic sclerosis and RF+ JIA • SLE and systemic sclerosis • RF+ JIA and Sjögren's syndrome • Polymyositis and Sjögren's syndrome

- Puffy, swollen hands ('sausage fingers'—diffuse swelling of the entire digit distinct from the articular swelling seen in JIA) and sclerodactyly.
- Raynaud's phenomenon.
- High titre speckled pattern ANA on immunofluorescence with antibodies to U1-RNP.
- A variety of formal diagnostic criteria have been proposed for MCTD in adults (e.g. Sharp's, Kasukawa, Porter's); none have been validated in children.
- Controversy still exists over whether MCTD is a discrete diagnostic entity because U1-RNP antibodies are also found in SLE, and follow-up of adult MCTD patients shows that many differentiate into SLE or SSc. Proponents of MCTD argue that antibodies to U1-RNP and MCTD have specific immunogenetic associations (e.g. HLA-DR4) suggesting a distinct pathogenesis.
- Clinical features and their frequencies (derived from synthesis of data from a number of case series) in juvenile onset MCTD are shown in Table 4.21.
- MCTD is one of the least common paediatric rheumatology diagnoses with a frequency of 0.1–0.5%.
- Mean age of onset of paediatric MCTD is 9–12yr.
- F:M ratio ~3:1.
- In children, evolution of MCTD is common. Over time arthritis, myositis, and SLE-like manifestations may transition to scleroderma-type features.
- Inflammatory manifestations (e.g. arthritis, myositis) respond better to immunosuppression and result in less permanent damage than scleroderma-type manifestations.
- There are conflicting observations from small case series of paediatric MCTD over whether SLE-like or sclerodermatous features are more common than in adult MCTD.
- Some studies report a more benign prognosis in paediatric MCTD compared to adult disease, but other series show the opposite.
- Long-term complications include renal disease, loss of range of movement in joints, restrictive lung disease, oesophageal dysmotility,

Table 4.21. Clinical features of MCTD

Manifestation	Frequency (%)*
Raynaud's phenomenon	91%
Arthritis	81%
Sclerodermatous skin changes/sclerodactyly	60%
Rash (may be lupus-type or JDM-type)	50–60%
Myositis	52%
Sicca symptoms/parotitis	40%
Interstitial lung disease	28%
Oesophageal dysmotility	15%
Thrombocytopenia	12%
Pericarditis	12%
Haemolytic anaemia	5%
Pulmonary arterial hypertension	5%

* Frequencies are derived from synthesis of data from a number of case series.

and cardiac disease. Pulmonary hypertension is less common than in adult patients.

Sjögren's syndrome overlap
- 1° Sjögren's syndrome is an autoimmune exocrinopathy characterized pathologically by focal lymphocytic infiltration of glandular tissue eventually leading to glandular destruction.
- Some patients have overlapping features of Sjögren's syndrome and other connective tissue diseases. The term 'Sjögren overlap' has been used to describe these patients.
- The syndrome manifests clinically as sicca symptoms (dryness of mucosal surfaces, particularly eyes and mouth).
- Extraglandular features such as arthralgia, hepatic involvement, and renal tubular acidosis may also occur.
- Both pSS and Sjögren overlap are very rare in children.

Overlap with organ-specific autoimmunity
- Systemic autoimmune disease may overlap with organ-specific autoimmune disease.
- SLE/autoimmune hepatitis (AIH) overlap is well described.
- AIH occurs in 9% of juvenile SLE patients (compared to only 1% of adult SLE patients).
- In juveniles AIH usually precedes the development of SLE; in adults the converse is true.

Investigations in patients with overlap syndromes:

- These depend on the clinical manifestations. However, consideration should be given to the following:
- Full immunological work-up at initial presentation to best characterize disease:
  - RF, ANA, ENA, dsDNA, ANCA, anticardiolipin antibodies and lupus anticoagulant, complement (C3, C4), immunoglobulins G, A, and M.
- Serial measurement of dsDNA & C3/C4; repeat ENA every 2yr as the autoantibody profile may evolve with time.
- TFTs and anti-thyroid antibodies.
- Coombs test.
- Muscle enzymes (CK, LDH, AST).
- Urine dip at all clinic visits; if abnormal request urine microscopy to look for casts, urine culture, and urine protein:creatinine ratio.
- MRI is a useful non-invasive tool for assessing myositis. Muscle biopsy remains the 'gold standard' but is painful and so often avoided in children.
- CXR.
- Barium swallow to assess for oesophageal dilatation/dysmotility.
- Lung function tests with gas transfer (depending on the age of the child) to identify interstitial lung disease—consider high resolution CT of the chest if abnormal.
- Echocardiography to estimate pulmonary artery pressure if pulmonary hypertension suspected.

Treatment

- Treatment is tailored to individual manifestations of the child's disease:
- *Arthritis*—NSAIDs, MTX, hydroxychloroquine, corticosteroids.
- *Rash*—hydroxychloroquine, topical treatments including corticosteroids and tacrolimus.
- *Raynaud's phenomenon*—calcium channel blockers (e.g. nifedipine), GTN patch, angiotensin II receptor blockers in addition to conservative measures.
  - IV epoprostenol or epoprostenol analogue (e.g. iloprost) may be used in severe cases with digital ischaemia.
- *Myositis*—steroids, AZA, MTX. IVIg, and cyclophosphamide may be used in severe cases. Other biological agents such as infliximab and rituximab may have a role.
- *Interstitial lung disease*—steroids, AZA, or MMF, or CYC.
- *Pulmonary arterial hypertension (PAH)*—this carries a poor prognosis. Consult a cardiologist with experience of PAH.

Iloprost administration: standard regimen is an infusion lasting 6h per day for 5 consecutive days. See also ➔ BSPAR guidelines for treatments uses in paediatric rheumatology, p. 472.

50 micrograms (0.5mL) iloprost is mixed with 49.5mL of normal saline in a syringe driver, giving a solution of 50mcg in 50mL. A fresh solution should be prepared daily.

Day1

- Commence at 0.5 nanogram/kg/min (1mcg = 1000ng).
- If tolerated, after 30min ↑ to 1 ng/kg/min.
- If tolerated, after further 30min ↑ to 1.5ng/kg/min.
- If tolerated, after further 30min ↑ to 2ng/kg/min. Run at this rate for the remaining 4.5h.

On subsequent days commence rate at the highest rate tolerated on the previous day.

Check P/BP/T prior to infusion, every 30min during infusion, and 1h post infusion.

Common side-effects: facial flushing, headaches, nausea & vomiting, diarrhoea, sweating, paraesthesia, erythema around infusion site, hypotension. If mild, reduce rate by 0.5ng/kg/min. If moderate/severe stop the infusion. It may be possible to re-start at the lowest rate following pre-medication with paracetamol and an antiemetic,

ND Iloprost is renally excreted: use ½ dose in patients on dialysis.

Antiphospholipid syndrome (APS)

Background

- APS is a multisystem autoimmune disease characterized by persistent positivity of antiphospholipid (aPL) antibodies in the presence of vascular thrombotic events, pregnancy morbidity, and other clinical manifestations.
- The APS may occur as an isolated clinical entity (primary APS) or in association with an underlying systemic disease (secondary APS), most commonly SLE.
- Paediatric 1° APS is very rare whilst the prevalence of 2° APS in children with SLE is estimated to be 9–14%.

Classification criteria

Preliminary criteria for the classification of paediatric APS are based on revised classification criteria for the diagnosis of APS in adults, and include:

- *Clinical criteria*—vascular thrombosis: 1 or more clinical episodes of arterial, venous, or small-vessel thrombosis, in any tissue or organ. Thrombosis must be confirmed by objective validated criteria (i.e. unequivocal findings of appropriate imaging studies or histopathology). For histopathological confirmation, thrombosis should be present without significant evidence of inflammation in the vessel wall.
- *Laboratory criteria* must be present on 2 or more occasions, at least 12 weeks apart and include:
  - Anticardiolipin (ACL) antibody of IgG and/or IgM isotype in serum or plasma: must be present in medium or high titre (i.e. >40 GPL or MPL, or >99th percentile).
  - Anti-β2 glycoprotein-I antibody of IgG and/or IgM isotype in serum or plasma: must be present in titre >99th percentile.
  - Lupus anticoagulant (LA) in plasma.

Paediatric APS is considered to be present if the clinical criterion and at least 1 of the laboratory criteria are met.

Pathogenesis

- Exactly how aPL antibodies cause thrombosis, and why some patients develop thromboses rather than pregnancy morbidity is currently unknown.
- One hypothesis postulates that pathogenic aPL antibodies target and bind cellular and platelet phospholipids in the presence of certain serum cofactors such as beta-2 glycoprotein I, leading to cellular activation and biological effects such as promotion of thrombosis.
- In addition, aPL antibodies cause an increase in expression of tissue factor (a critical pro-thrombotic intermediate in the clotting cascade) in both monocytes and endothelial cells.

Furthermore, platelet and complement activation as well as endothelial activation and a 'second hit' inflammatory signal may play a role, particularly in those with catastrophic APS (CAPS).

Clinical features

The clinical manifestations of APS in children include:

- *Vascular thrombosis:*
  - Most commonly this is deep vein thrombosis of the lower limbs.
  - More rare are thromboses in the superficial and upper extremity veins, inferior and superior vena cava, hepatic (Budd–Chiari syndrome) and portal veins, renal, adrenal, retinal, and intracranial veins.
  - Arterial thrombosis, resulting mainly in stroke (20% of all thrombotic events thromboses) and transient ischaemic attacks (11% of all thrombotic events), are less common. Other involved vessels include coronary, subclavian, mesenteric, renal, retinal, and pedal arteries. Of note is that arterial thrombosis is much more common in children than in adults.
- *Central nervous system symptoms*—chorea (always consider APS in the differential diagnosis of Sydenham's chorea), dementia, migraine, intracranial hypertension, neurocognitive deficits, psychosis and depression, epilepsy, Guillain–Barré syndrome, transverse myelopathy, and optical neuritis.
- *Cardiac manifestations*—valvulopathy (mitral/aortic valves), intracardiac thrombosis, coronary artery thrombosis, and cardiomyopathy.
- *Haematological disorders*—mainly thrombocytopenia and haemolytic anemia (direct Coombs testing is usually positive in the latter).
- *Skin manifestations*—livedo reticularis, cutaneous gangrene, skin ulcers, livedoid vasculopathy (an important occlusive vasculopathy mimicking vasculitis, although not vasculitic in nature), palmar and plantar erythema, anetoderma (focal loss of dermal elastic tissue, resulting in localized areas of flaccid or herniated saclike skin), Raynaud's phenomenon.
- *Renal manifestations* include:
  - Renal artery thrombosis.
  - Thrombosis in smaller-diameter renal vessels, resulting in areas of focal cortical, ischaemia and/or necrosis.
  - Thrombotic microangiopathy—most characteristic lesion of APS nephropathy, with distinctive microscopic and ultrastructural changes.
  - Thrombosis of the renal veins and inferior vena cava.
- *Pulmonary involvement* is rare in children with APS, but includes: pulmonary embolism, intra-alveolar haemorrhages, primary thrombosis of lung vessels, both major and minor, as well as pulmonary capillaritis, pulmonary hypertension.
- *Various GI manifestations* have been reported including intestinal and oesophageal ischaemia and infarction, ischaemic colitis, colonic ulceration, infarction of the liver, cholecystitis, and mesenteric, hepatic, and portal vein thrombosis.
- *Perinatal APS*—rare cases of perinatal thrombosis in infants born to mothers with APS or mothers with aPL antibodies have been reported, with the clinical presentation consisting of arterial and venous thromboses in multiple localizations. Although patients in this subgroup have diagnostic criteria of APS, their disease behaves differently, is transitory and does not recur, similar to patients with neonatal SLE.

Laboratory investigations

- Clotting screen:
  - The first clue to the presence of aPL antibodies is the finding of a prolonged APTT. If the clotting remains abnormal when the patient's plasma is mixed with normal pooled plasma, this is suggestive of the presence of an inhibitor, the LA.
  - The presence of LA is then confirmed with a phospholipid-sensitive functional clotting testing, such as the dilute Russell viper venom test (dRVVT). In part one of the test Russell viper venom directly activates factor X, but phospholipid is still required to generate thrombin, so in the presence of PL binding anticardiolipin antibodies (the LA), clotting is delayed. In the second part of the test the inhibitory effect of LA on phospholipids can be overcome by adding an excess of phospholipid to the assay. The clotting times of both the initial dRVVT assay and the second part of the test are used to determine a ratio of time with or without phospholipid excess. A ratio >1.2 is considered positive and implies that the patient may have aPL antibodies.
- Other tests for measuring aPL antibodies are the enzyme-linked immunosorbent assay (ELISA) which detects different isotypes of anticardiolipin antibodies and antibodies to many other phospholipids (phosphatidylserine, phosphatidylinositol, phosphatidylcholine).
- Another group of antibodies are directed against protein co-factors that bind the phospholipids, such as beta-2 glycoprotein-1 and annexin.
- Although there is some overlap between all these antibodies, it is important to use >1 test to detect them.

Treatment

The risk of thrombosis is low in asymptomatic children who are incidentally found to have positive aPL; high among those in whom thrombosis already occurred and extremely high in patients with CAPS.

- Aspirin at low doses (2–5mg/kg/once daily) has been used as prophylaxis in aPL-positive children with autoimmune diseases but without previous thromboses and in particular to prevent arterial thromboses.
- Hydroxychloroquine may be protective against the development of thrombosis in aPL-positive patients with SLE.
- Warfarin: lifelong treatment if one major thrombotic episode has occurred (such as pulmonary or femoral arterial thrombus) is recommended, aim for INR 2–3.

Dosing regimen for warfarin is:
- 200 micrograms/kg (max. 10mg) as a single dose on first day.
- Reduce dose to 100 micrograms/kg (max. 5mg) once daily for following 3 days. Note that:
  - If INR still below 1.4 use 200 micrograms/kg (max. 10mg) once daily, or
  - If INR above 3 use 50 micrograms/kg (max. 2.5mg) once daily, or
  - If INR above 3.5 omit dose.
- Dose is then adjusted according to INR, usual maintenance 100–300 micrograms/kg once daily (may need up to 400 micrograms/kg).

NB initial warfarinization should be covered with full heparinization to prevent warfarin-induced thrombosis due to inhibition of protein C and S which occurs at INR levels <2. Heparin is usually given in its low-molecular-weight forms (LMWH) subcutaneously at therapeutic doses. It will often take up to 10 days to adjust warfarin treatment to obtain the recommended INR. During this time LMWH treatment is assessed through monitoring anti-Xa levels to ensure a therapeutic range (0.5–1.0 anti-Xa units/ml plasma). This is of particular importance in children with renal or hepatic impairment and severely ill children. Note that LMWH is not as easy to reverse as unfractionated heparin.

In cases of 2° APS, treatment of the underlying condition should be initiated in addition to anticoagulation and anti-platelet therapy.

Outcome

In one study, of a large paediatric APS cohort at follow-up of 6.1yr:
• 19% developed recurrent thromboses, which usually occurred in a similar blood vessel type as initial thrombosis.
• 5% presented with life threatening widespread thrombotic disease suggestive of CAPS.
• 7% died mainly due to aPL-related thrombotic complications.

Catastrophic APS (CAPS)

• CAPS is a rapidly progressive life-threatening disease causing multiple organ thromboses and dysfunction in the presence of aPL antibodies, and is associated with an ↑ mortality despite treatment. The syndrome is characterized by a diffuse thrombotic microvasculopathy.
• The exact pathogenesis of CAPS remains unclear. One hypothesis postulates that clots continue to generate thrombin, fibrinolysis is depressed by an increase in plasminogen activator inhibitor type-1 (PAI-1), and there is consumption of the natural anticoagulant proteins such as protein C and anti-thrombin III. In addition, manifestations of the systemic inflammatory response syndrome are presumed to be due to excessive cytokine release from affected/necrotic tissues.
• Another specific characteristic of CAPS is that 60% of patients appear to have a triggering factor especially infections, the commonest identifiable trigger for CAPS and present in about 25% of cases.
• For treatment of CAPS seek *expert advice* and consider IVIg (2g/kg), Pulsed IV methylprednisolone, cyclophosphamide, and/or rituximab and plasma exchange, in addition to full anticoagulation and anti-platelet therapy as per APS.
• Despite treatment, mortality in CAPS is reported to be as high as 48%.

Further reading

Avcin T, Silverman ED. Antiphospholipid antibodies in pediatric systemic lupus erythematosus and the antiphospholipid syndrome. *Lupus* 2007; 16; 627.
Avcin T, Cimaz R, Rozman B; Ped-APS Registry Collaborative Group Lupus. The Ped-APS Registry: the antiphospholipid syndrome in childhood. *Lupus* 2009; 18:894–9.

Paediatric uveitis

Definition

- Uveitis is the term for intraocular inflammation, i.e. those layers internal to the sclera and cornea (see Fig. 4.17 for eye anatomy).
- The uveal tract is the vascular layer including the choroid, ciliary body, and iris (uvea = grape in Greek).
- The term uveitis referred to inflammation of the uveal tract but can also refer to inflammation of the retina and vitreous.

Aetiology

- The causes can be infectious and non-infectious (Tables 4.22 and 4.23).
  - Non-infectious uveitis has an approximate incidence of 4–7/100,000 children.
- The appearance and site of the inflammation may help to determine the cause, e.g. sarcoidosis is typically a granulomatous anterior or panuveitis (Table 4.24). The investigations to consider depend on the clinical presentation (Table 4.25).

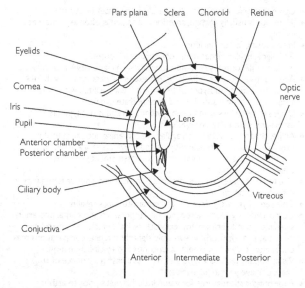

Fig. 4.17 Anatomy of the eye

Reproduced with permission from Uveitis Information Group (Scotland), http://www.uveitis.net/patient/glossary.php, accessed 09 Jan. 2017.

Table 4.22 Infectious causes of paediatric uveitis

Relatively common	Relatively uncommon but with geographical variation
• Toxoplasmosis gondii	• Lyme disease
• VZV	• Toxocara
• Herpes simplex virus	• Histoplasmosis
• CMV	• Ascaris
• Tuberculosis	• Echovirus
• Bartonella	• Fungal infection
	• Syphilis

Masquerade syndromes include:

• Leukaemia, retinoblastoma, intraocular foreign body, primary retinal detachment, retinal dystrophy, juvenile xanthogranulomatosis.

JIA associated uveitis

• JIA is the commonest systemic disease associated with paediatric uveitis.
• Reported prevalence of uveitis affecting children with JIA varies between 12–30%.
• Can occur before, or up to 7 years after, the onset of arthritis.
• JIA uveitis is usually chronic anterior uveitis and is often asymptomatic initially.
• Predisposing factors include:
  • Oligoarticular rather than polyarticular JIA onset.
  • Age at JIA onset <7yr (and especially <4yr), and ANA positivity.
• Acute anterior uveitis in JIA is almost exclusively associated with ERA rather than other subtypes of JIA, which are associated with chronic anterior or chronic anterior and intermediate uveitis.
• Uveitis is much less common in systemic JIA and is not typically associated with early onset RA.
• All JIA children should have regular eye screening according to the Royal College of Ophthalmologists and BSPAR (see ➲ Screening, pp. 148–51). Refer for ophthalmological assessment when JIA is diagnosed or suspected.
• Uveitis is measured by the amount of anterior chamber cells and flare in the slit lamp beam.
• Children <8yr rarely describe unilateral visual loss reliably.
• Complications include raised intraocular pressure, glaucoma, posterior synechiae, band keratopathy, cataract, retinal detachment, macular oedema, and hypotony. Irreversible sight threatening complications may occur after only a few weeks of uncontrolled eye inflammation.
• Visual impairment, to 20/50 vision or less, has an incidence of 0.18 cases per eye year in JIA uveitis.
• Poor prognostic features for vision include uveitis prior to arthritis, severe uveitis at presentation, and failure to achieve early remission.

Table 4.23 Non-infectious types of paediatric uveitis

No systemic disease association	Associated with systemic disease
Idiopathic uveitis: the most common type in population-based cohorts. In children <8yr of age idiopathic chronic anterior uveitis is by far the most common. In those with onset between 8–15yr of age intermediate uveitis is relatively more common, and in older patients acute anterior uveitis is the most frequent type, as in adults. Named uveitis syndromes are very rare in childhood: • Sympathetic ophthalmia—trauma to one eye causes uveitis in the other eye, typically multifocal choroiditis and panuveitis	**Common:** • Juvenile idiopathic arthritis (JIA)—typically chronic asymptomatic anterior uveitis. The most common systemic disease associated with paediatric uveitis worldwide • Enthesitis related arthritis (ERA)—usually acute anterior uveitis and often carry HLA B27 • Inflammatory bowel disease—anterior and intermediate uveitis • Kawasaki disease—an acute non-granulomatous bilateral uveitis which usually resolves without any specific ocular therapy and without visual complication • Sarcoidosis—anterior and pan uveitis. Granulomas of uvea frequent • Blau syndrome—if there is a family history of granulomatous disease consider this autosomal dominant genetic granulomatous condition involving arthritis, uveitis and dermatitis with a typical skin rash (*NOD2* gene; see ➜ pp. 316–20 sarcoid) • Tubulointerstitial nephritis uveitis (TINU)—bilateral anterior uveitis and acute interstitial nephritis; occasionally associated with deafness
	Less common
• Acute multifocal placoid pigment epitheliopathy • Fuch's cyclitis • Birdshot retinochoroidopathy	• Other childhood-onset vasculitides: GPA, PAN, scleroderma, SLE, Cogan's syndrome (atypical; typical Cogan's is associated with interstitial keratitis) • Behçet's disease—posterior and anterior uveitis is recognized. Rare to have onset of uveitis in childhood • Chronic inflammatory neurologic cutaneous and articular syndrome (CINCA)—uveitis and papillitis with chronic disc swelling • Other periodic fever syndromes • Vogt–Koyanagi–Harada syndrome—uveitis, vitiligo, poliosis (= ↓or absence of melanin in head hair, eyebrows, or eyelashes), neurological and auditory findings • Multiple sclerosis with intermediate uveitis is rare in childhood, although intermediate uveitis is common

Table 4.24 Anatomical classification of uveitis

Uveitis type	Inflammation site
Anterior uveitis	Anterior segment (i.e. iris ± ciliary body)
Intermediate uveitis	Vitreous and retina
Anterior and intermediate uveitis	Intermediate uveitis with significant anterior uveitis
Posterior uveitis	Retina or choroid only
Panuveitis	Anterior uveitis and posterior uveitis

Table 4.25 Suggested investigations in paediatric uveitis

Suggested first line investigations	Suggested second line investigations
• FBC, blood film • ESR, CRP • Renal function: plasma creatinine and consider formal GFR if abnormal • Immunoglobulins • ASO titre • ANA • Urine analysis for blood and protein; UA:UC if proteinuria on dip test • Mantoux and or Quantiferon (or equivalent gamma interferon release assay) • Case appropriate infection PCR/serology.	• Tissue biopsy—especially of rashes; other including renal biopsy • CXR • Chest CT • Serum ACE • ANCA • MRI/MRA brain • Selective visceral arteriography (particularly for PAN, see ➜ pp. 179–80 Vasculitis investigation) • Pure tone audiometry and assessment of vestibular function (Cogan's) • Many others—including specific genetic tests dependent on the clinical presentation • To pursue the diagnosis of infectious/malignant causes where the clinical diagnosis is in doubt: • PCR (including 16S and 18S ribosomal PCR as screening tests for bacterial and fungal infection respectively) and cytology of ocular fluids is usually necessary. • Serology for infectious agent may be helpful to exclude, but not diagnose, causes of ocular infection.

- Reducing JIA medication given for arthritis, e.g. MTX may result in a uveitis flare.
- Raised inflammatory markers in the absence of corresponding articular signs may represent ocular inflammation.
- JIA associated uveitis can persist into adulthood.

Treatment modalities in paediatric uveitis

Treatment balances the long-term risk of visual loss with the short- and long-term risks of treatment. In most cases these risks are not well established. About half of children with JIA uveitis do not suffer visual loss despite prolonged inflammation. Aggressive treatments should be used for those with a significant risk of permanent visual loss, and this risk (and the efficacy of available treatments) may change considerably over the course of disease. Treatment will depend on causes identified from the investigations previously described. For idiopathic and autoimmune/autoinflammatory causes, including uveitis associated with JIA:

Corticosteroids

- Topical corticosteroids are invariably used when the predominant site of inflammation is anterior, e.g. prednisolone 1% or dexamethasone 0.1% drops. They are not indicated when predominant site is intermediate or posterior. Cataracts are a side-effect of long-term use.
- Topical mydriatics are used to reduce the risk of synechiae formation in anterior uveitis.
- Topical glaucoma agents may be required to reduce intraocular pressure.
- Systemic corticosteroids are used for severe uveitis, e.g. intravenous methylprednisolone 20–30mg/kg/day for three days or high dose oral prednisolone followed by a reducing course over 4–6 weeks. Avoid long-term or frequent use due to side-effects.
- Periocular corticosteroids, e.g. orbital floor steroid injection, may be used where topical steroids are ineffective. Intravitreal steroids are occasionally used where risk of cataract and glaucoma are low.

Steroid sparing medications

- Methotrexate (MTX) 15mg/m^2 once weekly (SC or PO) is second-line treatment for JIA uveitis when topical steroids have not adequately controlled the inflammation.
- Mycophenolate mofetil, azathioprine, ciclosporin, tacrolimus.
- Evidence for use is from case series rather than controlled clinical trials.

Biologic medication

- Inhibitors of tumour necrosis factor alpha (anti-TNFα), adalimumab and infliximab, are used in JIA uveitis poorly controlled with MTX. Recent controlled clinical trials have demonstrated benefit of adalimumab in paediatric uveitis. Etanercept is not recommended for JIA uveitis— see ➔ Biologics, pp. 448–54.
- The interleukin 1 inhibitors anakinra and canakinumab have been used to treat uveitis associated with CAPS (which includes the severe variant chronic infantile neurological cutaneous arthritis, CINCA).

Standardizing uveitis measurement for research

- Currently there are no standardized criteria for measuring paediatric uveitis activity in clinical studies.
- Proposed standardized terms and grades for adult uveitis were published in 2005.
- Proposed outcome measures for prospective clinical trials in JIA-associated arthritis in 2012 are to be validated.

Further reading

Jabs DA, Nussenblatt RB, Rosen-baum JT, et al. Standardization of uveitis nomenclature for reporting clinical data. Results of the First International Workshop. Am J Ophthalmol 2005; **140**:509–16.

Heiligenhaus A, Foeldvari I, Edelsten C. Proposed outcome measures for prospective clinical trials in juvenile idiopathic arthritis-associated uveitis: a consensus effort from the multinational interdisciplinary working group for uveitis in childhood. Arthritis Care Res 2012;**64**:1365–72.

NHS England Interim Clinical Commissioning Policy: Adalimumab for Children with Severe Refractory Uveitis. November 2015. Reference: D12X02. ℬ https://www.england.nhs.uk/commissioning/wp-content/uploads/sites/12/2015/11/d12x02-paediatric-uveitis-anti-tnf.pdf

Periodic fever syndromes and autoinflammatory disease

Introduction to the periodic fever syndromes

The *periodic* fever syndromes/autoinflammatory syndromes are disorders of innate immunity. They are characterized by:

- recurring episodes of fever and constitutional upset, usually with normal health between attacks.
- systemic inflammatory symptoms affecting the:
  - serosal surfaces.
  - joints.
  - skin.
  - eyes.
- symptoms that are always accompanied by biochemical markers of inflammation such as raised ESR, CRP, and leucocytosis.

Most syndromes are compatible with near normal life expectancy, except for the risk of developing AA amyloidosis in later life. Despite similarities in symptoms, they have differing aetiologies, inheritance, attack durations, and clinical features.

The *hereditary* periodic fever syndromes are associated with mutations in genes involved in innate immunity and generally the onset is early in childhood and both sexes are equally affected. There are now almost 30 recognized syndromes. Many are extremely rare and the most recognized ones are described below (summarized in Table 4.26).

- Familial Mediterranean fever (FMF).
- TNF receptor associated period syndrome (TRAPS).
- Mevalonate kinase deficiency (MKD; also known as hyperimmunoglobulin D and periodic fever syndrome (HIDS)).
- Cryopyrin associated periodic syndrome (CAPS), subdivided into familial cold autoinflammatory syndrome (FCAS), Muckle Wells Syndrome (MWS) and chronic infantile, neurological, cutaneous and articular syndrome/neonatal onset multisystem inflammatory disease (CINCA/NOMID).
- Pyogenic arthritis, pyoderma gangrenosum and acne (PAPA) syndrome.
- Deficiency of IL-1 receptor antagonist (DIRA).
- Blau syndrome/early onset sarcoidosis (EOS).
- Deficiency of IL-36 antagonist (DITRA).
- Chronic atypical neutrophilic dermatosis with lipodystrophy and elevated temperature (CANDLE).
- Deficiency of adenosine deaminase 2 (DADA 2).
- STING-associated vasculopathy with onset in infancy (SAVI).
- NALP12 associated periodic syndrome (NAPS).
- Majeed syndrome.

There are now completely effective treatments for most patients with FMF, TRAPS, CAPS, and DIRA and although not always quite as effective, good treatments are available for the majority of the other syndromes.

Table 4.26 Hereditary periodic fever syndromes

Periodic fever syndrome	Gene	Mode of inheritance	Predominant ethnic groups	Usual age at onset	Potential precipitants of attacks	Distinctive clinical features	Typical duration of attacks	Typical frequency of attacks	Characteristic laboratory abnormalities	Treatment
FMF	MEFV Chromosome 16	Autosomal recessive (dominant in rare families)	Eastern Mediterranean	Childhood/ early adult	Usually none Occasionally menstruation, fasting, stress, trauma	Short severe attacks Colchicine responsive Erysipelas like erythema	1–3 days	Variable	Marked acute phase response during attacks	Colchicine Anti-IL1 therapies in refractory cases
TRAPS	TNRSF1A Chromosome 12	Autosomal dominant, can be de novo	Northern European but reported in many ethnic groups	Childhood/ early adult	Usually none	Prolonged symptoms	More than a week, may be very prolonged	Variable, may be continuous	Marked acute phase response during attacks. Low levels of soluble TNFR1 when well	Anti-IL1 therapies or etanercept. High-dose corticosteroids
HIDS	MVK Chromosome 12	Autosomal recessive	Northern European	Infancy	Immunizations	Diarrhoea and lymphadenopathy	3–7 days	1–2-monthly	Elevated IgD & IgA, acute phase response, and mevalonate aciduria during attacks	Anti-TNF, or anti IL1 therapies, or anti-IL6 therapies

	Gene / Chromosome	Inheritance	Ethnicity	Onset	Diurnal variation	Severity spectrum	Timing	Frequency	Acute phase response	Therapy
CAPS	*NLRP3* Chromosome 1	Autosomal dominant or sporadic	Northern European	Neonatal/infancy	Marked diurnal variation Cold environment but less marked than in FCAS	Severity spectrum including: Urticarial rash Conjunctivitis Sensorineural deafness Aseptic chronic meningitis Deforming arthropathy	Continuous often worse in the evenings	Often daily	Varying but marked acute phase response most of the time	Anti-IL1 therapies
PAPA	*PSTPIP1 (CD2BP1)* Chromosome 15	Autosomal dominant	Northern European (only 3 families reported)	Childhood	None	Pyogenic arthritis, pyoderma gangrenosum Cystic acne	Intermittent attacks with migratory arthritis	Variable, and may be continuous	Acute phase response during attacks	Anti-TNF therapy or anti IL-1 therapies
DIRA	*IL1RN* Chromosome 2	Autosomal recessive	Hispanic and European (few families reported)	Neonatal	None	Sterile multifocal osteomyelitis, periostitis, and pustulosis	Continuous	Continuous	Marked acute phase response	Anakinra (IL-1ra)
Blau syndrome	*NOD2 (CARD15)* Chromosome 16	Autosomal dominant	None	Infancy/ Childhood	None	Granulomatous polyarthritis, iritis, and dermatitis	Continuous	Continuous	Sustained modest acute phase response	Corticosteroids and anti-TNF

Disorders of unknown aetiology which shared some features with the inherited syndromes include:
- periodic fever, aphthous stomatitis, pharyngitis, and cervical adenitis (PFAPA) syndrome.
- Behcet's disease.
- Chronic recurrent multifocal osteomyelitis (CRMO).
- Systemic juvenile idiopathic arthritis (sJIA).

Inherited fever syndromes

Familial Mediterranean fever

Familial Mediterranean fever is commonest in Middle Eastern populations (prevalence 1/250 to 1/1000) but occurs worldwide. It is due to mutations in the *MEFV* gene on chromosome 16. The vast majority demonstrate recessive inheritance but disease is well recognized in heterozygotes and there are rare mutations which cause autosomal dominant disease.

Clinical features
- Attacks occur irregularly and may be precipitated by minor physical or emotional stress, the menstrual cycle, or diet.
- Attacks last 12–72 hours and the clinical features are:
  - fever.
  - aseptic peritonitis in 85%.
  - pleuritic chest pain in 40%.
  - erysipelas-like rash occurs in 20%.
  - meningitic headache rarely.
  - orchitis rarely.
  - joint involvement is rare and generally mild affecting the lower limbs.
- Acute attacks are accompanied by a neutrophil leukocytosis and a dramatic acute phase response.
- Protracted febrile myalgia is a very rare complication, characterized by severe pain musculature and can be accompanied by a vasculitic rash; it usually responds to high dose corticosteroid therapy.

Diagnosis
Diagnosis is supported by DNA analysis but remains clinical and centres on the history of recurrent self-limiting attacks of fever and serositis that are prevented by colchicine.

Treatment
- Colchicine has now been licensed by the US Food and Drug administration for the prophylactic treatment of FMF from the age of 4 years upwards.
- Continuous use prevents or substantially reduces symptoms of FMF in at least 95%, and almost completely eliminates the risk of developing AA amyloidosis.
- The mechanism of action of colchicine remains incompletely understood but most patients respond to between 250 mcg and 2 mg daily.

Long-term complications
- Life-long treatment is required but in general the long-term outlook is excellent with normal life expectancy.
- Prior to colchicine, 60% of Turkish patients developed AA amyloidosis; effective long-term colchicine prophylaxis should completely prevent this.
- Destructive arthritis is very rare.
- Growth, educational achievement, and fertility appear to be normal for both sexes once treated. In untreated disease recurrent attacks cause severe disruption to development, education, and family life.

Tumour necrosis factor receptor-associated periodic syndrome (TRAPS)

Tumour necrosis factor receptor-associated periodic syndrome (TRAPS) has an estimated prevalence of about 1 per million in Europe. It is an autosomal dominant disease and 64% have a family history. It occurs in many ethnic groups and median age at presentation is 4 years.

Clinical features
TRAPS attacks are often far less distinct than in FMF and may be precipitated by minor stress, travel, the menstrual cycle, or diet. Typical features are:
- Prolonged attacks lasting 1–3 weeks (symptoms are near continuous in 30%).
- ~90% of patients experience fever.
- 85% classically have arthralgia and myalgia often with centripetal migration.
- Abdominal pain occurs in 74% of patients.
- Rash (erythematous, oedematous plaques, discrete reticulate, or serpiginous lesions) occurs in 64% of patients.
- Other features include:
  - headache.
  - pleuritic pain.
  - lymphadenopathy.
  - conjunctivitis and periorbital oedema.
- Symptoms are accompanied by a marked acute phase response.

Diagnosis
- Genetic testing is central to diagnosis. One difficulty is interpretation of the significance of the common polymorphism, R92Q which is present in ~ 4% of normal population but can be associated with an inflammatory syndrome.

Treatment
- Acute attacks respond to high dose corticosteroids but this does not reduce the frequency of attacks.
- IL-1 blockade seems to be the most effective treatment. Recombinant IL-1 Ra (anakinra) is effective in ~ 90% cases but needs to be injected daily. Long-acting IL-1 blocking agents (anti-IL-1 monoclonal antibodies) are also effective.
- Etanercept is useful in some patients, but infliximab and other monoclonal antibodies to TNF may exacerbate attacks in some patients.

Long-term complications
- Life-long treatment is required but in general the long-term outlook is good.
- Without effective long-term treatment > 25% patients developed AA amyloidosis.
- Growth, educational achievement, and fertility appear to be near normal for both sexes with treatment. Otherwise the child's development, education and family life are severely compromised.

Mevalonate kinase deficiency (MKD)

Mevalonate kinase deficiency (MKD) also known as hyperimmunoglobulin D and periodic fever syndrome (HIDS) is an autosomal recessive disease. MVK is the enzyme after HMG CoA reductase, most mutations found in this syndrome reduce enzyme activity by >90%. Mutations resulting in near complete absence of enzyme activity cause mevalonic aciduria (MVA) with a much more severe phenotype. MKD is extremely rare; most patients are North European with a concentration in the Netherlands although it occurs in other ethnicities. Usually the onset of MKD is in the first year of life.

Clinical features
- Attacks occur irregularly and may be precipitated by vaccination, minor trauma, surgery, or stress.
- Attacks last 4 to 7 days.
- Attacks consist of:
  - fever.
  - unilateral or bilateral cervical lymphadenopathy.
  - abdominal pain with vomiting and diarrhea.
  - headache, arthralgia, large joint arthritis; erythematous macules and papules and aphthous ulcers are also common.
- History of high fevers or a full attack with vaccination.
- Sometimes less severe in adult life.

Diagnosis
- A high serum IgD, IgE, and IgA concentration are seen although these are not specific.
- Presence of mevalonic acid in the urine during attacks.
- A mutation in both alleles of the MVK gene can be identified in most patients.

Treatment
- Etanercept is useful in some patients.
- IL-1 blockade seems to be the most effective treatment anecdotally. Recombinant IL-1 Ra (anakinra) can either be used continuously or to abort attacks. A recent trial of canakinumab suggests long-term IL-1beta inhibition is very useful.
- Statins do not appear to be useful.
- Cure with allogeneic haematopoietic stem cell transplantation has been described; this treatment is reserved for those where all else has failed, however.

Long-term complications
- Symptoms may partially improve with age.
- AA amyloidosis has been reported but appears less common than in FMF, TRAPS, or CAPS.
- Metabolic consequences including retinitis pigmentosa, seizures. and intellectual impairment are described.

Cryopyrin associated periodic syndrome (CAPS)
CAPS comprises an overlapping severity spectrum ranging from mild to severe otherwise known as familial cold autoinflammatory syndrome (FCAS); Muckle Wells syndrome (MWS); and chronic infantile neurological, cutaneous, and articular syndrome (CINCA), which is known in the USA as neonatal onset multisystem inflammatory disease (NOMID). CAPS is associated with mutations in NLRP3 on chromosome 1q44, encoding a key component of the IL-1 activation complex, called the inflammasome. Dominant inheritance occurs in about 75% of patients with FCAS and MWS, whereas CINCA is usually due to de novo mutations. Most reported patients are Caucasian but cases have been described from South Asia and elsewhere. Onset of disease is usually in early infancy, often from birth, and there is no sex bias.

Clinical features
- In FCAS attacks of fever, urticarial rash, arthralgia, and conjunctivitis are precipitated by exposure to cold or damp conditions.
- In MWS attacks usually occur daily often in the afternoon and evenings although there may be a degree of cold exacerbation. Acute symptoms are fever, urticarial rash, arthralgia and myalgia, conjunctivitis, headache, and fatigue. The rash can be persistent. Deafness occurs later and is often missed in the early stages.
- In CINCA/NOMID there is continuous inflammation with additional severe chronic aseptic meningitis, raised intracranial pressure, uveitis, deafness and arthropathy.

Diagnosis
- Patients with FCAS and MWS have mutations in NLRP3. Mutations are present in only 50% of CINCA/NOMID patients and somatic mosaicism is increasingly recognized in sporadic cases.

Treatment
- The treatment of choice is IL-1 blockade with anakinra or with 2 other licensed therapies: fully human anti IL-1beta antibody, canakinumab or IL-1 Trap (rilonacept).

Long term complications
- AA amyloidosis occurs in ~ 25% of patients.
- Complications of chronic CNS inflammation—these are most severe in CINCA but are also seen in MWS.
  - Sensorineural deafness in 40%.
  - Blindness due to optic atrophy or uveitis.
  - Developmental delay.
- Arthropathy causes cartilage and bony overgrowth especially affecting the patella. Joint destruction can occur. In 17% clubbing of the finger nails is seen.

Pyogenic sterile arthritis, pyoderma gangrenosum and acne (PAPA) syndrome
- This is an exceptionally rare autosomal dominant disease caused by mutations in the proline serine threonine phosphatase-interacting protein 1 (PTSTPIP) gene encoding a protein also known as CD2 binding protein 1 (CB2BP1).
  - The underlying pathogenesis remains poorly understood although there is evidence that CD2BP1 interacts with pyrin.
- It is characterized clinically by severe acne and recurrent pustular sterile arthritis typically occurs after minor trauma.
- Early reports suggest that therapy with anakinra may be effective, especially for the skin lesions.

Deficiency of the IL-1 receptor antagonist (DIRA)
- This exceptionally rare autosomal recessive disease was first described in 2009 and only a handful of families are known.
- It is due to mutations in IL1RN resulting in a total deficiency of IL-1 receptor antagonist.
- It presents in the immediate neonatal period with a pustular rash, joint swelling, osteolytic lesions, and periosteitis typically affecting the distal ribs and the long bones.
- Treatment is anakinra with good responses seen in all cases treated so far.

Blau syndrome
- An exceptionally rare sarcoid-like autosomal dominant syndrome.
- Granulomatous infiltration of the skin, joints, and sometimes viscera associated with uveitis.
- Histologically it is indistinguishable from sarcoid.
- Associated with missense mutations in NOD2/CARD15.
- Treatment is with corticosteroids, anti-TNF, or other DMARDS.

DITRA
- An exceptionally rare autosomal recessive disease characterized by recurrent episodes of a generalized sterile pustular rash.
- Skin lesions appear psoriatic and accompanied by an acute phase response and fever.
- Due to mutations in IL36RN on chromosome 2. Loss of IL-36R antagonist results in unregulated signaling by IL-36 α, β, and γ.
- Early evidence suggests good response to treatment with anti IL-1 agents.

CANDLE
- An exceptionally rare autosomal recessive disease characterized by early onset, fevers, recurrent annular lesions, swollen violaceous eyelids, thick lips, progressive lipodystrophy, and arthralgia.
- Mutations in PSBM8 on chromosome 6 result in loss of function of proteasome and promote type 1 interferon signaling. Other proteasome and related mutations can also cause CANDLE.
- Early reports suggest benefit from Janus kinase (JAK) inhibition and clinical trials are underway.

DADA2

- This rare recessive disease presents as childhood onset polyarteritis nodosa (PAN), mild immunodeficiency, livedo racemose, and stroke. Other phenotypes include marrow failure, or Castleman's-like inflammation.
- Loss-of-function mutations in CECR1 encoding adenosine deaminase 2 (ADA2) cause reduced activity of ADA2 in plasma. ADA2 protein is produced by myeloid cells a growth factor for endothelial cells.
- There is preliminary evidence of benefit from anti-TNF therapies and analogy with ADA1 deficiency suggests a plausible role for allogeneic hematopoietic transplantation in selected cases. Gene therapy may be an option in the future.

SAVI

- This exceptionally rare autosomal dominant disease was first described in 2014 and is characterized by early-onset systemic inflammation, severe cutaneous vasculopathy, and lung disease.
- Gain-of-function mutation in TMEM173 (the gene encoding the stimulator of interferon genes, STING) induces type 1 interferon signaling.
- There is no established treatment, but JAK inhibitors are being trialled.

NAPS

- This exceptionally rare autosomal dominant disease was described in 2008 and causes episodes of fever with some reports of sensorineural deafness and cold-induced symptoms.
- Mutations in NLRP12 appear to reduce its inhibitory effect on NF-κB signaling.
- There is no established treatment.

Majeed syndrome

- This exceptionally rare autosomal recessive disease was described in 1989 and causes chronic, recurrent, multifocal osteomyelitis, congenital dyserythropoietic anemia with some reports of neutrophilic dermatosis.
- It is associated with mutations in LPIN2. Lipin2 protein is widely expressed and thought to play role in lipid metabolism. How mutations may cause an inflammatory phenotype is not known.

Periodic fever, aphthous stomatitis, pharyngitis and adenitis (PFAPA)

- This was first described in 1987 (as Marshall's Syndrome) and is of unknown aetiology. It is the most common periodic fever syndrome in the pediatric age group and does not appear to be a monogenetic disease.
- The diagnosis is clinical and is suggested by the presence of:
  - regular recurrent fever of early onset.
  - oral aphthous ulcers.
  - cervical lymphadenopathy.
  - pharyngitis.
- in the absence of evidence of recurrent upper respiratory tract infections or cyclic neutropenia.

Treatment
- Prednisolone.
- The first-line treatment of PFAPA is a single dose of corticosteroid, e.g. 1–2 mg/kg given at the start of the attack.
  - Tonsillectomy with around 50% success reported.
  - Long-term colchicine prophylaxis may ameliorate symptoms.
  - Cimetidine or anakinra may be useful but the response is unpredictable.
- In general the prognosis is good and most children will outgrow their symptoms by adolescence.

Chronic recurrent multifocal osteomyelitis (CRMO)

Background

- CRMO is an autoimmune/auto inflammatory disorder associated with non-infective painful inflammation of bones. It may also be called non-bacterial osteitis (NBO).
- Aetiology is unknown, but increasing evidence suggests a possible genetic component.
  - It may be associated with SAPHO syndrome (synovitis, acne, pustulosis, hyperostosis, and osteitis) or psoriasis (reported frequency of association with either varying from 7.5–23%).
  - It is also associated with sacroiliitis and inflammatory bowel disease.
  - The presence of HLA-B27 is increased (21% reported) suggesting an overlap between CRMO/SAPHO and spondyloarthropathies.
  - Some patients may develop persistent arthritis typical of enthesitis related arthritis.
- The diagnosis of CRMO is based on a combination of clinical, radiological, and histopathological features. The major and minor diagnostic criteria of NBO are included in Table 4.27.

Clinical presentations

- Predominantly a disease of young girls (mean age of 10yr) although occurs in both sexes and can occur de novo in adults.
- Typically, acute or insidious onset with unifocal or multifocal bone pain or swelling, nocturnal pain, and sometimes fever. Bony lesions may be associated with an asymmetrical inflammatory arthritis. Inflammatory markers may be raised and may be useful to follow disease activity. ANA is usually negative; and HLA B27 may be positive.

Table 4.27 Major and minor criteria for non-bacterial osteitis (NBO)

Major diagnostic criteria	Minor diagnostic criteria
Radiologically proven osteolytic/sclerotic bone lesion	Normal blood count, systemically well
Multifocal bone lesions	Mild/moderate elevation CRP or ESR
Palmoplantar pustulosis (PPP) or psoriasis	Observation time >6 months
Sterile bone biopsy with signs of inflammation and/or fibrosis, sclerosis	Hyperostosis
	Other autoimmune disease (excluding PPP or psoriasis)
	1st- or 2nd-degree relatives with autoimmune, auto-inflammatory disease, or NBO

NBO confirmed by 2 major criteria or 1 major and 3 minor criteria.

- Lesions can occur at any site; lower limbs are most frequently affected, followed by clavicle, spine, ribs, fibula, and mandible (median number of bony lesions is 3.5). Isolated swelling of the medial clavicle is common.

Management

- The main differential is exclusion of infection and malignancy and often requires multi-specialist input (including radiology, infectious diseases, orthopaedics, and paediatric rheumatology).
- X-ray may be non-specific (e.g. soft tissue swelling, localized osteopenia, periosteal reaction, or bony expansion); typically lytic and sclerotic lesions in the metaphyses of long bones and medial clavicles are observed (Fig. 4.18).
- Whole body MRI is a sensitive imaging modality for CRMO and is useful to define lesions, identify further 'silent' ones, and measure response to treatment.
- Radioirotope bone scan can detect 'hot spots' as evidence of inflammatory change.
- Bone biopsy may be necessary to exclude infection or malignancy.
- There are no validated disease activity scores in CRMO, but in practice, the degree of clinical involvement, pain scores, acute phase reactants, impact on physical function (e.g. CHAQ, see ⊃ p. 47), and imaging (especially MRI) are most helpful.
- Currently there is limited evidence for treatment with no RCT of treatments.
  - Antibiotics have not been shown to be effective.
  - NSAIDS may be effective for symptom control.
  - Pamidronate is often administered as first-line disease modifying agent pending further clinical trial data of other agents. Pamidronate helps reduce symptoms in acute CRMO. Efficacy may be related to anti-osteoclastic and/or anti-inflammatory activity. Regular infusions do not appear to reduce the frequency or severity of flares.
  - Corticosteroids can be useful particularly if there is associated arthritis or synovitis, and/or for severe, destructive disease (e.g. of the spine).
  - MTX has not been shown to reduce the severity or frequency of flares but may improve any associated arthritis.

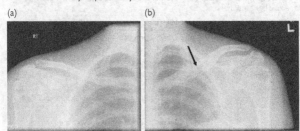

Fig. 4.18 Plain radiographs of (a) right and (b) left clavicle. Left clavicle shows cortical expansion and sclerosis (arrow).

- Anti-TNFα therapy has been used in severe cases unresponsive to pamidronate with clinical improvement reported in small case series.
- RCTs comparing treatment modalities are required: an RCT of pamidronate versus adalimumab is currently in set-up in the UK for children with CRMO.

Prognosis

- Varied disease course, from unifocal self-limiting lesions to chronic multifocal relapsing course over several years. May finally remit.
- Robust long-term follow up are data currently lacking, and prognosis reportedly varies widely:
  - 0–100% may have persistent disease as described by different authors.
  - Pathological fractures, most often of the vertebral body occurred in 49% of a German cohort.
  - Long-term skeletal deformity, particularly leg length discrepancy, may occur in up to 58% in one study.
  - Disease recurrence may occur as long as 6 years after the last episode of osteitis.
  - Difficulties with employment, education, and participation in sports have been reported in some cases.
- Persistence of disease is increased with greater number of initial bony lesions and in younger children (median duration of active disease 2–3yr).

Further reading

Jansson A, Renner ED, Ramser J, et al. Classification of non-bacterial osteitis. Rheumatology 2007; 46:154–60.

Fritz J, Tzaribatchev N, et al. Chronic recurrent multifocal osteomyelitis: comparison of whole-body MR imaging with radiography and correlation with clinical and laboratory data. Radiology 2009;252:842–51.

Eleftheriou D, Gerschman T, Sebire N, et al. Biologic therapy in refractory chronic non-bacterial osteomyelitis of childhood. Rheumatology 2010;49:1505–12.

Sarcoidosis

Background

- Idiopathic multisystemic inflammatory disease with non-caseating granulomata in affected tissues.
- The cause is unknown; aberrant host responses (under genetic control) to infection (undefined organism) remain the main hypothesis. Candidate genes may reside in loci that influence regulation of antigen presentation and/or T-cell function resulting in ↑ granulomata formation and fibrosis.
- There is an ↑ incidence of other autoimmune diseases in patients with sarcoidosis.

Epidemiology

- Prevalence varies worldwide and by age: primarily a disease of 20–40yr-olds. Twice as common in females.
- The disease is more common in Japanese and black children, although this racial distribution varies with geographic location. Sarcoid is seen more commonly in developed than underdeveloped areas.
- In Denmark, where the disease has a high prevalence, the incidence in children <15yr was 0.22–0.27 per 100,000/yr; 0.06 per 100,000 children aged <4yr; and ↑ gradually with age to 1.02 per 100,000 in children aged 14–15yr.

Genetics of sarcoidosis

- There is an ↑ incidence of sarcoidosis in certain families.
- An HLA association has been described including DQB1*0603, DQB1*0604, and DPB1*0201.
- In the USA, familial clusters observed in 19% of African Americans, compared to 5% of white families.
- Monozygotic twins are 2–4× more concordant for disease than dizygotic twins.
- Recent studies suggest a unique candidate gene *BTNL2* in the MHC II region on chromosome 6.
- Specific HLA genotypes appear to confer a predisposition to disease phenotype. For example, HLA-DQB1*0201 and HLA-DRB1*0301 are associated with acute disease and a good prognosis.

Early-onset sarcoidosis (EOS) and Blau's syndrome

- EOS refers to young children with disease onset in the first 5yr of life. These children differ from those with sarcoidosis of later presentation.
  - EOS typically presents with the classic triad of rash, arthritis, and uveitis (in that order), but without apparent pulmonary involvement or hilar lymphadenopathy.
  - EOS typically presents in the 1st year of life.
  - Uveitis, which occurs in more than half the children with EOS, is relatively less common in patients with later onset disease.
- Blau's syndrome—autosomal dominant granulomatous disease with an identical clinical phenotype to EOS.

- *EOS and Blau's syndrome represent the sporadic and familial forms respectively of the same disease* since both share genetic mutations in the nucleotide binding oligomerization domain 2 gene (*NOD2*, also referred to as the *CARD15* gene).
- The *NOD2* gene probably has no major effect on sarcoidosis susceptibility in older patients, however.
- Recent data from a prospective international cohort study of patients with Blau's syndrome and EOS containing 31 patients showed around half of patients developed expanded manifestations outside the classical triad including visceral involvement, recurrent fevers, and vasculitis.
- The same study revealed previously undiscovered dysplastic bony changes were commonly seen including camptodactyly, carpal dysplasia, abnormalities in distal radius and ulna, and abnormally shaped second metacarpal bone.

Clinical features

Multisystemic disease so presentation can vary greatly.

- *Multisystemic presentation*—older children usually present in a similar manner to adults with lymphadenopathy, pulmonary involvement, and systemic symptoms (fever, malaise, fatigue, and weight loss), in contrast to the presentation of EOS described previously.
- *Renal and biochemical findings:*
  - Renal involvement is rare in children and adults, and may be asymptomatic. Renal involvement is usually secondary to hypercalcaemia and/or hypercalciuria (occurring in ~30% of paediatric sarcoid cases) rather than renal infiltration with granulomata.
  - Polyuria, enuresis (2° nephrogenic diabetes insipidus from hypercalcaemia).
  - Hypercalcaemia ± hypercalciuria.
  - Hypercalciuria in the absence of hypercalcaemia.
  - Nephrocalcinosis and nephrolithiasis (only if hypercalciuria).
  - Bilateral enlargement of the kidneys.
  - Tubulointerstitial nephritis.
  - Rarely glomerular lesions: classically membranous glomerulonephritis, but crescentic nephritis also reported.
- *Pulmonary disease*—is the most commonly involved organ.
  - Chronic cough with or without dyspnoea.
  - Bilateral hilar lymphadenopathy with or without parenchymal involvement is the most common radiographic finding.
  - The hilar lymphadenopathy is usually symmetrical.
  - Parenchymal disease, pleural effusions, and atelectasis occur less commonly in children than in adults (25% of affected adults are affected with these).
  - Nearly 50% of all children with sarcoidosis demonstrate restrictive lung disease on pulmonary function tests.
  - An obstructive pattern 2° to intrabronchial granuloma or mediastinal lymph node airway compression may occasionally be observed.
- *Lymphadenopathy and hepatosplenomegaly*—lymphadenopathy, including retroperitoneal lymphadenopathy, is commonly observed, and can occur with or without hepatosplenomegaly.

- *Skin disease*—77% of young children; and 24–40% of older children:
  - Sarcoid should be considered in the differential diagnosis of unusual skin lesions in children.
  - Most common is a cutaneous eruption with soft, yellowish-brown flat-topped papules found most frequently on the face. Larger violaceous plaque-like lesions may be found on the trunk and extremities. Erythema nodosum is reported in 31%.
  - Other lesions include nodules and subcutaneous tumours, hyper- or hypopigmented lesions, and ulcers.
- *Eye disease*—it should be remembered that young children may be asymptomatic although blind in one eye at presentation. All of the following are described in sarcoid:
  - Uveitis—general term used to describe inflammation of the uvea (comprising iris, ciliary body, and choroid).
  - Iridocyclitis (inflammation of the iris and ciliary body),
  - Posterior uveitis—predominantly choroid but not iridocyclitis.
  - Lacrimal gland swelling, conjunctival granulomata.
  - Vitritis, chorioretinitis, optic neuritis.
  - Proptosis, interstitial keratitis.
- *Musculoskeletal disease*—affects 15–58% of affected children:
  - Arthralgia.
  - Arthritis, usually affecting multiple joints: boggy tenosynovitis with relatively painless effusion and little or no overlying erythema of skin. Erosive changes on x-ray usually absent.
  - Bone cysts (especially small bones of hand and foot).
  - Muscle involvement can occur but is unusual.
- *Neurological*—neurosarcoid is rare in children but is described. Encephalopathy and seizures; cranial nerve involvement; cerebral mass lesion (rare in posterior fossa); spinal cord involvement; aseptic meningitis; obstructive hydrocephalus.
- *Other*—parotid enlargement (with uveitis sometimes called 'uveo-parotid fever'); rectal prolapse; sicca syndrome; testicular mass; pericardial effusion; myocardial involvement, and granulomatous large and medium-size vessel vasculitis.

Differential diagnosis

- Infection causing granulomatous inflammation, including:
  - Tuberculosis, leprosy, histoplasmosis, blastomycosis.
- Chronic granulomatous disease (exclude with NBT test).
- Blau's syndrome.
- sJIA.
- Granulomatous small-vessel vasculitis including GPA (Wegener's granulomatosis) and EGPA (Churg–Strauss syndrome).
- Crohn's disease may rarely be confused with sarcoidosis.
- Lymphoma.
- Berylliosis: inhalation of beryllium has been associated with a granulomatous lung disease known as chronic beryllium disease (CBD).

Laboratory findings and investigations

No single test is diagnostic of sarcoid, and ultimately tissue diagnosis and the exclusion of other diseases that can mimic sarcoid is required. The historical Kveim–Siltzbach test, whereby intradermal injection of a splenic extract from a known sarcoid patient resulted in sarcoid granulomata in a suspected case, is antiquated, and the standard test reagent no longer available. Observed findings and useful investigations include:

- Leucopenia, thrombocytosis, eosinophilia relatively common, high ESR and CRP.
- Hypercalcaemia—varies from 2 to 60% of cases. The mechanism of this appears to be that abnormal pulmonary macrophages synthesize 1,25 (OH)$_2$ vitamin D from 25-hydroxy vitamin D, and are relatively insensitive to feedback by hypercalcaemia.
- Abnormal liver function.
- Raised UA:UC ratio, tubular function abnormalities.
- Raised serum angiotensin converting enzyme (sACE). Epithelial cells in the granulomas produce sACE, which thus may be elevated. This can also be used to monitor response to therapy, but is neither sensitive, nor specific.
- Recent studies have suggested that serum chitotriosidase concentrations may be a useful marker for monitoring disease activity in sarcoidosis but this remains a research tool at present.
- Mantoux test (to exclude TB). NB Sarcoid patients commonly demonstrate anergy (no response) to purified protein derivatives of *Mycobacterium tuberculosis* even if previously exposed.
- NBT test (alternatively a flow cytometric test of neutrophil oxidative metabolism using dihydrorhodamine) to exclude chronic granulomatous disease.
- Eye screen for uveitis.
- X-rays of affected bones and joints.
- CXR—standard screen for pulmonary sarcoid.
- ↑ sensitivity of detection of pulmonary involvement with high-resolution CT of chest.
- Pulmonary function tests including transfer factor.
- MRI of brain for suspected neurosarcoid.
- FDG-PET scanning may be useful in assessing the extent of organ involvement and planning diagnostic biopsy.
- Tissue biopsy—skin, lung, salivary glands, muscle. Occasionally renal biopsy.
- ECG and echocardiogram for suspected cardiac involvement. Cardiac MRI may also have a role in this context.

Treatment

- Acute transient disease requires rest and NSAIDs.
- Chronic and/or severe multisystemic disease requires corticosteroid therapy, e.g. 0.5–2mg/kg daily prednisolone, tapering over 2–3 months.
- An additional immunosuppressant agent may be required for persistent progressive sarcoidosis: MTX, AZA, or MMF.
  - An RCT of MTX in 24 adults with sarcoid demonstrated steroid sparing efficacy.

- Occasionally cyclophosphamide or ciclosporin have been used for more aggressive disease.
- Biologic therapy with anti-TNFα has been increasingly used, particularly for refractory uveitis.
- Ocular involvement usually responds to corticosteroid administered locally, or systemically.

Prognosis

- Guarded prognosis for young children with EOS—nearly all develop long-term morbidity from uveitis, polyarthritis, or other organ involvement.
- Older children have a variable prognosis, dependent on organ involvement, geography, sex, and race.
- A recurrence after >1yr of remission is uncommon, but can occur and may develop at any age and in any organ.
  - Long term follow up of 46 Caucasian Danish children reported 78% complete recovery; 11% still had chronic active disease with multi-organ involvement; 7% died; and 4% were recovered but with residual organ damage including unilateral loss of vision and abnormal chest radiography.
  - The presence of erythema nodosum was associated with a good prognosis, and CNS sarcoidosis was associated with a poor prognosis.
  - In patients without persisting active disease, health-related QoL scores were similar to the reference population.
  - In another series of 19 children followed-up for a mean of 21yr: 37% had persistent abnormalities on CXR, 68% had impaired lung function, and 63% had abnormal findings on echocardiography.
  - Follow-up of 41 children with pulmonary sarcoidosis in France, mostly of African ethnicity, showed that patients diagnosed before 10yr old were more likely to recover (50% vs 29%), and presented fewer relapses (29% vs 58%). At 4–5yr of follow-up, relapses were mostly observed for patients diagnosed after 10yr old. In this cohort pulmonary sarcoidosis usually presented as part of a multi-organ systemic inflammatory disease.

Further reading

Nathan N, Marcelo P, Houdouin V, et al. Lung sarcoidosis in children: update on disease expression and management doi:10.1136/thoraxjnl-2015-206825

Rose C, Pans, S, Casteels I, et al. Blau Syndrome: cross sectional data from a multicentre study of clinical, radiological and functional outcomes. Rheumatology 2015;54:1008-1016

Marcille R, McCarthy M, Barton J, et al. Long-term outcome of pediatric sarcoidosis with emphasis on pulmonary status. Chest 1992; 102:1444–9.

Milman N, Hoffman AL. Childhood sarcoidosis: long-term follow-up. Eur Respir J 2008;31:592–8.

Shetty AK, Gedalia A. Childhood sarcoidosis: a rare but fascinating disorder. Pediatric Rheumatology 2008;6:16.

Macrophage activation syndrome (MAS)

Introduction

MAS is the term used for 2° haemophagocytic lymphohistiocytosis (HLH) occurring in rheumatological diseases. It is potentially fatal with reported mortality rates of 8–22%.

Pathophysiology

- The exact pathophysiology remains unknown.
- The pathophysiology includes dysregulation of T lymphocytes, natural killer (NK) cells, excessive pro-inflammatory cytokine production, e.g. IFNγ, abnormal proliferation of macrophages, cytopenias, and coagulopathy.
- Macrophages phagocytose haematopoietic cells in the bone marrow.
- Proposed triggers for MAS include infections (see following list) and in the context of systemic JIA (sJIA) some medications, e.g. NSAIDs and biologics.
- But importantly, *MAS can also precipitated by persistently active inflammatory rheumatological disease alone.*
- Genetic overlaps between 1° (familial) HLH and 2° HLH are suspected in a minority of cases.

Potential infective triggers of MAS

- Epstein–Barr virus.
- VZV.
- Coxsackie virus.
- Parvovirus B19.
- Hepatitis A virus.
- *Salmonella enteritidis.*
- Enterococcus.

Diagnosis

- Early recognition and treatment is important to prevent significant morbidity and mortality.
- Diagnosis is often difficult because the features of MAS are similar to the underlying active rheumatological inflammatory disease (Table 4.28).
- The diagnostic criteria of the Histiocyte Society (Box 4.10) are the most universally recognized but have multiple limitations. The criteria are not absolute and need to be interpreted in the context of the clinical case. For example, in sJIA relative reductions of blood counts are more important than the absolute degree of cytopenia. Proposed criteria for diagnosing MAS in sJIA are under development.
- Diagnosis can be made in the absence of bone marrow haemophagocytosis, and in the absence of absolute cytopenia.

Box 4.10 Diagnostic guideline for haemophagocytic lymphohistiocytosis: HLH 2004 protocol

Establish the diagnosis if either (1) or (2) is fulfilled:
  (1) A molecular diagnosis consistent with HLH
  (2) Diagnostic criteria for HLH fulfilled (5 or more out of the 8 criteria):
  - (a) Fever
  - (b) Splenomegaly
  - (c) Cytopenias (affecting ≥ 2 of 3 lineages in the peripheral blood:
    - (i) Haemoglobin <9.0g/dL (in infants <4 weeks: haemoglobin <10.0 g/dL)
    - (ii) Platelets <100 × 10⁹/L
    - (iii) Neutrophils <1.0 × 10⁹/L
  - (d) Hypertriglyceridaemia and/or hypofibrinogenaemia: fasting triglycerides ≥3.0mmol/L (≥ 265mg/dL), fibrinogen ≤1.5g/L
  - (e) Haemophagocytosis in bone marrow, spleen, lymph nodes, or cerebrospinal fluid: no evidence of malignancy
  - (f) Low or absent NK cell activity (according to local laboratory reference)
  - (g) Elevated ferritin (≥500mcg/L)
  - (h) Soluble CD25 (i.e. soluble interleukin-2 receptor) above normal limits for age.

Adapted with permission from Henter JI, Horne A, Aricó M, et al. HLH-2004: Diagnostic and therapeutic guidelines for hemophagocytic lymphohistiocytosis. Pediatric Blood & Cancer, Volume 48, Issue 2, pp. 124–31, Copyright © 2007 John Wiley and Sons Ltd.

Rheumatological diseases which may be complicated by MAS

Commonly
- sJIA (most commonly).
- SLE.
- Kawasaki disease.

Less commonly
- JDM.
- Polyarticular JIA.
- PAN.
- SSc.
- MCTD.
- Sarcoidosis.
- Sjögren's syndrome.
- CINCA.

Characteristic clinical features

- Unremitting high fever.
- Hepatosplenomegaly.
- CNS dysfunction (irritability, disorientation, headache, seizures, coma).
- Purpuric rash or haemorrhages.

Table 4.28 Comparison of clinical and laboratory features of sJIA and MAS

Feature	sJIA	MAS
Fever pattern	Quotidian	Unremitting
Rash	Evanescent, maculopapular	Petechial or purpuric
Hepatosplenomegaly	Yes	Yes
Lymphadenopathy	Yes	Yes
Arthritis	Yes	No
Serositis	Yes	No
Encephalopathy	No	Yes
White cells and neutrophil count	High	Low
Haemoglobin	Normal or low	Low
Platelets	High	Low
ESR	High	Normal or sudden fall
Bilirubin	Normal	Normal or high
ALT/AST	Normal or slightly high	High
PT	Normal	Prolonged
PTT	Normal	Prolonged
Fibrinogen	High	Low
Ferritin	Normal or high	High or very high
D-dimers	High	Very high

Other clinical features
- Renal involvement.
- Lymphadenopathy.

Recognized haematological features
- Low haemoglobin.
- Low WCC and neutrophil count.
- Low platelets.
- Normal or falling ESR.
- Raised liver transaminases.
- Prolonged PT and PTT.
- Low fibrinogen.
- Very high ferritin (>500 microgrammes/L possible HLH, and >10,000 microgrammes/L very likely HLH).
- High D-dimers.
- Raised LDH.
- Low albumin.

- Raised triglycerides.
- Raised sCD25 and CD163.
- Low NK cell activity.
- Bone marrow haemophagocytosis.
- Abnormal perforin pathway tested by abnormal NK and CD8 T cell CD107a (LAMP1) granule release expression—although usually associated with 1° HLH these may also be a feature of 2° HLH in sJIA.

Important: laboratory values recognized to be falling or to be incongruous with the level of inflammation clinically evident may allow earlier recognition of developing MAS.

Management

1st-line—successful alone in almost 50% of cases:
- Supportive treatment—very important in all cases.
- Corticosteroid is the essential 1st-line treatment and should be started immediately with pulse high-dose methylprednisolone (30mg/kg/day with a maximum dose of 1g). This may be required for several days and is followed by maintenance oral prednisolone at least 1mg/kg/day or the equivalent corticosteroid intravenously depending on the patient condition.

2nd-line—chosen depending on progress and extent of multiorgan involvement:
- IVIg 1–2g/kg—also useful when diagnosis is unclear, i.e. whether this is true MAS or sepsis.
- Ciclosporin 3–5mg/kg/day PO or 1–2mg/kg/day IV – NB toxicity may be associated with posterior reversible encephalopathy syndrome (PRES).
- Etoposide 150mg/m² twice weekly (day 1 and 4) for the first 2 weeks, then once-weekly for another 6 weeks—effective; however, concerns exist regarding reported risk of 2nd malignancies. In patients with refractory disease therapy based on protocols for 1° HLH might be required.

Alternative 2nd-line management options with biologics—successful treatment has been reported however data are currently limited:
- Anakinra 2mg/kg (maximum 100 mg) once daily SC injection. Published experience mostly favourable. Higher doses have been used anecdotally, mainly for MAS 2° to sJIA—seek expert advice.

Primary immunodeficiency and rheumatological disease

Primary immunodeficiency disorders (PID) are characterized by:
- Unusual susceptibility to (and recurrent) infections presenting from birth/early childhood.
- Dysregulation of immune functions resulting in:
  - Autoimmunity, mediated by auto-reactive B or T lymphocytes, which could be either organ-specific (e.g cytopenias, endocrinopathies) or systemic (e.g. SLE, vasculitis, etc.), or as
  - Autoinflammatory disorders (see ➲ pp. 303–12) with episodes of seemingly unprovoked inflammation, mediated by disturbed innate immune system, without presence of auto-reactive B or T lympho-cytes (Fig. 4.19).
  - In reality, it is increasingly recognized that immunodeficiency, autoin-flammation, and autoimmunity may all coexist.
- The field of immune dysregulation disorders has undergone unprecedented and fascinating development over the last few years, and the rapid 'new gene' discovery (thanks to next-generation sequencing) continues to provide more evidence for monogenic nature of many of these disorders.
- Rheumatological features of PID include:
  - arthritis/arthralgia.
  - vasculitis and/or 'vasculopathy'.
  - fever.
  - early onset enteropathy.
  - interstitial lung disease (ILD)
  - skin involvement (e.g. blisters; panniculitis, granulomatous, others).
  - hepatosplenomegaly and lymphadenopathy.
  - organ-specific autoimmunity including cytopenias.
  - raised inflammatory markers.
  - autoantibodies.

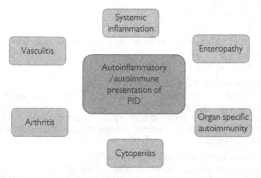

Fig. 4.19 Immune dysregulation as presentation of PID.

- Before the gene defects were known (and for quite a few this is still the case), many of these complex disorders with features of autoinflammation, autoimmunity, and immunodeficiency were referred to as either 'IPEX-like' or 'ALPS-like' (see below).
- Specific anti-inflammatory biologic DMARDs (e.g. anti-IL-1, -IL-6, -TNF-a agents, etc.) and/or B and T lymphocyte depletion agents (e.g. anti-B cell and/or anti-CD52 monoclonal antibodies, etc.) are efficacious in some instances, although the balance between immunodeficiency and autoimmunity /autoinflammation has to be considered on an individual basis (see ➲ autoinflammatory disease, pp. 303–12).
- New treatment targets (e.g. JAK-STAT cytokine pathway, PI3K pathway) are being identified and explored, and allogeneic haematopoietic stem cell transplantation (HSCT) has proven successful in many of these conditions (see below).

When to 'think of' PID tips for daily practice

'SLE-like/JDM-like' phenotype

Classical complement activation pathway, early component deficiencies (C1-4; C1 esterase INH)
- Early childhood onset vasculitis and/or discoid LE.
- Functional complement testing essential: e.g. functional tests of classical and alternative complement pathways (discuss with immunology lab regarding availability).
  - HSCT (for C1q-deficiency; in contrast to most other complement components are made in the liver, C1Q predominantly derived from leucocytes).

Chronic granulomatous disease (CGD)
- Discoid lupus, colitis/inflammatory bowel disease.
- Absent/reduced neutrophil oxidative burst and/or nitro-blue tetrazolium test (NBT).

Aicardi-Goutieres Syndrome (TREX1; SAMHD1; and other newly-described genes) (see below)
- Familial 'chilblain' SLE.
- Interferon 'signature'.

SPENCDI (ACP5)- spondyloenchondrodysplasia with immune dysregulation (see below)
- Interferon 'signature'.

PRKCD (protein kinase C-delta) deficiency
- Early-onset lupus with skin rash and cytopenias; may respond well to B-cell depletion e.g. with rituximab.
- Recurrent infections, hepatosplenomegaly, lymphadenopathy.
- B cell immunodeficiency (Common variable immunodeficiency –CVID) present in some.

Autoimmune lymphoproliferative syndrome (ALPS)
- Hepatosplenomegaly, lymphadenopathy, cytopenias.
- Raised serum B12 levels, hypergammaglobulinaemia.

- Increased (>2%) double negative T cells (DNT; CD3+/CD4-/CD8-); NB: DNTs may also be elevated in sporadic SLE so this is not entirely specific; consider genetic screening for ALPS, and functional assays of apoptosis.

Macrophage activation syndrome (MAS) (see ➔ pp. 321–4)

Primary (familial) haemophagocytic lymphohistiocytosis (F/HLH)

- 'Classically' due to mutations of genes involved in perforin-related cytolysis (*perforin, syntaxin-11, UNC 13-D, UNC 18-2*), intracellular vesicle trafficking (*Chediak-Higashi, Griscelli, Hermansky-Pudlak*) and/or signalling (lymphoproliferaive syndromes-*SH2DIA; XIAP; ITK*)
  - XIAP (X-linked lymphoproliferative disease):
    —Early onset enteropathy, arthritis, erythema nodosum, periodic fevers, uveitis.
  - Other/numerous PIDs:
    —HSCT.

NLRC4 (gain of function)-related MAS/syndrome of enterocolitis and autoinflammation

(newly described NLRC4 inflammasomopathy)

- Early onset rash, arthralgia.
- Cold-induced urticarial.

Issues with fever—'no fever' (with infection) vs. 'too much fever' (without infection)

- Patients bearing mutations of genes coding for different molecules of the innate immune system (e.g. *NEMO, IRAK4, MyD88*), are characterized by:
  - 'Peculiar' absence of inflammatory response (no fever or rise in CRP) in the light of an overwhelming, usually bacterial infection.
  - Recurrent, life-threatening bacterial (*S. pneumoniae* in particular), mycobacterial, and/or viral infections, and variable features of ecto-dermal dysplasia (NEMO)
  - CD62-ligand shedding assay (absence of) may point towards diagnosis.
  - Specific antibody deficiency (to Pneumococcus), variable B/T cell immunodeficiency:
    —HSCT.
- In contrast, the gain-of-function mutations of the genes involved in the same process (i.e. of IL-1 production, via intracellular 'inflammasomes' such as *NLRP3*) cause unprovoked and on-going inflammation (see ➔ chapter on autoinflammation, pp. 303–12).

Chronic (non-septic) arthritis (inflammatory arthropathy), usually associated with fever, vasculitis (and/or 'vasculopathy'), enteropathy, and/or cytopaenias

'Classical' PID syndromes

- Thrombocytopaenia with low MPV, eczematous dermatitis (*Wiskott-Aldrich syndrome*).
  - HSCT.
- Facial features, congenital heart disease, hypocalcaemia (*DiGeorge syndrome*).

- Recurrent sino-pulmonary/joint infections, cytopenias (haemolytic anaemia and/or thrombocytopenia), intestinal nodular lymphoid hyperplasia, autoimmune hepatitis, lymphoid interstitial pneumonia; hypogammaglobulinaemia (*X-Linked Agammaglobulinaemia/XLA; Common variable immunodeficiency/CVID*).
  - HSCT (in some CVID).
- Cytopenias, cholangitis, autoimmune hepatitis (*CD40L deficiency/ XL-HIgM Sy*).
  - HSCT.

Severe combined immunodeficiency /SCID ('leaky' mutations, i.e. not complete loss of function; less severe, some function still 'leaks through' into the phenotype) and various combined (T cell) immunodeficiencies (CID)

- Granulomatous lesions, cytopenias, hepatosplenomegaly, lymphadenopathy.
- Viral infections (CMV FRV)
- Low/absent 'naïve' T cells (early thymic emigrants).
  - HSCT.

New disease entities—monogenic immune dysregulation syndromes
Below listed are some of the newly described disorders with features of both rheumatic disorders and immunodeficiency/immune dysregulation, and readers are strongly encouraged to refer to the recent reviews for more specific details.

DADA2 - Deficiency of adenosine deaminase 2 (CECR1)

- Mimic of polyarteritis nodosa (see ➜ autoinflammation, pp. 303–12). Early-onset stroke, livedo reticularis, recurrent fever, hepatosplenomegaly, arterial hypertension, ophthalmologic manifestations, myalgia, leg ulcers, Raynaud phenomenon, subcutaneous nodules, purpura, digital necrosis.
- Variable B cell immunodeficiency:
  - anti-TNFα effective in majority of patients.
  - HSCT (if no response to other treatments).
  - gene therapy in the future?

STAT3 (gain of function)—mediated early-onset lymphoproliferation and autoimmunity (signal transducer and activator of transcription 3)

- 'ALPS-like'; 'IPEX-like'.
- IDDM, autoimmune enteropathy, autoimmune thyroiditis, ILD, atopic dermatitis.
- Features of systemic JIA, scleroderma.
- Short stature, eczema, dental anomalies, cytopenias, hepatitis, alopecia.
- Recurrent and/or severe infections.
- Variable 'combined' immunodeficiency.
  - HSCT.

CTLA-4 (cytotoxic T lymphocyte antigen 4) haploinsufficiency with autoimmune infiltration

- Diarrhoea/enteropathy, granulomatous lymphocytic ILD, hepatosplenomegaly, lymphadenopathy, cytopenias, thyroiditis, arthritis, autoantibodies.

- Extensive CD4T cell infiltrates in intestines, lungs, bone marrow, CNS, kidneys, and liver.
- Progressive loss of circulating B cells, hypogammaglobulinaemia.
  - HSCT.

PI3K-pathway related immunodeficiency with lymphoproliferation (PIK3CD/ PIK3R1) (phosphoinositide 3-kinase)
- Recurrent sinopulmonary infections and diffuse lymphadenopathy, splenomegaly bronchiectasis, inflammatory bowel disease, ITP.
- Arthritis (JIA- like), systemic inflammation/increased inflammatory markers.
- Variable 'combined'/B cell immunodeficiency (CVID phenotype).
  - HSCT.

PLCG2 (phospholipase Cγ2)-associated antibody deficiency and immune dysregulation (APLAID)
- Early-onset recurrent blistering skin lesions, cellulitis, nonspecific interstitial pulmonary disease, arthralgia, inflammatory eye and bowel disease.
- Granulomatous rash, sinopulmonary infections, autoantibodies.
- Allergy (asthma, eczema, rhinitis, conjunctivitis, drugs/food).
- B and NK cell immunodeficiency, hypogammaglobulinemia (CVID phenotype).

LUBAC—linear ubiquitin assembly complex (HOIL-1; HOIP; Serpin) deficiency (innate immune regulator)
- Early-onset systemic inflammation, hepatosplenomegaly, lymphadenopathy.
- Lymphangiectasia.
- Amylopectin-like deposits in myocytes.
- Combined immunodeficiency.

IL-10 pathway deficiency (IL-10/IL-10R)
- Early onset inflammatory bowel disease, respiratory infections.
- Arthritis.
  - HSCT.

IPEX—immunodysregulation, polyendocrinopathy, enteropathy, X-linked
- Absent/afunctional peripheral regulatory T cells (CD4/CD25/Foxp3).
- Early onset recurrent fever, eczematous dermatitis.
  - HSCT.

APECED-Autoimmune polyendocrinopathy, candidasis, ectodermal dystrophy (APS1—autoimmune polyendocrinopathy type 1)
- Loss of central tolerance/mutations in *AIRE* (autoimmune regulator).
- Autoantibodies to Th-17 cytokines (IL-17/IL-22)
- Early onset recurrent fever, skin rash, hepatitis, enteropathy, arthritis.

ALPS (see above)

LACC1—associated monogenic systemic JIA (laccase (multicopper oxidoreductase) domain-containing 1)
- Characteristic fever, erythematous maculopapular rashes, chronic polyarthritis, leukocytosis, thrombocytosis, elevated inflammatory markers.
- Unresponsive to treatment with NSAIDs, systemic corticosteroids, methotrexate, and biological agents (anti-TNF, anti-IL-6, or rituximab).

COPA (coatomer subunit a)—associated interstitial lung disease and arthritis
- ILD/pulmonary hemorrhage, arthritis, autoantibodies (ANA, ANCA, RF).
- Immune complex-mediated renal disease.

New disease entities—Mendelian type I interferonopathies
- Some of these disorders are characterized by up-regulation of type I interferons, the 'interferon signature', and are classified both as new PIDs (Mendelian type I interferonopathies) and autoinflammatory disorders (see ➲ pp. 303–12).
- Inhibiting type I interferon up-regulation by altering JAK-STAT cytokine pathway is one of the promising new treatments for these conditions (see ➲ pp. 303–12).

Aicardi-Goutieres Syndrome (see above)

SPENCDI - spondyloenchondrodysplasia with immune dysregulation ACP5, encoding tartrate-resistant acid phosphatase (TRAP)
- Axial bone dysplasia, cerebral calcifications.
- Immune dysregulation (AIHA, thyroiditis).
- SLE.

SAVI—STING-associated vasculopathy with onset in infancy TMEM173 (GOF), encoding stimulator of interferon (IFN) genes (STING)
- Early onset vasculopathy.
- Interstitial lung disease.

Proteasome-associated autoinflammatory syndromes (PRAAS; often referred to as CANDLE syndrome)
- CANDLE= **c**hronic **a**typical **n**eutrophilic **d**ermatosis **l**ipodystrophy and **e**levated temperature.
- PSMB8, 4 and 9 and other proteasome components deficiency.
- Neutrophilic dermatosis, panniculitis, lipodystrophy.
- Fevers and joint contractures.

ISG15 (IFN responsive gene) deficiency
- Basal ganglia calcifications akin to AGS.
- Lack of response to IFNγ, recurrent, severe mycobacterial infections.

Further reading

Torgerson TR. Immunodeficiency Diseases with Rheumatic Manifestations. *Pediatr Clin N Am* 2012;59:493–507.

Picard C, Al-Herz W, Bousfiha A, Casanova J-L, Chatila T, Conley ME, et al. Primary Immunodeficiency Diseases: an Update on the Classification from the International Union of Immunological Societies Expert Committee for Primary Immunodeficiency 2015. *J Clin Immunol.* 2015;35:696–726.

de Jesus AA, Canna SW, Liu Y, Goldbach-Mansky R. Molecular Mechanisms in Genetically Defined Autoinflammatory Diseases: Disorders of Amplified Danger Signaling. *Annu. Rev. Immunol.* 2015; 33:26.1–26.52.

Boisson B, Quartier P, Casanova J-L. Immunological loss-of-function due to genetic gain-of-function in humans: autosomal dominance of the third kind. *Curr Opinion Immunol* 2015;32:90–105.

Crow YJ. Type I interferonopathies: Mendelian type I interferon up-regulation. *Curr Opinion Immunol* 2015;32:7–10.

Mucopolysaccharidoses (MPS) and mucolipidoses (ML)

- Rare progressive storage disorders with a spectrum of clinical features (Table 4.29) varying from facial dysmorphism, bone dysplasia, hepatosplenomegaly, neurological and cardiorespiratory abnormalities, developmental regression, and a severely reduced life expectancy at the severe end of the clinical spectrum to an almost normal clinical phenotype with longer life span in patients presented more attenuated disease.
- MPS are due to a reduction of activity in lysosomal enzymes which break down glycosaminoglycans (GAGs)—long chains of carbohydrates that help build bone, cartilage, tendons, corneas, skin, and connective tissue.
- Over time GAGs in three different forms—dermatan sulfate (DS), heparan sulfate (HS), and keratan sulfate (KS)—accumulate in the cells, blood, and connective tissues resulting in the progressive skeletal dysplasia, dwarfism, marked coarsening of the facial features.
- In addition, deposition of GAG leads to corneal clouding and neurological deterioration.
- ML is due to multiple enzyme deficiencies secondary to failure of targeting of these enzymes to the lysosome.
- Phenotypic variability (heterogeneity) is very much a feature of MPS disease and within each specific enzyme deficiency there is a very wide spectrum of clinical effects.

Differential diagnosis

- Arthrogryposis.
- Juvenile polymyositis and dermatomyositis .
- Scleroderma and systemic sclerosis.
- Juvenile idiopathic arthritis.
- Skeletal dysplasia.
- Osteogenesis imperfecta.

Investigations

- Prenatal:
  - Chorionic villus biopsy at around 12th week of pregnancy.
  - Amniocentesis: measuring the enzyme activity in cultured amniotic cells in the 15th to 16th week of gestation or GAGs in cell-free fluid.
- Postnatal:
  - Urinary glycosaminoglycan as screening test (GAG)
  - White blood cell enzymes assay and cultured cells.
  - Urine oligos and blood gastrin in mucolipidoses.
  - Mutation analysis—possible for all disorders listed.
- Imaging:
  - Skeletal survey—dysostosis multiplex.
  - Large skull with thickened calvaria, premature suture closure, j-shaped sella turcica, and shallow orbits.
  - Short, thickened, and irregular clavicles.

Table 4.29 Classification and clinical features of mucopolysaccharidoses (MPS) and mucolipidoses (ML)

Types	Name	Inheritance	Enzyme defect	Clinical manifestations
MPS				
IH	Hurler	AR	alpha-L iduronidase	Corneal clouding, coarse facies, dysostosis multiplex, hernia, kyphosis, hepatomegaly, severe mental retardation
IHS	Hurler/Scheie	AR	alpha-L iduronidase	Joint contractures, corneal clouding, valvular abnormalities, carpel tunnel syndrome, hernia
IS	Scheie	AR	alpha-L iduronidase	Mild organ and skeletal involvement
II	Hunter	X linked	Iduronate sulfatase	Coarse facial features, skeletal deformities (such as claw hand), joint stiffness, retinal degeneration, hydrocephalus, mental retardation
IIIA	Sanfilippo	AR	Heparan N-sulfatase	Subtypes are not distinguishable clinically, hyperactivity, mental deterioration, developmental delay, coarse hair, hirsutism, mild hepatosplenomegaly, and enlarged head. Severely disturbed social behaviour occurred later in life (e.g. uncontrollable hyperactivity, destructive physical aggression)
IIIB	Sanfilippo	AR	Alpha-N-acetylglucosaminidase	
IIIC	Sanfilippo	AR	Acetyl CoA:alpha-glucosaminide acetyltransferase	
IIID	Sanfilippo	AR	N-acetylglucosamine 6-sulfatase	
IVA	Morquio	AR	N-acetylgalactosamine-6-sulfate sulfatase	Skeletal involvement with spondyloepiphyseal dysplasia, genu valgum, short stature, spinal curvature, odontoid hypoplasia, ligamentous laxity and atlantoaxial instability. Normal intelligence.

(Continued)

Table 4.29 Contd.

Types	Name	Inheritance	Enzyme defect	Clinical manifestations
VI	Maroteaux-Lamy	AR	N-acetylgalactosamine-4-sulfatase	Corneal clouding, coarse facies, joint stiffness, skeletal deformities, heart valvular disease, and normal intelligence
VII	Sly	AR	Beta-glucuronidase	Severe form with hydrops fetalis and hepatosplenomegaly in the neonatal period. Corneal clouding, coarse facies, macrocephaly, metatarsus adductus, prominent sternum, pelvic hypoplasia, hepatosplenomegaly, and hernias.
IX		AR	Hyaluronidase	Mild short stature and multiple periarticular soft-tissue masses
Mucolipidoses				
ML I	Sialidosis I	AR	Neuraminidase	Myoclonus and ataxia associated with a macular cherry-red spot, dementia in later life
ML II	I cell	AR	1Phosphotransferase (mutation in GNTAB gene alpha sub unit)	Course facies, hepatomegaly, severe skeletal dysplasia from birth
ML III	Pseudo-Hurler polydystrophy ML III alpha/beta	AR	1Phosphotransferase (mutation in GNTAB gene either alpha or beta subunits)	Hepatosplenomegaly, dysostosis multiplex, cardiac valve lesion
ML III	Pseudo-Hurler polydystrophy ML III gamma	AR	1Phosphotransferase (mutation in GNPTG gene)	Learning impairment, cardiac valvular lesion skeletal disease
ML IV		AR	Unknown (mutations in MCOLN1)	Motor impairment, severe mental retardation, retinal degeneration, corneal clouding, iron deficiency anaemia and achlorhydria with elevated blood gastrin levels

1UDP-N-acetylglucosamine: lysosomal hydrolase N-acetylglucosamine-1-phosphotransferase (GNPTAB) enzyme deficiency—enzyme requires the action of 2 genes GNTAB and GNPTG. Mutations in GNTAB are associated with ML II and ML III ML III alpha/beta and mutations in GNPTG cause ML III gamma.

- Short, wide, and trapezoid shaped proximally pointed metacarpals.
- Oar-shaped ribs.
- Anterior hypoplasia (with anterior beaking) of the lumbar vertebrae with kyphosis (often termed a gibbus).
- Poorly formed pelvis with small femoral heads and coxa valga.
- Enlarged diaphyses of long bones and irregular metaphyses.
- Abnormal spacing of teeth with dentigerous cysts.
- MRI scan: craniocervical stenosis and instability, enlarged perivascular spaces, white matter change, cerebral atrophy, arachnoid cysts.
- Echocardiogram: valvular heart disease, ventricular wall thickening.
- Neurophysiology:
  - Electroretinography: retinal degeneration.
  - Nerve conduction study: Carpal tunnel syndrome.
- Audiology:
  - Conductive and neuro-sensory hearing loss.

Management

Apart from MPS I, specific treatment is limited for MPS and ML that involve the central nervous system. In such patients management has been limited to a supportive one in improving quality of life for the child, although much research aimed at addressing the brain involvement is underway.

Early identification and diagnosis (Fig. 4.20) of the condition is essential and follow-up will require the involvement of multi-agency expertise in specialties including paediatrician specialized in metabolic disorders, orthopaedic surgeon, ENT surgeon, neurologist, physiotherapist, occupational therapist, cardiologist, and rheumatologist.

Enzyme replacement therapy (ERT)

- *Laronidase* therapy increases catabolism of GAGs, which accumulate with MPS I. Laronidase therapy has shown to improve walking capacity, pulmonary function, joint range of movement, stabilize or decrease sleep apnoea, and improve quality of life.
- *Idursulfase* is a purified form of human iduronate-2-sulfatase. It is used in MPS II, Hunter syndrome. The weekly infusion has shown improvement in walking capacity with reduction of size of liver and spleen as well as reduction (but not normalization) of urinary GAG levels in phase III trial.
- *Galsulfase* is a recombinant form of galactosamine 4 sulphate sulphatase. It is used as ERT in MPS VI (Maroteaux-Lamy syndrome) with result of improvements in walking and stair climbing capacity and reductions of urinary GAG excretion.
- *Elosulfase Alfa* is a recombinant form of the human N-acetylgalactosamine-6-sulfatase enzyme and it is the ERT for MPS IVa, Morquio A syndrome. There is improvement in walking and climbing capacity and trend to improvement in quality of life with less dependency on wheelchair usage.

All these ERTs are administered by weekly intravenous infusions.

Haematopoietic stem cell transplantation

- Offered to severely affected MPSI patients (Hurler Disease) and clearly improves lifespan; however, some skeletal manifestations remain. Outcomes relate to age at transplant and donor enzyme levels.

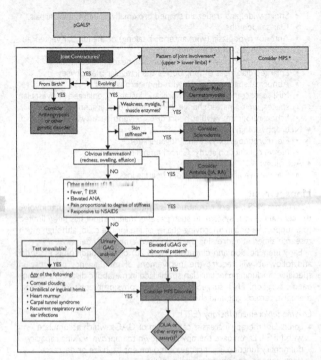

Fig. 4.20 Suggested approach to joint contractures. IDUA, Iduronidase alpha-L.

Reproduced with permission from Chan M, et al. Assessment of musculoskeletal abnormalities in children with mucopolysaccharidoses using pGALS. *Pediatric Rheumatology*, Volume 12, Issue 32, Copyright © 2014, Chan et al. Adapted with permission from Cimaz R et al., Joint contractures in the absence of inflammation may indicate mucopolysaccharidosis. *Pediatric Rheumatology*, Volume 9, Issue 18, Copyright © 2009 Cimaz et al.

Hearing and vision

- Hearing aids, grommet placement, and visual aids are beneficial.
- Corneal grafting if clouding is severe.

Respiratory

- Sleep apnoea may necessitate treatment with high pressure BiPAP with supplementary oxygen.
- Airway surgery may help manage the multi-level airway involvement.
- Tracheostomy.
- Central nervous system.

- Ventriculoperitoneal(VP) shunting is indicated in moderate to severe hydrocephalus.
- Carpal tunnel syndrome with surgical decompression of median nerve.

Cardiovascular
- Valve replacement surgery is rarely required. Bacterial endocarditis prophylaxis may be necessary.
- Routine evaluation of ventricular function, wall thickness.

Orthopaedic
- Soft tissue surgery with release of contractures.
- Corrective osteotomy: valgus deformity.
- Cervical spinal decompression and/or fusion: kyphosis or atlantoaxial subluxation.

Chromosomal abnormalities and associated musculoskeletal morbidity

- Children with chromosomal problems may have significant musculoskeletal (MSK) problems.
- These are often overlooked, especially in the presence of learning difficulties, developmental delay, and other complex needs where the child cannot communicate symptoms and observed motor problems may be ascribed to neurological or other cause.
- Examples of the most common conditions and associated MSK morbidity are given in Table 4.30. The frequency of MSK abnormalities in these conditions is often poorly defined.

Table 4.30 Chromosomal conditions and musculoskeletal (MSK) problems

Chromosomal condition	MSK abnormalities	MSK presentations and clinical features
Down's syndrome (Trisomy 21) Learning difficulties, upslanting palpebral fissures, epicanthic folds, brachycephaly, cardiac abnormalities	Inflammatory arthritis: • Poly or oligo articular • Psoriatic • Small and large joints Cervical spine instability: • Atlanto axial • Occipital cervical Hip dislocation/ subluxation General hypotonia: • Joint hypermobility • Pes planus (flat feet) • Patella dislocation • Scoliosis Other: • Short stature • Metatarsus primus varus • Brachydactyly	Limp, leg-length discrepancy, motor delay. May express no pain, instead behavioural changes, e.g. reluctance to hold hands, reversion to earlier stage of development, morning stiffness. Joint swelling, ↓ or 'normal' range of movement *(remember these children are normally markedly hypermobile therefore an observed 'normal' range of joint movement, especially if symmetrical, may actually signify loss of movement)* Associated psoriatic rash ±nail pitting Asymptomatic, neck pain, limited neck mobility/ torticollis, sensory deficit, hyper-reflexia, spasticity Limp, antalgic gait, motor delay Clumsiness, poor-coordination, generalized hypotonia, front of feet pointing away from each other, may be asymptomatic Big toe bending inwards Short fingers

(Continued)

Table 4.30 Contd.

Chromosomal condition	MSK abnormalities	MSK presentations and clinical features
DiGeorge syndrome (22q11 deletion) Immunodeficiency T-cell dysfunction, IgA deficiency hypocalcaemia, facial, pharyngeal, and cardiac abnormalities	Inflammatory arthritis Micrognathia and retrognathia Scoliosis, short stature	Limp, leg-length discrepancy, motor delay. Pain, joint swelling, ↓ range of movement Malocclusion, difficulty brushing teeth Feeding difficulties, dentist recognizes problem. Postural shift, altered function, back pain
Turner's syndrome (X0) Webbed neck, low hair line, horseshoe kidney, lymphoedema	Inflammatory arthritis: poly or oligo Cubitus valgus Clinodactyly, brachydactyly Blunt fingertips Micrognathia Short stature	Limp, leg-length discrepancy. Pain, joint swelling, ↓ range of movement Wide carrying angle at elbows Curved 5th fingers Short fingers Small jaw, malocclusion
Trisomy 8 Learning difficulties thick lips, deep-set and prominent ears, pectus excavatum (mild clinical features often associated with mosaicism)	Joint contractures—camptodactyly, clinodactyly Scoliosis Absent patella Micrognathia	Restricted joints—e.g. fixed flexion deformity of interphalangeal joint of little fingers Curved 5th fingers Postural shift Small jaw, malocclusion
18p syndrome Learning difficulties, IgA deficiency	Inflammatory or non-inflammatory arthritis of large joints Short stature	Limp, leg-length discrepancy, pain, morning stiffness, joint swelling, ↓ range of movement
Cystic fibrosis (CF)—see ➜ pp. 349–53 Mutations for CF transmembrane conductance transporter, chromosome 7 Detected on screening, failure to thrive, chronic respiratory symptoms, malabsorption	Arthralgia Inflammatory arthritis: • Oligo or polyarticular • Relapsing Hypertrophic pulmonary osteoarthropathy	Troublesome joint pain, occasionally related to ciprofloxacin use Limp, pain, joint swelling, ↓ range of movement Can be associated with erythema nodosum Joint pain and swelling. Consider in long-standing CF and marked finger clubbing.

(Continued)

Table 4.30 Contd.

Chromosomal condition	MSK abnormalities	MSK presentations and clinical features
Neurofibromatosis (NF) NF1 gene— chromosome 17 2 or more of the following: ≥6 café au lait spots, ≥2 neurofibromata, axillary or inguinal freckling, optic glioma, ≥2 Lisch nodules, osseous dysplasia on the sphenoid bone or cortex of a long bone, 1st-degree relative with NF	Scoliosis & kyphosis Short stature Pseudoarthrosis of the tibia or forearm Bone/soft tissue hypertrophy	Usually presents before 10yr of age, May be an incidental clinical finding, back pain, postural shift Bowing of leg or arm Asymmetrical limb length/ macrodactyly
NF2 gene—long arm chromosome 22 Usually presents in adults but childhood cases are reported. May present with VIII nerve masses, family history NF2, presence of ≥2 neurofibroma, meningioma, glioma, schwannoma, juvenile posterior capsular lenticular opacity	Spinal tumour	Difficulty walking, pain, postural shift, loss or altered function, neurological signs

- It is important to consider other differentials including metabolic disorders and skeletal dysplasias (see ➜ pp. 362–70) especially in the presence of contractures.
  - Most chromosomal problems are also associated with hypermobility, dysmorphism, and short stature.
- Inflammatory arthritis in these children is managed in a similar way to JIA (see ➜ p. 162, and Table 4.31) and requires input from an experienced MDT.
  - The use of MTX and biologics in this patient group requires caution as some conditions are prone to malignancy (e.g. Down's syndrome) and anecdotally, these children appear less tolerant of MTX. However, most patients derive benefit from these agents where indicated, and the presence of a chromosomal abnormality per se is not a contraindication to the use of DMARDS or biologics for inflammatory arthritis in this context.

Table 4.31 Chromosomal conditions and MSK problems: an overview approach to management

MSK problem	MSK radiological investigations & features	Management
Inflammatory arthritis	If clinical uncertainty, US or contrast-enhanced MRI to identify joint effusions & synovial enhancement. Plain films are of limited use until long-standing arthritis has caused significant joint damage such as joint space narrowing and erosions	Referral to a paediatric rheumatology MDT for confirmation of diagnosis, medical treatment and access to ophthalmology for uveitis screening Consider broad spectrum of autoimmune disorders
Cervical spine instability	Cervical spine plain radiograph—as showing ↑ atlanto-dental interval on lateral flexion/extension view (normal <8yr <4mm, >8yr <3mm) MRI may show ligamentous swelling suggestive of instability. CT may show malalignment of vertebrae in the neutral position	Close surveillance, neurosurgical referral Advice to avoid contact sports and to wear a neck collar when travelling in a car
Hip dislocation/ subluxation	Hip plain radiograph—flared iliac wings, hip dysplasia and or dislocation Hip US may be useful in younger children	Referral to orthopaedics
Abnormal foot positioning	Radiology of limited use	Referral to orthotics/ podiatry or orthopaedics.
Scoliosis	Spinal plain radiograph	Referral to orthopaedics or spinal surgeon
Hypermobilty	Radiology of limited use	Referral to hypermobility MDT —physiotherapy and occupational therapy
Joint contractures	Radiology of limited use	Referral to physiotherapy & occupational therapy Consider orthopaedic referral to improve function if severe
Abnormal finger positions, e.g. camptodactyly/ clinodactyly	Radiology of limited use	Referral for occupational therapy for hand function assessment and aids

Table 4.31 Contd.

MSK problem	MSK radiological investigations & features	Management
Micrognathia Jaw malocclusion	Orthopantomogram may show malalignment of the teeth and small mandible	Referral to orthodontics or maxillary facial surgeons depending on severity
Short stature		Ensure plotted on appropriate growth chart (e.g. Turner's and Down's syndromes). Referral to endocrinologist for growth hormone consideration (e.g. in Turner's syndrome)

Further reading

Cimaz R et al; Joint contractures in the absence of inflammation may indicate mucopolysaccharidosis. Pediatric Rheumatol.2009; 9:18

Manger B. Rheumatological manifestations are the key in early diagnosis of mucopolysaccharidosis type I. Eur Musculoskeletal Rev 2008:1–6.

Chan M, Sen E, Hardy E, et al. Assessment of musculoskeletal abnormalities in children with mucopolysaccharidoses using pGALS. Ped Rheum Online 2014 12:32. ℘ http://www.ped-rheum.com/content/12/1/32

Down syndrome and musculoskeletal problems

Down syndrome is a chromosomal disorder caused by full trisomy 21 (94%), mosaicism (2.4%), or translocations (3.3.%). It has an estimated incidence of 1/1000–1100 live births/year worldwide.

Joint laxity, which may be associated with delayed ambulation, is almost universal in children with Down syndrome. This, combined with hypotonia, also a feature of Down syndrome, has significant and widespread functional impact, and contributes to the increased risk of a number of musculoskeletal disorders[1]. Conversely however, over-attributing motor difficulties to low tone and hypermobility may lead to missed pathology and misdiagnoses.

The foot and Down syndrome

Overall laxity of the feet has been reported in 88% of children with Down syndrome. Pes planus is common, and was almost universal in a large cohort of Down syndrome children (Fig. 4.21)[2]. Digital deformities also occur, such as hallux valgus. Young people with Down syndrome have an inability of the heel bone to come out of eversion, resulting in multiple postural changes contributing to inability of many children with Down syndrome to sustain good strength when standing and build good core musculature. Therefore physiotherapy will also yield unsatisfactory results as you can't build on a poor foundation! With poor foot alignment whilst performing exercises, failure or delay of achieving a strong kinetic chain is inevitable as during the exercises the muscles may not even fire.

Young people with pes planus and incorrect footwear are at risk of callus formation over pressure points, repetitive ligamentous injury, and development of bone spurs[3]. Screening by a paediatric podiatrist experienced in Down syndrome should be early, routine, and ongoing, to allow for timely detection and management of foot deformities. Podiatric interventions and good footwear will help to encourage a more 'normal' foot posture, in turn improving posture and quality of life, which are underestimated and neglected[4]. However, in severe cases orthopaedic review and surgical intervention may be required.

The spine and Down syndrome

Cervical spine instability is a well described orthopaedic condition associated with Down syndrome. It involves either the occiput-C1 level (atlanto-occipital instability) or the C1-C2 level (atlanto-axial instability). Cervical spine instability was reported in 1% of the cohort described (Fig. 4.20). The literature states that 10–30% of all people with trisomy 21 may have radiological findings of instability, but most are asymptomatic with only 1–2% developing symptomatic instability. Most commonly signs and symptoms of symptomatic instability progress over time, but complications from spinal cord compression can worsen suddenly. While serious complications are rare, death can occur. Interestingly, low correlation between radiological findings and symptoms has been observed, emphasising the need for a high index of suspicion if symptoms develop. Currently there is no screening

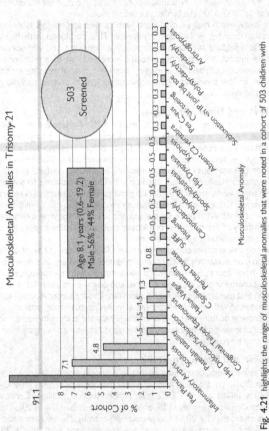

Fig. 4.21 highlights the range of musculoskeletal anomalies that were noted in a cohort of 503 children with Down syndrome, age 0.6–19.2 years[3].

Musculoskeletal Anomalies in Trisomy 21

503 Screened

Age 8.1 years (0.6–19.2)
Male 56%; 44% Female

% of Cohort

91.1
7.1
4.8
1.5 1.5 1.5 1.3 1
0.8
0.5 0.5 0.5 0.5 0.5
0.5 0.5 0.5
0.3 0.3 0.3 0.3 0.3 0.3 0.3

Pes Planus
Inflammatory Arthritis
Scoliosis
Hip Dislocation/Subluxation
Patellan stability
Congenital Talipes Equinovarus
Hallux Valgus
Spine Instability
Perthes Disease
SUFE
Incising
Camptodactyly
Polydactyly
Spondylolisthesis
Hip Dysplasia
Kyphosis
Absent C2 vertebra
Pes C/vus
Subluxation at IP Joint Big toe
Stir-rooting
Polysyndactyly
Syndactyly
Arthrogryposis

Musculoskeletal Anomaly

> **Box 4.11 Red Flag signs & symptoms for C-spine instability**
> - Neck pain
> - Abnormal head posture
> - Torticollis
> - Reduced neck movements
> - Deterioration of gait and/or frequent falls
> - Increasing fatigability on walking
> - Deterioration of manipulative skills.

procedure which can predict those at risk. In particular cervical spine x-rays in children have no predictive validity for subsequent acute dislocation/subluxation at the atlanto-occipital/axial joints. In an attempt to reduce morbidity and mortality from cervical spine instability, the Down Syndrome Medical Interest Group (DSMIG UK) developed basic surveillance essential for people with Down syndrome, revised in 2012. Box 4.11 highlights warning signs that parents, relatives, carers, and all healthcare professionals should be aware of.

Assessment for scoliosis should be routine and on-going in all children with Down syndrome. Vigilance is required in particular for those that may be at risk of thoracic curves secondary to early thoracotomies from congenital heart surgery. Spondylolisthesis may also occur and present with the classic symptoms of low back pain and radiculopathy.

The hip and Down syndrome

Hip hypermobility is common in Down syndrome. Five to eight percent of children with Down syndrome will develop hip abnormalities. Radiographic studies demonstrate that, in comparison with a normal acetabulum, the acetabulum of a patient with Down syndrome is deep, more horizontally placed, and has increased anteversion, whilst the proximal femur has a normal neck-shaft angle and a moderate increase in anteversion[5]. With associated hypotonia, it is therefore not surprising children with Down syndrome develop hip dislocation/subluxation (1.5%). Perthes Disease (0.8%) and slipped upper femoral epiphysis (0.5%) are also reported to occur[2]. The most common presenting sign for hip pathology is a limp, which may often be painless. Hip x-rays should therefore always be performed in a child with Down syndrome presenting with a limp.

The knee and Down syndrome

Patella instability has been reported to occur in Down syndrome to varying degrees, from mild subluxation to complete dislocation. Altered gait may be a sign of patella instability and a decreased range of motion of the knee may be noted. Orthoses or even corrective surgery may be required.

Inflammatory arthritis and Down syndrome

Inflammatory arthritis occurs, but is greatly under-reported or misdiagnosed. It was first described in the literature in 1984, when the term 'arthropathy of Down syndrome' was coined[6]. There are no published population surveys establishing the prevalence and incidence rates of Down's arthropathy, but previous crude estimates suggest that the incidence was as much as 3 to 6-fold greater than JIA in the general paediatric population. Prevalence has been estimated to be 8.7/1000[7,8]. Alarmingly, more recent studies of Down's arthropathy suggest the prevalence is in fact higher and 18–21 times more common than JIA[2]. It is unknown whether arthritis in children with Down syndrome represents JIA and its subtypes, or is a unique arthropathy in light of the genetic and immunologic abnormalities associated with Down syndrome.

Clinical features

A polyarticular pattern of disease, with predominance in the wrists and small joints of the hands (Fig. 4.22) is most commonly seen. The clinical features match the JIA subgroups, rheumatoid factor negative polyarthritis, or the asymmetrical small joint involvement typical of psoriatic arthritis. There have been no reports of a systemic-onset arthritis or uveitis occurring in Down's arthropathy cases.

Delay in diagnosis and pain expression in Down syndrome

The average time to diagnosis of Down's arthropathy is 1.7 years (range 0.2–4.9 years) compared with 0.7 years (range 0.2–2.4 years) in the JIA population[2]. Children are presenting with significant joint damage as a result of delayed diagnosis and therefore delayed instigation of appropriate treatment. Reasons for this delay are multifactorial such as many children may be non-verbal. A significant contributory factor is the altered expression of pain observed in children with Down syndrome. They express pain more

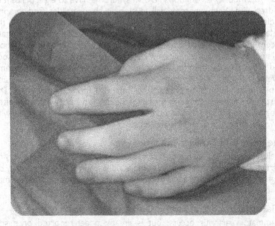

Fig. 4.22 Inflammatory arthritis affecting the Proximal-Inter-Phalangeal (PIP) and Meta-Carpo-Phalangeal (MCP) Joints of the hand of a child with Down syndrome and arthritis

slowly and less precisely than a child without Down syndrome[9]. Children with Down's arthropathy often adapt to pain with reported observations such as slowing mobility, reluctance to hold a parental hand, or behavioural change. When assessing a child with Down syndrome, careful consideration of possible interpretations of the history and a thorough clinical examination will aid correct and timely diagnosis of Down's arthropathy.

Radiological features

Radiological changes are seen with higher frequency in Down's arthropathy than JIA. These changes include erosions, joint space narrowing, subluxations, osteopenia, and acro-osteolysis. Down's arthropathy is potentially a more aggressive and erosive disease than JIA, but the observed findings with regards to radiological changes could also be attributed to the significant delay in diagnosis of Down's arthropathy.

Investigation and treatment

Investigation and management of Down's arthropathy is as per normal clinical practice for JIA. Multi-disciplinary team care should be paramount. Treatment is often complicated by drug-associated side-effects, in particular methotrexate-related nausea.

Conclusion

Early, regular and continuous musculoskeletal assessment of children with Down syndrome is paramount to management of musculoskeletal conditions. The aim is to avoid children presenting with irreversible, preventable joint damage and disability due to delayed or incorrect diagnosis and management of these very treatable conditions.

Key messages

- When a child with Down syndrome presents with a limp they should always be referred for a hip x-ray.
- A high index of suspicion for pathology should be employed when assessing a child with Down syndrome presenting with change and/or deterioration in function and mobility.
- Inflammatory arthritis in children with Down syndrome is common and potentially erosive and debilitating if left undetected and untreated.
- Variability exists in the basic biomechanics of the musculoskeletal system in children with Down syndrome in terms of motor control, coordination, and skill.
- Multidisciplinary team assessment and management should be regular and ongoing to ensure these children reach their potential with regards to motor function.

References

1. Jacobsen FS, Hansson G. Orthopaedic disorders in Down's syndrome. Current Orthopaedics 2000; 14: 215–222
2. Foley C, Killeen OG 2015; In Press
3. Rigoldi C, Galli M, Mainardi L, Crivellini M, Albertini G. Postural control in children, teenagers and adults with Down syndrome. Research in Developmental Disabilities. 2011;32:170–175
4. Concolino D, Pasquzzi A, Capalbo G, Sinopoli S, Strisciuglio P. Early detection of podiatric anomalies in children with Down syndrome. Acta Paediatrica 2006; 95: 17–29

5. Shaw ED, Beals RK. The hip joint in Down's syndrome. A study of its structure and associated disease. *Clinical Ortopaedics* 1992; 278: 101–107

6. Yancey, CL. Zmijewski, C. Athreya, BH and Doughty, RA. Arthropathy of Downs syndrome. Arthritis Rheum 1984; 27(8): 929–34

7. Padmakumar, B. Evans, LG. Jones and Sills, JA. Is arthritis more common in children with Down syndrome? Rheumatology 2000; 41: 1191–1193

8. Juj, H and Emery, HJ. The Arthropathy of Down syndrome: an underdiagnosed & under-recognised condition. J Pediatr 2009; 154(2): 234–8

9. Hennequin M, Morin C, Feine JS. Pain expression and stimulus localisation in individuals with Down's syndrome. Lancet. 2000; 2;356(9245):1882–7

Arthritis and other musculoskeletal features associated with cystic fibrosis

• Many patients (reported as 13%) with cystic fibrosis (CF) will have musculoskeletal complaints; with increasing prevalence of rheumatic symptoms with age, CF lung disease severity, and infection with *Pseudomonas aeruginosa* and *Aspergillus fumigatus*.

• CF arthropathy is reported in 2–8.5% of patients and hypertrophic osteoarthropathy in 2–7% of patients.

• Undoubtedly patients with chronic lung disease are more likely to be physically deconditioned and this tends to associate with generalized musculoskeletal pain and being prone to mechanical/non-inflammatory musculoskeletal complaints.

• The different rheumatological features associated with CF are summarized in Table 4.32.

Table 4.32 Rheumatological features associated with CF

	Clinical features	Investigations	Management
Transient recurrent arthritis Affects 5–10% Increasing with age May be related to presence of circulating immune complexes	Episodic joint swelling lasting 1–10 days May be related to exacerbations of CF Mostly monoarticular/asymmetric-knees most common Can be accompanied by skin rash-erythema nodosum purpura and overlying erythema reported	Acute phase reactants may be raised Amylase: rare association with pancreatitis, panniculitis and arthritis Increased frequency of RF and anti CCP positivity related to level of lung disease and frequency of CF exacerbations ANA usually negative	No trials available to support any particular management strategy NSAIDs; and/or short courses of glucocorticoids may be helpful
Persistent arthritis	Subgroup of patients with transient arthropathy may go on to develop persistent arthritis indistinguishable from JIA Typically polyarthritis affecting small joints of hands and feet Can be associated with destructive joint disease	RF positivity more commonly observed than in transient recurrent arthritis	No trials available to support any particular management strategy Benefits of DMARDS need to be balanced against the risks of immunosuppression Case report level evidence available for the use of MTX or ETN in CF-associated arthritis with beneficial effect on lung function Some concerns with use of MTX in adults with pre-existing pulmonary disease and RA due to risk of developing MTX-related pneumonitis. Shared care with respiratory team essential

Condition	Features	Investigations	Management
Hypertrophic pulmonary osteoarthropathy	Associated with severity of CF and disease duration. Digital clubbing. Long bone tenderness. Periosteal reactions of tubular bone. Non inflammatory effusions in joints mainly symmetrical. Can also get skin thickening/acne/hyperhydrosis	Radiographs: Periosteal reaction and cortical bone thickening	Management of underlying lung condition: chest physiotherapy and antibiotics. NSAIDs. Glucocorticoids. Pamidronate. Changes can reverse following lung transplantation
Metabolic bone disease (osteoporosis/osteopenia/osteomalacia/renal osteodystrophy)	Increased risk in patients on frequent glucocorticoids and with reduced physical activity levels. Vit D/Ca deficiency.	Serum calcium, PO_4, ALP, PTH, and 25OH Vitamin D levels. DEXA screening guidelines: Children age 8 years or greater with other risk factors (i.e. ideal body weight <90%, FEV1 <50% predicted, glucocorticoids 5mg/day or more for 90 days/year or longer; delayed puberty, or previous history of fractures)	Careful attention to bone health including Vitamin D (target 75–150 nmol/l) and calcium supplementation as indicated. Use of bisphosphonates as indicated by DEXA
Drug-induced arthropathy	Cartilage damage in patients on fluoroquinolones (ciprofloxacin). Low level of evidence for association. Pain after 3–8 weeks of treatment		Pain typically resolves up to 2 weeks after discontinuation of medication

Table 4.32 Contd.

	Clinical features	Investigations	Management
Vasculitis	Usually cutaneous Palpable purpuric rash Cerebral and renal involvement also reported Can be a poor prognostic sign	Increased rate of non-specific ANCA (e.g P-ANCA) that are not usually pathogenic	Response to glucocorticoids
Secondary (AA) amyloidosis	Associated with increased pulmonary and systemic inflammation, and more of a concern in those who now have an increased life expectancy Case reports in adolescents: renal, liver, spleen and thyroid involvement	Low threshold for renal biopsy in patients with persistent proteinuria	Case report of two patients supporting the use of colchicine
Sarcoidosis	Reported in 3 patients with CF Unclear if definite link	Exclude infectious mimics of granulomatous inflammation, e.g. tuberculosis	Treatment tailored to individual requirements as per severity of organ involvement

Further reading

M A Turner, E Baildam, L Patel, and T J David. Joint disorders in cystic fibrosis. *J R Soc Med*. 1997; **90**(Suppl 31):13–20.

Botton E1, Saraux A, Laselve H, *et al*. Musculoskeletal manifestations in cystic fibrosis. *Joint Bone Spine* 2003;**70**:327–35.

Garske LA, Bell SC. Pamidronate results in symptom control of hypertrophic pulmonary osteoar-thropathy in cystic fibrosis. *Chest* 2002;**121**:1363–4.

Inflammatory bowel disease and musculoskeletal features

Introduction

- Musculoskeletal (MSK) symptoms in inflammatory bowel disease (IBD) are common and include arthralgia, myalgia, peripheral arthropathy, enthesitis, sacroiliitis, and spondylitis.
- Non-inflammatory MSK pain can be the result of deconditioning and general debilitation in IBD.
- Glucocorticoid and chronic disease-related osteopenia and hypertrophic osteoarthropathy may also result in MSK pain.
- Inflammatory arthropathy is uncommon.
- Features of arthropathy may occur before, during or after the presentation of clinical features suggestive of IDD.
- 20–30% of IDD presents in childhood and is more likely to have extra intestinal manifestations of which arthropathy is the commonest.

Definitions

- *Ulcerative colitis (UC)*—diffuse mucosal inflammation limited to the colon.
- *Crohn's disease (CD)*—patchy transmural inflammation affecting any part of the GI tract.
- *Indeterminate colitis (IC)*—10% of children with IBD affecting the colon cannot be classified as there are some features of both conditions.
- *Arthropathy of inflammatory bowel disease*—any non-infectious arthropathy occurring before or during the course of UC, IC, or CD.
- Clinical features, see Table 4.33.

Table 4.33 Clinical features of IBD at presentation

Symptoms or sign	CD (%)	IC (%)	UC (%)
Common symptoms			
Abdominal pain	72	75	62
Diarrhoea	56	78	74
Bleeding	22	68	84
Weight loss	58	35	31
Lethargy	27	14	12
Anorexia	25	13	6
Arthropathy	7	4	6
Other symptoms			
Nausea/vomiting, constipation/soiling, psychiatric symptoms, amenorrhea			

Epidemiology

- Collective incidence of IBD <16yr olds in UK is 9.37 per 100,000/year (60% CD, 28% UC and 12% IC). Mean age at presentation: 11.9yr (58% are boys, 4% are <5yr). 25% of all IBD presents in children and young people.
- Family history—29% have a ≥1 relative with IBD (greatest in those presenting before 3yr old).
- Arthralgia and myalgia are common (1/3 of patients and often coincide with disease activity)—this may reflect the incidence of MSK pain in healthy adolescents.
- Incidence of arthropathy in IBD variable (2.4–21%) and there is no observed difference between UC and CD. Most common EIM of IBD.

Extra intestinal manifestations (EIM)

- These may present before (6%), during, or after the presentation of IBD (at least one EIM in 29% 15 years following diagnosis).
- Anal fistula/anal abscess (CD), aphthous ulceration, growth failure/delayed puberty (CD), osteoporosis, erythema nodosum/rash/pyoderma gangrenosum (CD), liver disease, appendicitis, uveitis.
- Perianal disease and extra intestinal manifestations are more common in the paediatric onset disease.

Peripheral arthritis

- Oligoarthritis affecting knees and ankles most common—most likely to reflect IBD activity.
- Occasionally affects multiple joints, including small joints of hands and TMJs. Independent of IBD activity and more persistent.
- Onset of arthritis does not correlate with activity of IBD and may occur before, during, or unrelated to flare of bowel disease.
- Persistent arthritis is more likely to reflect poor control of bowel disease.
- Arthritis is rarely persistent, progressive, or erosive.

Sacroiliitis and spondyloarthropathy (axial skeletal involvement)

MSK symptoms with back pain and generalized idiopathic (non-inflammatory) pain are common in IBD and important to distinguish from inflammatory back pain.

- May begin as a peripheral inflammatory arthritis and progress to involve sacroiliac joints, hips, and lumbosacral spine.
- Disease does not reflect activity of IBD, and may be progressive despite good control of IBD.
- Associated with the presence of HLA B27.
- May progress to ankylosing spondylitis (3–7%) with no difference between UC and CD for the prevalence of axial spine involvement.

Diagnosis and investigation

See: Guideline for the investigation and management of IBD in children in the United Kingdom (℘ http://bspghan.org.uk/).

Diagnosis of arthropathy in IBD is clinical and supported by radiology.

A high level of suspicion from a history suggestive of arthritis accompanied by any of the listed presenting clinical features of IBD. Consider IBD in the child with arthritis when:
• Intolerant of NSAIDs.
• Presence of anaemia, raised acute phase reactants, and low albumin.

Investigations
• Faecal calprotectin (FC). Sensitive measure for detecting IBD. Not specific and raised in infection, coeliac, and other bowel inflammation. If low suspicion on basis of symptoms and serological markers: FC <50µg/g NPV of 96%, therefore further investigations unlikely to be needed. In known IBD FC levels may be useful to monitor disease activity.
• Perinuclear antineutrophil cytoplasmic antibodies (pANCA) and anti-*Saccharomyces cerevisiae* antibodies (ASCA), may help distinguish between UC and CD (pANCA 68% of UC, ASCA 81% of CD).
• Endoscopy and biopsy: gold standard for diagnosis, position, and extent of disease.
• MRI of sacroiliac joints and spine help distinguish non-specific MSK pain from true sacroiliitis and spondylitis—x-rays are not helpful in the adolescent as the epiphyses do not fuse until mid-20s.

Management
• Multidisciplinary approach to management including physiotherapy.
• Primary approach is to control underlying inflammatory bowel disease. In addition:
  • Mild disease/first line for peripheral and axial disease: note that NSAIDS may lead to flare of active IBD.
  • Moderate disease: Sulfasalazine, mesalazine or methotrexate with intra-articular steroids.
  • Axial disease or resistant peripheral arthritis: anti-TNF such as infliximab and adalimumab (etanercept is not effective at controlling IBD) use of other agents demonstrate benefit in adults (gobilimumab and certazilumab).
  • Biosimilars suggested to have equal efficacy in adult RA, their use is increasing in paediatric diseases for cost saving.
  • Other agents such as rituximab and usterkinumab may be of benefit in refractory cases.
• Benefit from anti-TNF may not be sustained.
• Choice of medication should consider other extra-intestinal manifestations such as uveitis.

Further reading
Guideline for the investigation and management of IBD in children in the United Kingdom (⅏ http://bspghan.org.uk/).
Guariso G, Gasparetto M, Visonà Dalla Pozza L et al. Inflammatory bowel disease developing in paediatric and adult age. *J Pediatr Gastroenterol Nutr* 2010;51(6):698–707. doi: 10.1097/MPG.0b013e3181da1db8.
Saha A, Tighe MP, Batra A How to use faecal calprotectin in management of paediatric inflammatory bowel disease. *Arch Dis Child Educ Pract* Ed doi:10.1136/archdischild-2014-307941.
Sheth T, Pitchumoni CS, Kiron MD Management of musculoskeletal manifestations in inflammatory bowel disease. Gastroenterol Res Pract. 2015;2015:387891. doi: 10.1155/2015/387891.

Chapter 5

Bone diseases, skeletal dysplasias, and collagen disorders

Metabolic bone diseases

Primary osteoporosis

Osteogenesis imperfecta (OI)

- Principal features are bone fragility and low bone mass leading to fractures and bone deformity with growth retardation.
- Ligamentous laxity, dentinogenesis imperfecta, and blue scleral hue are variable features. 90% of OI dominantly inherited due to defects in the type I collagen genes *COL1A1* and *COL1A2*. Small number due to defect in IFITM5/BRIL promoter region mutation.

Idiopathic juvenile osteoporosis

15–20% due to heterozygous mutations in low-density lipoprotein receptor related protein 5 (*LRP5*) gene, rest unknown. Typically presents pre/early puberty with metaphyseal and vertebral crush fractures.

Rare disorders presenting in the neonatal period with fractures

All have other features that help distinguish them from OI. These disorders include:

- Akinesia.
- Spinal muscular atrophy with arthrogryposis.
- Neurofibromatosis.
- Cytomegalovirus inclusion disease.
- Caffey's disease.
- I-cell disease (mucolipidosis II).

Bone active treatment is with bisphosphonates to ↑ bone mass, reduce bone pain, and improve vertebral size and shape:

- Infants and those with more severe disease, or where growth will soon cease more often receive IV therapy—pamidronate 9–12mg/kg/yr (see ➋ Guidelines, pp. 490–1). Some now receive zoledronic acid 0.025–0.05mg/kg at 6–12 month intervals.
- Oral therapy in milder cases with risedronate (1–2mg/kg/week) is safe and effective. Other bisphosphonates are used but the evidence base is less clear.
- Denosumab (anti-RANK ligand, antiresorptive) in phase 2/3 clinical trials.

Secondary osteoporosis

Inflammatory conditions (e.g.)

- *Inflammatory bowel disease*—bone loss and fractures more common in Crohn's disease than in ulcerative colitis, before and after starting glucocorticoids.
- *Juvenile arthritis*—up to 7% of children with inflammatory joint disease have vertebral crush fracture prior to use of glucocorticoids. Main clinical feature is back pain.
- *Cystic fibrosis*—bone mass loss after 1st decade with concomitant ↑ in fracture risk.

Use of glucocorticoids
- ↑ fracture risk when taking oral glucocorticoids irrespective of underlying condition.
- Complex actions on skeleton—reduce cortical bone turnover leading to retention of older, more heavily mineralized bone that ↑ DXA-measured bone mass; loss of trabecular bone, leading to ↑ risk of fractures in vertebrae.
- Resolution of risk 3–6 months after steroid cessation.

Disuse
- *Cerebral palsy*—long bone fractures occur in major bones during handling; bones are narrow with thin cortices.
- *Duchenne muscular dystrophy*—low bone mass 2° to disuse and corticosteroids; fractures occur whilst still mobile, but ↑ in frequency once boy becomes immobile. Bone loss ↑ when steroid dose higher.
- *Epidermolysis bullosa*—bone loss due to immobility.

Endocrine disturbance
- *Anorexia nervosa*—low bone mass may not be apparent in childhood/adolescence;—low bone mass consistently reported in adult women who were anorexic as teenagers.
- *Cushing's syndrome*—low bone mass and fractures reported; vertebral crush fractures resolve on treatment of underlying disorder.
- *Turner's syndrome*—no evidence of low bone mass or fractures until young adulthood.

Haematology/oncology
- Acute leukaemia—↑ fracture risk and bone loss both at diagnosis and during treatment.
- Post chemotherapy for childhood cancer. Studies suggest that chemotherapy alone does not lead to ↑ later fracture risk;—risk is ↑ in those receiving radiotherapy.
- Thalassaemia.
- Post haematopoietic stem cell transplantation.

Osteomalacia/rickets
- Clinical features—bowed limbs, metaphyseal swelling, bossed forehead, pain.
- Vast majority are due to lack of vitamin D, resulting from poor sunlight exposure or dietary inadequacy; more common in darker-skinned individuals living in colder climates.
- Vitamin D deficiency results in myopathy and musculoskeletal aches and pains; infants are usually miserable. Investigations: serum Ca, PO_4, ALP, PTH, and 25OH vitamin D.
- The threshold for deficiency in asymptomatic individuals is debated widely; a typical cut-off is 25mmol/L 25OH vitamin D. Above this, either treatment or supplementation (200–400U/d) is given. Sufficiency is generally accepted as being >75mmol/L.
- Treatment is with ergo/cholecalciferol daily for 2 months. <2yr 3000U/day; 2–10yr 6000U/day; 10yr 10,000U/day.

- Inherited forms of rickets often associated with ↑ circulating FGF-23, which promotes phosphaturia and inhibits renal production of the vitamin D metabolite 1,25 dihydroxyvitamin D; this group includes X-linked hypophosphataemic rickets, and children with McCune–Albright syndrome/polyostotic fibrous dysplasia. Replacement with oral phosphate in divided doses (40–50mg/kg) and 1,25 dihydroxyvitamin D or 1-α calcidol (30–50ng/kg); anti-FGF23 antibody entering phase 3 clinical trials.
- Hypophosphatasia: new enzyme replacement treatment—asfotase alfa—for severely affected infants and children substantially reduces mortality and morbidity.

Osteopetrosis

- Increased bone mass due to failure to resorb bone.
- Severe cases present with bone marrow failure and incipient blindness at 3–6 months—urgent decompression of optic nerves may be required.
- Some respond well to bone marrow transplantation.
- Milder forms present later in life—nerve compression and poor fracture healing are significant problems.

Skeletal dysplasia

- Achondroplasia – various new therapies targeting downstream signaling from FGFR3 in phase 2/3 studies.

Avascular necrosis

- Commonest site affected is the femoral head (other sites described in ➐ The osteochondroses, pp. 371–4).
- Thought to be due to interruption to blood supply to the femoral head.
- Affects approximately 1 in 1000 children, ♂ more than ♀ (4:1), usually between 3–12yr. 5–10% of cases are bilateral.
- Presenting features—deep hip or referred pain to the knee especially with exercise, may present with limp.
- Diagnosis is by radiograph; however, MRI results in earlier detection.
- Treatment—conservative in early disease. Surgical intervention may be required.
- Prognosis—relatively good in the very young and with early detection. Older children and those with significant deformities of the femoral head develop premature osteoarthritis.

Bone densitometry

- DXA is most commonly used to assess bone density, but cannot measure tissue depth; hence adjustment procedures are often applied to account for body size.
- No simple algorithm is available that fully corrects this problem.

- Small children will have lower values than large children; hence adjusting for body size seems logical, but may be confounded when the underlying disease affects growth. Sequential measurements (usually twice annually) assessed alongside a growth chart are helpful in assessing bone mass trajectory in response to therapy.
- Indications for the use of DXA in 1° and 2° osteoporosis in children, along with comprehensive supporting evidence, are given on the International Society for Clinical Densitometry (ISCD) website: ⅆ http://www.iscd.org/visitors/pdfs/ISCD2007OfficialPositions-Pediatric.pdf.

Skeletal dysplasias

Background

A group of several hundred clinically and genetically heterogeneous disorders causing generalized abnormalities of bone growth and/or bone modelling. Due to advances in DNA sequencing technologies, the molecular basis of many skeletal dysplasias is now known. The majority are rare with one of a small number (<10) conditions present in most affected individuals. Usually present with 1 or more of:

- Short stature (usually disproportionate).
- Bone deformity/joint malalignment.
- Joint (or generalized bone) pain or limitation of movement.
- Abnormal gait.
- Recurrent fractures.
- Significant family history

Healthcare needs, associated features, prognosis, and recurrence risks in other family members are dependent on specific diagnosis.

Assessment

History

- Pre- and post-natal growth pattern—age at which abnormalities first noted (a subset of skeletal dysplasias are lethal in the perinatal period).
- Age of onset and progression of symptoms.
- Associated features including abnormalities of vision, hearing, teeth, palate, development, neurological function.
- Effect on physical and psychosocial functioning.
- Three-generation family history including, parental heights, evidence of short stature, early onset 'arthritis', low trauma fractures, joint replacement at young age, and consanguinity.

Examination

- Height, weight, head circumference.
- Skeletal proportion—span, where possible sitting height (subischial leg length = height − sitting height) or upper and lower segments (US, LS) and US/LS.
  - LS measured from symphysis pubis to floor, US = height − LS.
  - Centile charts are available for sitting height and subischial leg length. US/LS normally >1.0 until age 10yr, 1.0 at 10yr, <1.0 after 10yr (see ℘ http://www.castlemeadpublications.com).
  - If limbs are short it is important to note which segment(s) are affected: i.e. if the proximal segment (shoulder to elbow, or hip to knee) is short, e.g. in achondroplasia—*rhizomelic* shortening; middle segment (elbow to wrist, knee to ankle)—*mesomelic*; distal segment (hands, feet)—*acromelic*; or all segments—*micromelic*.
- Hands and feet—brachydactyly, polydactyly, talipes, joint limitation/deformity.
- Joint function, spine (assess for kyphosis, scoliosis, lumbar lordosis), gait.

- General examination—including particularly vision, hearing, palate, teeth, heart, abdominal organomegaly, dysmorphic facial features and development.

Investigation

- Radiological skeletal survey—discuss exact composition with local radiologist but likely to include:
  - Anterior–posterior (AP) and lateral skull.
  - PA chest.
  - AP and lateral spine.
  - AP pelvis and bilateral hips.
  - AP 1 upper limb and 1 lower limb.
  - AP of left hand and wrist (both if hands affected).
  - Other views as clinically indicated—consider views of cervical spine in flexion and extension where there is significant spine involvement.
- Biochemical assessment including vitamin D levels if abnormal bone density or metaphyseal abnormalities (nutritional rickets is frequently misdiagnosed as a metaphyseal dysplasia).
- Metabolic investigation if features of storage disorder (coarse facies, organomegaly, dysostosis multiplex, developmental delay).
- Chromosome analysis (array CGH, karyotype)—if associated malformations and/or cognitive developmental delay.
- If diagnosis is uncertain, or if a molecular diagnosis would alter the management, then genetic testing may be indicated. May also be indicated if prenatal diagnosis in future pregnancies is requested. Discuss with clinical genetics.

Differential diagnosis

- Most skeletal dysplasias result in disproportionate short stature with specific clinical and radiographic features:
  - Expert assessment of x-rays may be required (discuss with radiology or European Skeletal Dysplasia Network: ℘ http:www.esdn.org).
  - Radiographic changes may not be present in infancy and may disappear after puberty;—previous x-rays may be helpful.
- Consider other causes of short stature—endocrine, chronic illness, syndromic, constitutional delay of growth and puberty particularly if short stature is proportionate & delayed bone age ± non-skeletal features (including cognitive delay).
- Consider overall diagnostic group (Table 5.1). Common diagnoses only are described (for full classification of skeletal dysplasias / more information see Warman et al., Further reading,).

Management

- MDT including rheumatology, orthopaedics, radiology, clinical genetics, physiotherapy, occupational therapy, ear nose throat, paediatrics, neurosurgery.
- Diagnosis will help identify likely natural history and healthcare needs. Anticipatory management important,—e.g. kyphosis in achondroplasia, retinal detachment in spondyloepiphyseal dysplasia congenita (SEDc).
- Surgical intervention is not always required.

Table 5.1 Skeletal dysplasias

Clinical/ radiographic group	Clinical features	Radiological features	Inheritance/molecular genetics	Other features
Short limbs/'normal' trunk				
Achondroplasia/ hypochondroplasia	• Short limbs (rhizomelic) • Macrocephaly • Thoraco-lumbar kyphosis in infancy, lordosis later • Trident hand • ↓Elbow extension • Tibial bowing	• Large calvaria, ↓size foramen magnum • ↓ Interpedicular distance, short pedicles • Flat, round iliac bones, notch-like sacroiliac groove • Short tubular bones • Brachydactyly	AD—mostly new-dominant with unaffected parents Mutations in FGFR3	Risk of hydrocephalus and foramen magnum stenosis in early years. Lumbar stenosis in adulthood Obstructive sleep apnoea common Achondroplasia/ hypochondroplasia may be difficult to differentiate clinically
Pseudoachondroplasia	• Short limbs (micromelic) • Brachydactyly • Extreme joint hypermobility • Normal head size/shape • Kyphoscoliosis • Waddling gait • Knee deformity (wind swept)	• Delayed epiphyseal ossification, flat irregular epiphyses • Biconcave vertebrae, later platyspondyly, anterior vertebral tongue • Brachydactyly	AD—many new dominant Mutations in COMP	Not related to achondroplasia Present with waddling gait and later hip and knee pain. At risk of cervical spine instability Overlaps with severe multiple epiphyseal dysplasia
Dyschondrosteosis	• Madelung deformity of upper limbs with limitation of pronation supination • Mesomelic shortening • Radial, tibial bowing • May present as 'isolated' familial short stature	• Madelung deformity • Bowing of forearm and lower leg bones	AD Deletion or mutations in SHOX	Very variable phenotype Growth velocity may increase on treatment with hGH Important to differentiate from familial short stature

Short trunk with 'normal' limbs

Spondyloepiphyseal dysplasia congenita (SEDc)	• Short spine and neck, barrel chest, pectus carinatum, genu valgum • Hands and feet clinically normal • Flattened midface • ± Myopia, cleft palate, club feet	• Delayed ossification of skeleton, absence of various ossification centres (e.g. pelvis, vertebral bodies, femoral head and neck) • Odontoid hypoplasia, kyphoscoliosis • Coxa vara	AD Mutations/deletion/duplication of COL2A1 Spectrum of allelic disorders includes Kniest dysplasia, AD spondyloarthropathy, stickler syndrome COL2 type, achondrogenesis II, hypochondrogenesis	Motor development may be delayed, but cognitive development normal Small thorax may cause respiratory complications Risk of atlanto-axial dislocation and spinal cord compression High myopia associated with retinal detachment
Progressive pseudorheumatoid arthropathy of childhood (spondyloepiphyseal dysplasia tarda with progressive arthropathy)	• Short trunk • Progressive large joint contracture • Contracture of small joints of hands and feet with soft tissue swelling	• Platyspondyly, ± scoliosis • Enlarged epiphyses initially. Later develop cystic lesions with flattening • Enlarged epiphyses and metaphyses of bones of hands and feet with osteoporosis but no periostitis	AR Mutations in WISP3	An important differential for JIA especially where there is a family history Differentiating factors include platyspondyly and the absence of erosions and periostitis Progressive joint contracture and osteoarthrosis may lead to decreased mobility and the need for joint replacement
Brachyolmia	• Short trunk, scoliosis, mild short stature • Clinically and genetically heterogeneous • Types 1–3	• Platyspondyly • Short ilia • ± longitudinal striations of metaphyses of large long bones (e.g. femur)	Heterogeneous Both AR and AD forms documented Type 1: AR Type 2: AR Type 3: AD, TRPV4	Type 1: corneal opacities Type 2: calcification of falx cerebri Type 3: severe kyphoscoliosis

Table 5.1 Contd.

Clinical/ radiographic group	Clinical features	Radiological features	Inheritance/molecular genetics	Other features
Short trunk with short limbs				
Kniest dysplasia	• Short limbs, joint enlargement, ↓joint mobility • Dorsal kyphosis, ilumbar lordosis, thoracic scoliosis • Flattened midface, depressed nasal bridge, • ± cleft palate, myopia, deafness, clubfeet	• Platyspondyly, anterior wedging of vertebral bodies • Broad, hypoplastic ilia • Broad, short femoral necks • Delayed ossification of capital femoral epiphyses • Short tubular bones, broad metaphyses, deformed epiphyses	AD, mutations in COL2A1 (most are deletions resulting in truncated type II collagen)	Complications include chronic otitis media, retinal detachment, cataracts, joint contractures, early arthrosis
Diastrophic dysplasia	• Wide phenotypic variability • Short limbs • Multiple joint contractures • Proximal hypermobile thumbs ('hitchhiker thumb': deformity of 1st metacarpal) • Clubfeet • Cysts of external ear (in first 12 weeks of life), subsequently cauliflower deformity of pinnae • Progressive kyphoscoliosis • ± cleft palate	• Flat dysplastic epiphysis with wide metaphyses • Delta-shaped distal femoral/ radial metaphyses • Short, wide, long bones • Deformities of metacarpals, metatarsals, and phalanges • Progressive thoraco-lumbar kyphoscoliosis, cervical kyphosis	AR Mutations in DTDST	Perinatal and infant mortality ↑ Risk of medullary compression from cervical kyphosis (present at birth but usually resolves by ~7yr Clubfeet often difficult to manage and resistant to surgical correction Joint contracture is progressive and may recur after surgical release

Epiphyseal disorders

| Multiple epiphyseal dysplasia (MED) | • Very variable phenotype
• Joint pain
• Hypermobile joints, especially in hands
• ↓Mobility, waddling gait | • Delayed epiphyseal ossification
• Flattened irregular epiphyses
• Mild irregularity and flattening of vertebrae in severe cases | Mostly AD Mutations in:COMP MATN3 Col9A1/A2/A3 Rare AR form Mutations in: DTDST | Poor correlation between phenotype and genotype. Very variable even within families
Overlaps with mild pseudoachondroplasia severe end of MED spectrum |

Metaphyseal dysplasias

| Metaphyseal dysplasia, Schmid type | • Bowed legs, waddling gait
• Normal epiphyseal development
• Brachydactyly
• Lordosis | • Short tubular bones
• Broad irregular metaphyses hips worse than knees
• Coxa vara, short femoral necks
• Brachydactyly
• ± mild platyspondyly | AD Mutations is COL10A1 | May be difficult to differentiate clinically and radiographically from rickets. Always check biochemistry including vitamin D levels |

Table 5.1 Contd.

Clinical/radiographic group	Clinical features	Radiological features	Inheritance/molecular genetics	Other features
Cartilage–hair hypoplasia	• ↓length at birth • Fine, sparse hair/eyebrows/lashes • Brachydactyly with hypermobile hands • ↓Elbow extension • Ligamentous laxity • Recurrent infections (children) secondary to ↓in vitro T-cell function • Particularly at risk from varicella infection • Hirschsprung's disease	• Short tubular bones • Metaphyseal dysplasia of tubular bones knees more than hips • Mild platyspondyly • Brachydactyly with cone-shaped epiphyses	AR Mutations in RMRP	Risk of cervical spine instability. All features variable including severity of immunodeficiency Probable ↑ risk of malignancy in adulthood, e.g. lymphoma.
Skeletal dysplasias with ↓bone density				
Osteogenesis imperfecta	• Recurrent low trauma fracture • Bone deformity • Blue sclerae and dentinogenesis imperfecta may be present • Back pain • Very variable phenotype with multiple types based on clinical features	• Generalized hypomineralization • Wormian bones in skull	Mostly AD Mutations in COL1A1/2 Very rare AR forms	Vital to differentiate from non accidental injury. Requires expert assessment. Both diagnoses may be present Management of severe OI revolutionized by use of IV bisphosphonates

Skeletal dysplasias with ↑ bone density

Osteopetrosis	• Very variable phenotype • Severe infantile • Intermediate childhood onset • Mild late onset • Low trauma fractures • Cranial nerve impingement • Bone marrow failure • Early dental decay and loss	• Generalized increase in bone density especially at skull base • 'Bone within a bone' • 'Rugger jersey' spine	AR—severe neonatal form Mutations in: CLCN7 TCIRG1 OST AD—later onset forms Mutations in: CLCN7 LRP5	Mutation analysis is important in neonatal forms as it may determine suitability for definitive treatment by BMT. Urgent assessment is required Neurosurgical assessment required
Camurati-Engelmann Disease (Progressive Diaphyseal Dysplasia)	• Proximal muscle weakness • Limb pain • Waddling gait	• Hyperostosis of one or more long bones (diaphyses > metaphyses > (rarely) epiphyses • Hyperostosis does not affect spine • Periosteal involvement • Endosteal bony sclerosis	AD. Reduced penetrance. Mutations in TGFB1	Skull involvement may occur (headaches). Pain is a significant feature—treated with steroids Cranial nerve deficits, including facial palsy, hearing and vision loss, and other neurological sequelae may be present.

AD, autosomal dominant; AR, autosomal recessive.

- Pain is a major feature of many bone dysplasias and is often poorly controlled:
  - Pain may be the presenting feature, e.g. joint pain in multiple epiphyseal dysplasia (MED), generalized bone pain in Camurati–Engelmann Disease disease:
    —May not respond to usual analgesics.
    —Appropriate physiotherapy may be more helpful.
  - Steroid treatment can be very effective in, e.g. Camurati–Engelmann disease.
- Most bone dysplasias are heritable—discuss with family; offer referral to clinical genetics.
- Support available for family from several organizations (see Useful contacts below).

Further reading

Bonafe L, et al. Nosology and classification of genetic skeletal disorders: 2015 revision. *Am J Med Genet Part A* 2015; **167A(12)**:2869–92.

The 2010 Nosology tables are also available online at the International Skeletal Dysplasia Society web site (℧ www.isds.ch)

Wright MJ, Irving MD. Clinical management of achondroplasia. *Arch Dis Child* 2012;**97(2)**:129–34.

Useful contacts

European Skeletal Dysplasia Network—online diagnostic resource: ℧ http://www.esdn.org.
Little People of America—support organization: ℧ http://www.lpaonline.org.
Restricted Growth Association—support organization: ℧ http://www.restrictedgrowth.co.uk

The osteochondroses

Definition

- Historically, the term 'osteochondrosis' or 'osteochondritidis' has been applied to a heterogeneous group of conditions characterized by a disturbance in endochondral ossification in an area in which previously growth had been normal.
- Changes have been observed in relation to many growth centres, both epiphyseal and apophyseal and several sites are associated with eponyms.
- Osteochondritis dissecans (OCD) is a separate entity, as are the two conditions of Blount's disease and Legg–Calve–Perthe's disease. (Table 5.2). Also see ➔ Metabolic bone disease, pp. 358–61.

Aetiology

- The initial event (or combination of events) that leads to the disorder in endochondral ossification is unknown and hence these conditions are considered idiopathic in origin. Both a vascular and a traumatic aetiology have been proposed.
- The vascular theory is certainly part of the process in Legg–Calve-Perthes (LCP) disease *and*
- Repetitive microtrauma is implicated in OCD and Osgood–Schlatter's amongst others.

Pathology

- Histologically, in the osteochondritides, the affected area shows many of the features of ischaemic necrosis of the bone within the epiphysis and the apophysis (*not* the cartilage).
- Necrosis (often with collapse of the dead bone).
- Revascularization with fragmentation of the bony epiphysis/apophysis.
- Invasion with granulation tissue.
- Osteoclastic resorption of dead bone.
- Osteoid replacement along necrotic trabeculae.
- Formation of mature lamellar bone.

It is important to remember that the cartilaginous articular surface is not involved.

- In OCD, the process is more localized and frequently leads to articular cartilage damage and subsequent incongruity.
- Segmental necrosis may lead to fracture and collapse of the small portion of involved epiphyseal bone.
- The loss of bony stability increases the stresses on the articular cartilage which may then fissure and then fracture with potentially physical separation of an osteoarticular fragment: the bony fragment is usually no more than a few mm in size.
- Once separated this fragment may continue to grow as the articular cartilage is nourished by the synovial fluid: this fragment now acts a loose body within the joint.
- When the history, clinical examination, and imaging are typical then bone biopsy is *not* required.

Table 5.2 The osteochrondroses

	Eponym	Site
Lower limb	Kohler	Navicular
	Freiberg	2nd metatarsal head (or $3^{rd}/4^{th}$)
	Sever	Calcaneal apophysis
	Osgood–Schlatter	Tibial apophysis
	Sinding–Larsen–Johansson	Inferior pole of the patella
Upper limb	Panner	Capitellum
	Keinboch	Lunate
Spine	Scheuermann	Vertebral end plates
Others	*Blount	Proximal tibial physis
	Legg–Calve–Perthes	Proximal (capital) femoral epiphysis
	**Osteochondritis dissecans	Knee (distal femoral condyle and patella), talus, capitellum

* Most paediatric orthopaedic surgeons consider these two conditions as separate entities—
the natural history is more severe, the outcome often poor, and the management strategies
significantly more aggressive.

** Most paediatric orthopaedic surgeons consider OCD as a separate entity—the natural history
is more severe, the outcome less favourable, and the management strategies may be more
aggressive to prevent later degenerative joint disease.

Clinical features
- Overall, the natural history for the osteochondroses is distinct from OCD, and with the exception of LCP disease and Blount's is well defined and often associated with a predictably good outcome.
- The specific symptoms vary from site to site, apophyseal or physeal location, and with age of onset of the condition.
- Symptoms are often activity related but can be exacerbated by both exercise and immobility.
- Symptoms and signs may include:
  - Local or referred pain.
  - Swelling and symptoms of inflammation such as tenderness and warmth.
  - Joint stiffness, with or without a limp.

Features on plain radiographs
The exact features vary with the anatomical site involved but some plain XR features are common:
- Early signs include a change in size and shape of the bony epiphysis or apophysis, with increased density and/ or irregularity. Often the whole epiphysis/apophysis is involved.
- Later, bone resorption is seen as fragmentation.
- With continued re-ossification the radiographic appearances may return to near-normal.

- In *OCD lesions*, the bony changes may be limited to irregularity of the surface of the bony epiphysis in 'classical' areas such as the lateral aspect of the medial femoral condyle.

Features on MR imaging

- The MRI features vary depending on the stage of the disease process and the site of involvement but bone oedema is common as is relative cartilage 'overgrowth'.
- In OCD lesions, if there is fracture of the articular cartilage overlying the small bony lesion, instability of this fragment can be predicted if synovial fluid is seen tracking down the fracture line. With delay in revascularization, the small bone fragment and the larger associated cartilaginous 'cap' may lift off and/or separate completely.
- If the osteochondral fragment separates completely it may be seen as a loose body within the joint and its site of origin is seen as a 'crater' with no articular cartilage overlying the bone. In time the defect is often filled with fibrocartilage.
- MRI and/or bone scans can be useful in excluding other pathologies (see ➲ Pitfalls, p. 374).

Natural history and treatment recommendations

Most true osteochondroses are benign, self-limiting processes; treatment is usually symptomatic and conservative. Symptoms may take some time to resolve and with apophyseal lesions this may not occur until after physeal fusion at skeletal maturity. Beware of 'over-treatment'. Management includes the following:

- Family/patient education.
- Relative rest from exercise;—encourage sporting 'warm up and cool down'.
- Analgesic and/or anti-inflammatory medication as required.
- In selected cases physiotherapy, support bandaging, bracing (perhaps in Scheuermann's disease) may help.
  - Treatment of Blount's and Legg–Calve–Perthes requires referral to an orthopaedic surgeon.
- The management of OCD lesions can be more complex and orthopaedic referral should be considered particularly if symptoms such as locking, sharp pain, and 'giving way' of the joint with signs of an effusion are present. Surgical options include:
  - Pinning *in situ* for the lesion that is not separated (often with biodegradable pins).
  - Drilling to enhance revascularization (retrograde or antegrade to protect the physis and/or the articular cartilage).
  - Replacement and fixation of the loose fragment.
  - Removal of a loose body.
  - Debridement of craters/ulcers if the fragment has been 'lost'.
  - In the adolescent or skeletally mature patient with knee problems, consideration of techniques such as ACI or MACI (autologous chondrocyte implantation or matrix-induced ACI) to improve the congruity of the articular surface with the aim of reducing the risk of degenerative disease in the long term.

Pitfalls

- Children are not used to 'chronic' pain and parents do not like to see their child limping. For both it can be a depressing/frustrating time.
- If the child has a 'disease' label, then parents expect treatment for it and it is unfortunate that most of the eponyms imply that the osteochondrosis is a disease state rather than an essentially benign condition that disrupts normal growth temporarily.
- Remember that some of the radiological features described such as fragmentation of the calcaneal apophysis (in Sever's disease) and the tibial tubercle (in Osgood–Schlatter's) are frequently seen in normal, asymptomatic children.
- It is important to determine whether or not the radiographic features are a 'red herring': does the clinical history and examination match the imaging results?
- The *differential diagnosis* must always include tumour (benign or malignant, primary or metastatic) and infection particularly if the symptoms of pain and swelling are unilateral.

Take home messages

- OCD, LCP, and Blounts disease are *not* typical osteochondritides: all require orthopaedic review.
- Do not over treat the simple osteochondroses—particularly those affecting apophyses.

Heritable disorders of connective tissue

A number of inherited disorders of connective tissue may present to paediatric rheumatology services with biomechanical pain related to musculoskeletal features.

- The majority of these conditions are recognizable by their clinical features.
- It is important to identify those patients with conditions that may predispose to potentially preventable causes of morbidity and mortality.
- A physiotherapy-led multidisciplinary approach with attention to strengthening areas of weakness and pacing activities is effective for patients with significant musculoskeletal symptoms.
- Emerging new therapeutic drug approaches are being used in Marfan syndrome to limit cardiovascular complications.

Marfan syndrome

Background
- Inherited disorder of fibrillin transmitted as an autosomal dominant trait.
- Incidence 1:5000, pan-ethnic, no sex predilection.
- Marfan syndrome is fully penetrant with variable expression.

Pathophysiology
- Caused by mutations in fibrillin-1 gene (*FBN1*), located on chromosome 15.
- Fibrillin-1 is a glycoprotein which aggregates to form complex extracellular structures called microfibrils which are essential for elastic fibre maintenance in postnatal life.
- Abnormal microfibrils weaken the aortic wall and other structures such as the suspensory ligament of the lens, ligaments, lung airways, and spinal dura.
- Recent studies suggest that abnormalities in *FBN1* lead to dysregulation of transforming growth factor-beta (TGF-β) and that many of the multisystem manifestations including cardiovascular complications relate to excess TGF-β signalling.
- Severe neonatal Marfan syndrome is associated with a cluster of mutations between exons 24–32 of *FBN1*, but there are no other established correlations between genotype and phenotype.

Clinical features
A diagnosis of Marfan syndrome is based on the revised Ghent nosology.
- Systemic features and differential diagnosis are shown in Tables 5.3 and 5.4.
- In the absence of family history, Marfan syndrome is diagnosed when there is:
  - Aortic root dilatation or dissection (z score >2) *and* ectopia lentis.
  - Aortic root dilatation or dissection *and FBN1* mutation.
  - Aortic root dilatation or dissection *and* ≥7 points on systemic features score.
  - Ectopia lentis *and FBN1* mutation known to be associated with aortic root dilatation or dissection.

Table 5.3 Scoring system for systemic features of Marfan syndrome (Revised Ghent nosology).

Feature	Points	Feature	Points
Wrist or thumb sign*	1	Pneumothorax	2
Wrist and thumb sign	3	Dural ectasia	2
Pectus carinatum	2	Protrusio acetabuli	2
Pectus excavatum or chest asymmetry	1	Reduced upper:lower segment ratio and increased armspan:height ratio and no severe scoliosis	1
Hindfoot deformity	2	Scoliosis or thoracolumbar kyphosis	1
Pes planus	1	Reduced elbow extension	1
Facial features 3/5 from: dolichocephaly, enophthalmos, downslanting palpebral fissures, malar hypoplasia, retrognathia	1	Skin striae	1
Myopia >3 dioptres	1	Mitral valve prolapse	1

* The thumb sign is positive if the thumb, when completely opposed within the clenched hand, projects beyond the ulnar border.

Maximum score = 20 points. ≥7 points indicates systemic involvement. The wrist sign is positive if the distal phalanges of the 1st and 5th digits of 1 hand overlap when wrapped around the opposite wrist.

Reproduced with permission from Loeys BL, Dietz HC, Braverman AC, et al. The revised Ghent nosology for the Marfan syndrome. Journal of Medical Genetics, Volume 47, Issue 7, pp. 476-48. Copyright © BMJ Publishing Ltd 2009.

- In the presence of family history Marfan syndrome is diagnosed when there is ectopia lentis or ≥7 points on systemic features score or aortic root dilatation/dissection.
- *Caveat*: when the diagnosis of Marfan syndrome is made without a known mutation in *FBN1*, discriminating features of vascular Ehlers-Danlos syndrome (vEDS), Shprintzen–Goldberg syndrome (SGS), or Loeys–Dietz syndrome (LDS) must not be present (Table 5.4) *and* appropriate diagnostic tests performed if indicated.
- Patients <20yr with borderline aortic root measurements and a family history of Marfan syndrome or a known *FBN1* mutation are defined as having potential Marfan syndrome and require close cardiology follow-up to detect progressive aortic root dilatation.
- Patients with musculoskeletal features typical of Marfan syndrome without further organ involvement are classified as having a Marfanoid habitus.
- Neonatal Marfan syndrome is not a separate entity but represents the most severe end of the Marfan syndrome spectrum.

Table 5.4 Differential diagnosis of Marfan syndrome

Differential diagnosis	Gene	Discriminating features
Loeys–Dietz syndrome (LDS)	TGFBR1/2	Bifid uvula/cleft palate, arterial tortuosity, hypertelorism, diffuse aortic and arterial aneurysms, craniosynostosis, clubfoot, cervical spine instability, thin and velvety skin, easy bruising
Shprintzen–Goldberg syndrome (SGS)	FBN1 and others	Craniosynostosis, mental retardation
Congenital contractural arachnodactyly (CCA)	FBN2	Crumpled ears, contractures
Weill–Marchesani syndrome (WMS)	FBN1 and ADAMTS10	Microspherophakia, brachydactyly, joint stiffness
Ectopia lentis syndrome (ELS)	FBN1, LTBP2 ADAMTSL4	Lack of aortic root dilatation
Homocystinuria	CBS	Thrombosis, mental retardation
Familial thoracic aortic aneurysm syndrome (FTAA)	TGFBR1/2, ACTA2, MYH11	Lack of Marfanoid skeletal features, livedo reticularis, iris flocculi
Arterial tortuosity syndrome (ATS)	SLC2A10	Generalized arterial tortuosity, arterial stenosis, facial dysmorphism

Investigations
- A high rate of new mutations means a clinically useful genetic screening test has not been developed.
- ECG and echocardiogram are indicated in patients with Marfanoid habitus to identify potential cardiac involvement.

Management
- Antihypertensive treatment with β-blockers to delay or prevent aortic root dilatation and dissection is the current standard of medical care.
- Elective aortic graft surgery is recommended for patients with an aortic diameter of ≥5cm or rapidly progressive dilatation.
- Losartan is an angiotensin II receptor blocker which has also been shown to block TGF-β signalling. Recent animal studies and one case series of 18 children with progressive aortic root dilatation unresponsive to standard therapy suggest that Losartan may reduce or halt progression of aortic root dilatation in these patients.

Ehlers–Danlos syndromes (EDS)

- Ehlers–Danlos syndrome (EDS) comprises a heterogeneous group of disorders. Each subtype has a separate and different genetic cause where this is known. Many similar features are seen between subtypes, with skin, joints, blood vessels, and internal organs variably affected.
- The subtypes with known genetic causes are shown in Table 5.5 with information on clinical features.
- Early diagnosis is essential to enable appropriate management particularly in vEDS where all patients should be under the care of a specialist cardiology team.
- Young children with classical EDS benefit from skin protection against injury. The use of customized shin pads is particularly valuable in preventing skin damage and consequent atrophic scarring. These children should be made known to their local plastic surgery team for expert suturing when injury occurs.
- A highly specialized service for patients with atypical and complex EDS is available in Sheffield (eds.sheffield@nhs.net) and London www.lnwh.nhs.uk/services/a-z-services/e/ehlers-danlos-syndrome-national-diagnostic-service/.
- Patients who present with biomechanical pain and are found to have joint hypermobility and soft, mildly extensible skin have previously been classified as EDS type III or 'hypermobile type EDS' (see ➌ chapter on hypermobility, p.126); the label may cause unnecessary anxiety for patients and families and current UK practice is to describe these patients as having joint hypermobility and biomechanical pain. Bowel symptoms and autonomic dysfunction including postural orthostatic tachycardia syndrome (POTs) is frequently described in this group.
- Conditions that may mimic EDS are listed in Box 5.1.

Osteogenesis imperfecta

- Children with mild subtypes of osteogenesis imperfecta (OI) are usually of average stature and have a history of minimal trauma fractures.
- Family members with OI type 1 have been identified who have never sustained a fracture and these patients may present with hypermobility and musculoskeletal symptoms.
- Clinical and laboratory discriminating features are shown in Table 5.6.

Table 5.5 Types of Ehlers-Danlos syndrome

Villefranche classification	Clinical features	Inheritance pattern	Molecular genetic and other testing
Classical	Marked skin hyperextensibility + atrophic widened cutaneous scars + generalized joint hypermobility are typical signs. Additional signs: easy bruising with haemosiderin staining, subcutaneous spheroids, molluscoid pseudotumours. Stretch marks tend to be absent.	Autosomal dominant	COL5A1, COL5A2 Electron microscopy of skin shows numerous large collagen flowers
Hypermobile	Generalized joint hypermobility assessed by the Beighton score (a score of 5 or more). Smooth velvety skin, chronic pain, autonomic dysfunction including bowel symptoms and POTs	Autosomal dominant	Unknown
Vascular	Arterial dissection and rupture, intestinal rupture (mainly colon), thin translucent skin with visible vessels. Easy bruising is often presenting sign in childhood (which may raise child protection concerns), acrogeria, congenital talipes, pneumothorax, small joint hypermobility, uterine rupture in pregnancy.	Autosomal dominant	COL3A1 Electron microscopy of skin shows marked variability in collagen fibre diameter
Kypho-scoliotic	Kyphoscoliosis, eye involvement with glaucoma sometimes leading to globe rupture, skin signs the same as classical EDS, increased risk of vessel rupture.	Autosomal recessive	Lysyl hydroxylase 1 (PLOD1) [Also urine testing for pyridinoline/deoxypyridinoline ratio]
Arthro-chalasic	Congenital bilateral hip dislocation, severe joint hypermobility with recurrent dislocations, skin hyperextensibility, easy bruising	Autosomal dominant	Targeted COL1A1, COL1A2; this condition is extremely rare

Table 5.5 *Contd.*

Villefranche classification	Clinical features	Inheritance pattern	Molecular genetic and other testing
Dermato-sparactic	Redundant sagging fragile skin, delayed closure of fontanelles, blue sclerae, umbilical hernia, short stature.	Autosomal recessive	Procollagen N-proteinase (ADAMTS2) Electron microscopy shows hieroglyphic fibrils; this condition is extremely rare
Subtype identified after Villefranche	**Clinical features**	**Inheritance pattern**	**Molecular genetic and other testing**
Tenascin-X deficient	Marked skin hyperextensibility, pronounced joint hypermobility and severe bruising, scarring is normal.	Autosomal recessive	TNXB
EDS with scoliosis, myopathy, hearing impairment	Similar features to kyphoscoliotic EDS, sensory neural hearing impairment may be a feature. Generalized hypotonia at birth usually improves in infancy.	Autosomal recessive	FKBP14
Musculo-contractural EDS	Progressive kyphoscoliosis, adducted thumbs in infancy, club foot, arachnodactyly, fragile skin	Autosomal recessive	CHST14 Very rare condition

Box 5.1 Conditions mistaken for EDS

Osteogenesis imperfecta
Loeys–Dietz syndrome
Skeletal dysplasias
Mucopolysaccharidoses
Cutis laxa
Pseudoxanthoma elasticum
Ulrich congenital muscular dystrophy
Bethlem myopathy

Table 5.6 Disorders predisposing to bone fragility which can be associated with joint hypermobility (see ➔ Metabolic bone diseases, pp. 358–61)

Type and inheritance	Discriminatory features	Other features	Laboratory
Osteogenesis imperfecta type I AD	Blue sclera Hypermobility, especially of small joints Wormian bones in 70% Generalized osteopenia on DEXA	Kyphoscoliosis Arcus cornea Hearing impairment Metatarsus varus Easy bruising Fractures from minimal trauma Opalescent dentine	Reduction in synthesis of type I procollagen Abnormalities in COL1A1
Osteogenesis imperfecta type IV AD	White sclera Fractures from minimal trauma Short stature Wormian bones in 50–70%	Progressive long bone deformity Joint hypermobility Opalescent dentine	COL1A1 or COL1A2 mutations which reduce collagen stability

Further reading

Loeys BL, Dietz HC, Braverman AC, et al. The Revised Ghent Nosology for the Marfan syndrome. *J Med Genet* 2010; **47**:476–85.

Sobey G, Ehlers–Danlos syndrome: how to diagnose and when to perform genetic tests. *Arch Dis Child* 2014; **100**(1):57–61.

Infection and immunization

Tuberculosis and mycobacterial disease

There are 3 main scenarios which clinicians treating children with rheumatic diseases may be confronted with:
1. Primary musculoskeletal TB
2. Latent TB infection (LTBI) and reactivation of LTBI as a result of drug-induced immune-suppression.
3. Reactive immunological phenomena associated with *Mycobacterium tuberculosis* (MTB) and/or antimycobacterial therapy.

Primary musculoskeletal TB

Epidemiology and pathophysiology
- There are an estimated 1.3 million cases of TB annually in children, resulting in 450,000 deaths.
- Overall notification rates for TB in children have been rising in Europe over the last decade, mostly due to a significant rise in Eastern Europe and some specific areas such as London, whilst notification rates for Western Europe including the UK in general have been declining.
- Musculoskeletal TB is rare in developed countries and epidemiological data is scarce especially in the paediatric population. 2–5% of children with TB have musculoskeletal involvement. In untreated primary MTB infection the average risk of developing bone lesions for all children under the age of 5yr is 1–2% within 2yr.
- TB is caused by MTB, rarely by *M. bovis* (see Fig. 6.1).
- During the formation of the primary complex and for some months after, in many individuals bacilli escape intermittently into the bloodstream and may lodge anywhere in the body, but particularly in the central nervous system (CNS), bones, or the kidneys.
- If circumstances favour the organism rather than the host (i.e. young age or poor nutrition), then the cells of the reticulo-endothelial system do not control the disease and haematogenous spread leads to a localized lesion or multiple lesions (miliary disease).
- Bone or joint disease is usually the result of lymphohaematogenous spread from a primary focus, usually pulmonary. Rarely, direct invasion by extension from adjacent lymph nodes or the lung may cause spinal disease. Lesions can be found within 3 months but usually occur within 1–3yr of the primary infection and hence evidence of concomitant pulmonary involvement is not always found.
- Infection develops in the metaphyses; bone may be destroyed eroding through into the adjacent joint space and epiphyseal growth plates are at risk of damage.
- In spinal TB, 3 different patterns of vertebral body infection have been described—anterior, paradiscal, and central. Subsequent spread involves intervertebral discs and narrowing of the disc space.
- Abscesses frequently develop in advanced disease, following tissue planes from vertebrae into the retropharyngeal space, lung, psoas sheath, perineum, or gluteal region, or may extend posteriorly into the spinal canal.
- Healing is by formation of fibrous tissue and calcification may be seen.

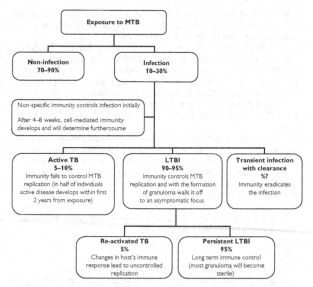

Fig. 6.1 Pathogenesis of TB following exposure to MTB in immune-competent individuals.

Clinical presentation
- Often indolent and non-specific leading to significant diagnostic delay.
- Manifestations of musculoskeletal TB include spondylitis, extra-axial osteomyelitis, septic arthritis and other rarer manifestations.
- *TB spondylitis* ('Pott's disease') accounts for 50% of TB involvement of the musculoskeletal system in adults although data is unclear in children. Thoracic and lumbar lesions are most common. Pain is the presenting symptom producing alteration of gait or posture secondary to muscle spasm. Young children unable to localize the pain may cry when moved or picked up, or refuse to sit or walk. Vertebral collapse may results in kyphosis. Paraplegia is usually due to spinal cord compression either by oedema, abscess, granulation tissue or sequestra.
- *Extra-axial osteomyelitis* is responsible for 20% of musculoskeletal TB and is most commonly a single focus process in the immune-competent host. However, an immunosuppressed state and young age predispose to multifocal TB. The infection in children commonly involves the metaphysis of femur and tibia, skull, and small bones of hands and feet (i.e. dactylitis). Osteomyelitis can be associated with septic arthritis and overlying soft tissue abscess or can occur without joint involvement (more often in the long bones or in dactylitis). Soft tissue swelling is

seen, followed by a non-tender mass attached to bone. Dactylitis usually presents as painless or mildly painful swelling mostly involving the proximal phalanges or the metacarpal bones.

- *Septic arthritis*, although rare, is particularly relevant due to its frequent mono-articular nature (90% of cases), common involvement of large weight-bearing joints, and insidious manifestations rendering it difficult to differentiate from oligo-articular JIA. Onset is gradual with joints initially becoming swollen, then developing limitation of movement, stiffness, and alteration of gait. Involvement of the small joints of hands and fingers are also often described in children and immune-suppressed patients.
- Because of the rarity of musculoskeletal TB in Western countries, there are no current recommendations to rule out TB in children presenting with mono-arthritis. However, unusual features such as proliferative synovitis with subtle signs of inflammation, peri-articular abscesses and draining sinuses, and/or lack of response to intra-articular steroids should prompt investigations to rule out TB.
- *Other musculoskeletal manifestations* including tenosynovitis, bursitis, and muscle abscesses are rarer and often a result of continuous spreading from adjacent bony and articular lesions.

Diagnosis
See Fig. 6.2.
- The triad of a history of TB contact, positive Mantoux test or interferon-γ release assays (IGRA), and suggestive CXR changes is highly suggestive for a diagnosis of TB.
- Plain skeletal x-ray survey is often abnormal and therefore essential and cost-effective. Typical x-ray features include:
  - Lytic lesions with poorly defined edge.
  - Absent or minimal reactive sclerosis.
  - Juxta-articular osteopenia, narrowing of joint space, and adjacent soft tissue involvement.
  - In dactylitis there is usually enlargement of the bone with periosteal thickening and destruction of the spongiosa giving a cystic appearance ('spina ventosa').
  - In spinal involvement, disc space narrowing, anterior vertebral scalloping, or variable degrees of destruction with kyphosis can be seen.
- Definitive diagnosis relies on culture of the organism. Open biopsy or fine needle aspiration of bone, synovial fluid aspiration and/or synovial biopsy obtain specimens. Microscopy for acid fast bacilli and culture for MTB must be specifically requested as these tests are not routinely performed on microbiology culture samples. The differential diagnosis is broad and includes bacterial and fungal infection, syphilis, bone tumours including sarcomas and sarcoidosis.

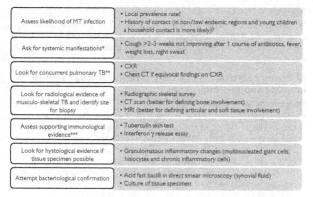

Fig. 6.2 Diagnosis of musculoskeletal TB.*Systemic manifestations will be absent unless disseminated TB or concurrent pulmonary involvement.** The coexistence of pulmonary TB is reported in 30–50% of cases. If a pulmonary lesion is identified, attempt specimen collection (sputum in older children, gastric aspiration and/or nasopharyngeal aspirate in young children) and detection of acid fast bacilli in direct smear microscopy and culture; these yield a positive result in only 20–50% of cases.*** Both TSTs and IGRAs lack sensitivity to reliably distinguish between TB and LTBI in a patient with TB-like illness. Either test is therefore an adjunct to other tests for diagnosing TB disease. A recent UK study failed to show that IGRA are more sensitive than TST>15 mm in diagnosing active TB but confirmed that combining both tests identified more than 90% of culture-confirmed cases.

Treatment

- Due to the difficulty in obtaining bacteriological confirmation of TB in children, treatment should be started if the clinical picture and histology are consistent without waiting for the results of cultures, and should be completed even if the culture results are negative unless an alternative aetiology is identified.
- The standard regimen recommended by NICE (2011 guidelines) to treat active musculoskeletal TB in all ages is 6 months of isoniazid and rifampicin initially plus pyrazinamide and ethambutol for the first 2 months.
- Surgery in spinal TB is indicated only if needed to establish a diagnosis or in those with active disease and neurological deficit requiring decompression. Drainage may be useful in joint involvement to relieve pressure. Radical resection/bone grafting may be considered if there is destruction of ≥2 vertebral bodies.
- Bed rest and immobilization are no longer recommended.

Prognosis

In contrast to bacterial infections, MTB does not produce proteolytic enzymes that destroy cartilage. Therefore, a good response to treatment and return to normal function is to be expected if the diagnosis is made early.

LTBI and reactivation of LTB as a result of drug-induced immune-suppression

Epidemiology and pathophysiology

• Following exposure to MTB, in over 80% of people, the immune system kills and removes the bacteria from the body, whilst most of the remaining individuals (with the exception of the small minority—around 5%—in whom active TB develops following initial contact) will develop LTBI, hosting live MTB in the absence of clinical manifestations (Fig. 6.1). In LTBI, MTB enters a state of non-replicating persistence or low replication contained by a highly organized infiltrate called a granuloma constituted by mycobacteria-containing macrophages surrounded by activated lymphocytes.

• Tumour necrosis factor (TNF) plays multiple roles in the host's ability to respond to and control infection with MTB, including responsibility for granuloma formation and maintenance.

• MTB is kept at bay long term in most immunocompetent individuals. However MTB remains viable and a change of the host's immune response, such as immune-suppression with TNF antagonists may lead to granuloma disintegration and uncontrolled replication of MTB producing TB disease.

• A consensus statement on the risk of TB in relationship to TNF antagonists by the Tuberculosis Network European Trials Group (http://www.ncbi.nlm.nih.gov/pubmed/20530046) can be summarized as follows:

  • The risk of TB in adults with RA treated with TNF antagonists (including the newest golimumab and certolizumab pegol) is increased up to 25 times (although the disease itself and the use of non-biological immunosuppressants are likely to contribute to the risk).

  • The risk of TB may be increased in children exposed to TNF antagonists although follow-up studies report very few cases. This may be because children treated with biologics have so far been mainly in countries with a very low risk of TB.

  • TNF antagonists efficacious against granulomatous conditions (Crohn's disease and sarcoidosis), such as infliximab and adalimumab, are more likely to cause TB reactivation than etanercept.

  • TB cases have also been reported in adults in association with the use of tocilizumab but no TB risk is reported for anakinra, rituximab or abatacept.

Clinical features and diagnosis
- As screening for LTBI is currently recommended for all candidates prior to starting anti-TNF therapies, paediatric rheumatologists have to manage children with positive immunodiagnostic tests for TB in absence of clinical symptoms.
- Due to the risk of reactivation of LTBI, it is also important to be aware of presentations of TB in the immune-suppressed host. Although most reported TB cases in RA patients treated with anti-TNF are pulmonary, there is an increased frequency of multifocal articular and bone lesions.

Diagnosis
- Immunodiagnostic tests for TB, either tuberculin skin tests (TSTs) such as Mantoux and/or the T-cell based interferon-γ release assays (IGRAs), measure adaptive immune response to MTB infection and neither of them distinguish active TB disease from LTBI. However, in the absence of a gold standard for the detection of LTB, these immunodiagnostic tests are used as proxy marker for LTBI.
- A positive TST (i.e. Mantoux) indicates a cellular immune response to MTB antigens.
  - TST induration >5mm indicates infection in individuals without BCG vaccination and ≥15mm with BCG (in the UK).
- IGRAs measure interferon γ released by T cells (QuantiFERON-TB Gold) or the T cells releasing interferon γ (T-SPOT TB) in response to MTB-specific antigens. Both include a positive control and a negative control to help differentiate a true negative response from anergy (i.e. in immune-suppressed patients).
- IGRAs compared to TSTs are more specific (i.e. do not cross-react with BCG strains and environmental mycobacteria), and are likely to be more accurate in diagnosing LTBI in immunosuppressed patients than TSTs.
- There are current no published guidelines on how to best screen children prior starting anti-TNF alpha. Most paediatric rheumatology local guidelines are modelled on adult recommendations which suggest a chest radiograph with either a tuberculin skin test or an IGRA.
- Simultaneous use of TST and IGRAs in children may provide additional, more accurate information; however, as there are insufficient data to recommend one test over the other, local policies vary. Treatment should be offered if either test is positive.
- A history of significant past exposure or untreated tuberculosis should be an indication for preventive chemotherapy even when tests for latent infection are negative.
- As the TB risk persists despite negative initial screening, a high index of suspicion for TB should be maintained during the entire treatment and regular monitoring to detect new TB infection in anti-TNF-treated patients should also be considered.

Treatment

- Preventive chemotherapy should be offered to all individuals receiving TNFα antagonists in the presence of evidence of LTBI.
- Recommended prophylactic treatments for LTBI (all ages) in the UK include 3 months of rifampicin and isoniazid or 6 months of isoniazid.
- Ideally LTB treatment should be completed before TNFα antagonist treatment is initiated; however, some experts suggest it can be safely initiated after at least 4 weeks of treatment for LTBI has been completed.
- Reactivated TB disease in association with immunosuppression is treated in the same way as primary TB (depending on the clinical presentation).
- Whilst active TB needs to be adequately treated before starting anti-TNF, patients on anti-TNF who develop symptoms of TB infection may continue with their anti-TNF (whilst receiving full anti-mycobacterial treatment) if clinically indicated.

Reactive immunological conditions (in association with MTB infections and anti-mycobacterial therapy)

- Erythema nodosum is a well-recognized hypersensitivity reaction to MTB.
- Poncet's disease, a rare aseptic reactive polyarthritis, is usually seen in the context of active pulmonary TB. Other hypersensitivity reactions to MTB include ocular manifestations such as conjunctivitis and phlyctenular keratoconjunctivitis (redness, tearing, and foreign body sensation) and interstitial keratitis.
- Drug-induced lupus has been described in association with isoniazid and rifampicin therapy. Reactive phenomena tend to resolve with discontinuation of the offending drug.

Further reading

Sandgren A, *et al.* Childhood tuberculosis in the European Union/European Economic Area, 2000 to 2009. *Euro Surveil.* 2011 Mar 24; 16(12).

Marais BJ. Tuberculosis in children. J Paediatr Child Health 2014 Oct, 50(10): 759–67.

Tebruegge M, et al. Diagnostic tests for childhood tuberculosis –past imperfect, present tense and future perfect? *Pediatr Infect Dis J.* 2015 Jun, 22.

Solovic, I., et al. The risk of tuberculosis related to TNF antagonist therapies: a TBNET consensus statement. *Eur Respir J.* 2010 Nov; 36(5): 1185-206

Shim TS. Diagnosis and treatment of latent tuberculosis infection due to initiation of anti-TNF therapy. *Tuberc Respir Dis* 2014 Jun; 76 (6): 261–8.

NICE, *Tuberculosis: clinical diagnosis and management of tuberculosis and measures for its prevention and control.* ℘ https://www.nice.org.uk/guidance/cg117 and updated ℘ http://www.nice.org.uk/guidance/ng33 (January 2016)

Tuberculosis and musculoskeletal manifestations—clinical aspects

TB and anti-tuberculous drugs may involve the musculoskeletal (MSK) system in a variety of ways:
- Primary TB of bones/joints:
  - Peripheral: arthritis, osteomyelitis, including dactylitis.
  - Central: osteomyelitis of vertebrae, sacroiliitis.
- Immunological phenomena:
  - Skin: erythema nodosum.
  - Eyes: uveitis.
  - Joints: Poncet's disease.
- Immunosuppressive drug induced TB reactivation:
  - Screening for TB pre-biologics.
- Anti TB drug-induced arthropathy:
  - Pyrazinamide.
  - Quinolones.
  - Ethambutol.

Tuberculosis of joints

Arthritis
- Usual pattern of joint involvement—monoarticular.
- Large weight-bearing joints—most commonly knees and hips. Rare case reports for other joints—talonavicular, tibiotalar, interphalangeal, intermetatarsal joint.
- Pain, swelling, reduced range of motion, limp over days to weeks are common presenting features.
- Long-standing cases results in atrophy of proximal muscles, limb length discrepancy.
- Presentations can mimic oligoarticular JIA.
- Multifocal osteoarticular TB—rare, suspect multi drug resistance.
- Clinical clues to diagnosis—single joint involvement in a high risk background setting (endemic area, travel to endemic area, contact with TB case).
- Additional clues—systemic features of TB: fever, night sweats, weight loss. However, absence of these features does not exclude TB.
- Most valuable clue to diagnosing TB arthritis is a high index of suspicion.
- Differential diagnoses to consider—JIA (oligoarticular subtype), pyogenic arthritis, reactive arthritis, Perthe's disease, slipped capital femoral epiphysis.

Dactylitis
- Also called spina ventosa, in view of the specific deformity of the digits.
- Most common age group—less than 10 years.
- TB involvement of phalanges, metacarpals, and metatarsals
- Painless / mildly painful insidious swelling of digits.
- Hand more commonly involved than foot.
- Usually single bone affected.

- If present then suspect an immune compromised state with multifocal involvement.
  - Primary immune deficiency reported with TB dactilitis—severe combined immunodeficiency.
  - Secondary immune deficient states–HIV infection.
  - Low vitamin D levels—implicated in creating immune deficient state predisposing to TB Dactilitis.
- Differential diagnoses—pyogenic infections, psoriatic arthritis.

Osteomyelitis
- Non-specific clinical presentation with pain, localized swelling, disability of involved limb, often brought to attention by minor trauma.
- Lower limbs more commonly affected, with frequently involved sites being distal femur, proximal tibia, proximal femur, various bones of the foot.
- May involve proximal and distal radius, infrequently ribs and mandible.
- Rarely multiple bones may be involved simultaneously.
- Underlying constitutional features of tuberculosis-like fever, weight loss, if present may point to the diagnosis.
- MRI and CT scan can identify and localize lesions; however, biopsy is mandatory for definitive diagnosis.
- Extended treatment with antituberculosis drugs for 12–18 months with judicious surgical intervention usually leads to complete resolution.

TB spine
- Osteomyelitis of vertebrae:
  - Myriad clinical presentations—painful mass, spinal deformity (kyphosis), cold abscess, paraspinal muscle spasm, spinal instability, and most ominous are varying degrees of neurological deficits.
  - Likely to occur in conjunction with other sites of tuberculous involvement.
  - Constitutional features more likely than in other forms of TB of MSK system—night cries, restless sleep, low to moderate grade fever, weight loss.
  - Always look for contiguous areas of involvement—upper lobe of lung, cervical lymph nodes in cervical TB, mediastinal lymph nodes in thoracic/thoracolumbar TB.
  - Site of spinal involvement—lumbar (56%), thoracic (49%), thoracolumbar (13%).
  - Cervical spine involvement is uncommon but reported–atlantoaxial dislocation is the dreaded complication.
  - High suspicion and early diagnosis followed by appropriate treatment minimizes long-term morbidity and potential mortality.

Sacroiliitis
- Uncommon site and often missed.
- Can be associated with tuberculous spondylitis.
- Clinical presentation—subacute, rarely acute onset of low back pain, stiffness, radicular pain, buttock pain. Usually unilateral.
- Sacroiliac tenderness and positive sacroiliac pain provocation tests on examination.

- Differential diagnoses—pyogenic infections, sacroiliac joint dysfunction, and juvenile spondyloarthropathy.

Immunological phenomena

Erythema nodosum
- Delayed (Type 4) hypersensitivity reaction to various infectious and non-infectious antigens, including mycobacterial protein.
- May indicate underlying inapparent systemic tuberculosis.
- Acute, nodular, erythematous, poorly defined eruptions, 2–6 cm in diameter, usually confined to extensor aspects of legs, but may occasionally occur on thighs and arms.
- Low grade fever, arthralgias, joint swelling (commonly ankle joint), can be accompanying features.
- The arthritis is non-destructive with sterile, acellular synovial fluid.
- May be associated with other immunological tuberculous phenomena (e.g phlyctenular conjunctivitis).
- Self-limiting condition, does not require specific treatment; however, mandates use of anti-tuberculosis therapy for clearing the underlying infection.

Uveitis
- Ocular tuberculosis—a re-emerging health issue.
- Tuberculous uveitis—mimics other causes of uveitis.
- Patterns of involvement:
  - Acute anterior uveitis.
  - Intermediate uveitis.
  - Posterior uveitis.
  - Pars planitis.
- Ophthalmologic findings (bilateral granulomatous anterior uveitis, choroiditis, and certain types of retinal vasculitis are suspicious for tuberculous origin; however, are not diagnostic).
- Excellent response to anti tuberculosis therapy—and useful to confirm diagnosis.

Poncet's disease
- Also known as tuberculous rheumatism.
- Predominantly a clinical diagnosis.
- Aseptic, reactive polyarthritis, in the presence of active tuberculous focus elsewhere in the body.
- More common feature of extra pulmonary tuberculosis.
- Erythema nodosum considered as a hallmark association; however, the incidence is low (6% in a case series).
- Acute to subacute onset of symmetrical joint involvement, most commonly affecting knees and ankles, followed by wrists and small joints of hands and feet.
- Axial involvement—extremely rare, but known.
- Dramatic and usually complete response to anti tuberculous treatment, with a benign non-chronic, non-destructive outcome.

TB reactivation with antirheumatological drugs and pre-biologic screening

- Use of certain anti rheumatic drugs may be associated with reactivation of latent tuberculosis; more so in endemic high risk populations.
- Methotrexate—most widely used first line DMARD and an unlikely culprit for reactivation of tuberculosis.
- Use of concomitant steroids with methotrexate can increase the risk.
- Biologic medications, specifically anti TNF alpha agents (etanercept, infliximab, adalimumab, golimumab, certolizumab)—more likely to cause TB reactivation.
- Pre-biologic screening for latent TB with tuberculin skin test, CXR (alternatively QuantiFERON-TB Gold testing in BCG-vaccinated patients) is recommended prior to starting TNF alpha inhibitors (see ➌ Tuberculosis and mycobacterial disease, pp. 384–90).
- In the event of positive testing, treatment with single anti tuberculosis drug to be initiated, and TNF inhibitor therapy can be started after 1 month

Pyrazinamide, quinolone and ethambutol-induced arthropathy

- Crystal arthropathy induced by anti-tuberculosis drugs—poorly recognized adverse effect.
- Interference with the renal uric acid clearance is the pathogenetic factor.
- Full spectrum of manifestations ranging from arthralgias to true gout may occur.
- Incidence is directly related to duration of treatment and serum uric acid levels.
- Onset usually within 6–8 weeks of treatment initiation.
- Non-deforming, non-erosive arthralgias affecting knees, shoulders and ankles most common.
- Synovial fluid aspiration and analysis can help to determine the presence of crystals.
- Symptoms usually respond within a matter of days to aspirin/NSAIDs:
  • Oral NSAIDs may be prescribed as a 7–10 day course.
  • In case of persistent inflammation, intra-articular joint injection with corticosteroids may be warranted.
- Discontinuation of inciting drug is usually not required.
- Quinolone-induced arthropathy—frequently reported adverse effect.
  • Spectrum ranging from arthralgia not requiring any specific treatment, to tendinitis and tendon rupture, most commonly of Achilles' tendon.
  • Clinical or radiological evidence of objective arthritis secondary to quinolones has been infrequently reported.

Rheumatic fever

Introduction

- Acute rheumatic fever (ARF) is an autoimmune consequence secondary° to infection with Group A *Streptococcus* (GAS), causing a sub-acute generalized inflammatory response and an illness that mainly affects the heart, joints, brain, and skin.
- ARF results from a complex interplay between susceptible hosts, virulence of GAS strain, and environmental features (Fig. 6.3).
- The prognosis of rheumatic fever is solely determined by the cardiac sequelae. Cardiac involvement leads to rheumatic heart disease. People who have had ARF previously are at higher risk of subsequent episodes which may cause further cardiac valve damage.
- Arthritis occurs early and more frequently in large joints. Lower extremities are generally affected initially followed by upper extremities. It is often but not always transient and self-limiting.

Epidemiology

- The mean annual incidence is 19/100,000; a higher incidence of >10/100,000 was reported in Eastern Europe, the Middle East, and Asia. The incidence peaks in childhood. In the indigenous population in Australia annual incidence in 5–14 year olds is reported as 194/100,000, although criteria used for diagnosis in this population are slightly broader than the Modified Jones Criteria (see Box 6.1). A far lower incidence is found in Western Europe and North America; the difference is probably due to improved hygiene standards. In Western Europe and North America, periodic outbreaks occur rather than the endemic form.
- RHD is the most common form of acquired paediatric heart disease in the world and thus is the leading cause of cardiac death in the first 5 decades of life. Notably, Kawasaki disease is now the commonest cause of acquired paediatric heart disease in developed countries including the UK and North America (see ➋ Chapter 4, Kawasaki disease, pp. 190–5).

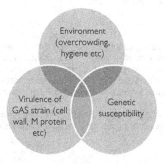

Fig. 6.3. ARF pathogenesis.

Box 6.1 Summary of the Modified Jones criteria
The Modified Jones criteria are broken into major and minor criteria.

The major criteria include:
- Carditis: clinical and subclinical
- Arthritis (must be a polyarthritis for low risk populations; monoarthritis also counts if high-risk population)
- Arthralgia (high risk populations only)
- Chorea
- Erythema marginatum
- Subcutaneous nodules

The minor criteria include:
- Polyarthralgia for low risk populations; and monoarthralgia or polyarthralgia for high risk populations
- A fever greater than 38.5°C for low risk populations or greater than 38.0°C for high risk populations
- ESR ≥60 mm and/or CRP ≥30 mg/L (low risk populations); and ESR ≥30 mm and/or CRP ≥30 mg/L (high risk populations)
- Prolonged PR interval, unless carditis is already scored as a major criterion

Source: data from Gewitz MH et al. Revision of the Jones Criteria for the Diagnosis of Acute Rheumatic Fever in the Era of Doppler Echocardiography: A Scientific Statement from the American Heart Association. *Circulation*, Volume 131, Issue 20, pp. 1806–181, Copyright © 2015 American Heart Association, Inc.

- Worldwide, an estimated 5–30 million children and young adults have chronic RHD and 90,000 patients die from this disease each year.

Revised Jones Criteria
- The previously accepted Modified Jones Criteria have been revised by the American Heart Association in 2015. These are referred to as the Revised Jones Criteria. They now take into account population risk of ARF and echocardiography findings.
- Population risk is defined as low if:
  - ARF incidence is < 2/100,000 in school-age children.
  - RHD prevalence is <1/1000 across all age groups.
- Evidence of preceding streptococcal infection (increased or rising anti-streptolysin O titre or other streptococcal antibodies (anti-DNASE B); positive throat swab for Group A ß-haemolytic *Streptococcus*; positive rapid Group A streptococcal carbohydrate antigen test in a child whose clinical presentation suggests a high probability of group A streptococcal pharyngitis).
- Initial diagnosis of ARF requires 2 major criteria or 1 major and 2 minor; recurrent ARF requires 2 major or 1 major and 2 minor or 3 minor.

- Subclinical carditis is identified on echocardiography. Echocardiography is now recommended in all patients with suspected ARF. The recent AHA review gives details of what echocardiography findings should be considered as subclinical carditis (Boxes 6.2, 6.3, and 6.4).

Management

Antibiotic treatment of GAS infection

Penicillin is the antibiotic of choice. GAS resistance to penicillin has not been reported.

- Oral penicillin (for doses check BNFC) should be commenced in all cases while diagnosis is being established.
- Oral narrow spectrum cephalosporin, e.g. cephalexin or erythromycin (for doses check BNFC) in cases with reliably documented penicillin allergy. Be aware that macrolide resistant rates in GAS are high in some areas and local microbiology advice may be required.
- A full 10 day course of antibiotics is required to reliably eradicate GAS.
- IM benzathine penicillin G for patients in whom compliance is doubtful, given as a single IM injection.

Box 6.2 Doppler findings in rheumatic valvulitis

Pathological mitral regurgitation (all 4 criteria met):
- Seen in at least 2 views.
- Jet length ≥ 2cm in at least 1 view.
- Peak velocity > 3 m/s.
- Pansystolic jet in at least 1 envelope.

Pathological aortic regurgitation (all 4 criteria met):
- Seen in at least 2 views.
- Jet length ≥ 1cm in at least 1 view.
- Peak velocity > 3 m/s.
- Pansystolic jet in at least 1 envelope.

Arthritis/arthralgia
- Controlled trials show response to salicyclates or NSAIDS, often within hours but almost always within 3 days.

Carditis/heart failure
- Diuretics/fluid management for mild-moderate heart failure.
- ACE inhibitors for more severe failure, particularly if aortic regurgitation present.
- There are few trials looking at the benefit of anti-inflammatory agents (aspirin, glucocorticoids, IVIG) for carditis associated with ARF. Most date from the 1950s–1960s. There is no proven benefit but evidence is lacking. Both aspirin and glucocorticoids are recommended by the WHO for the treatment of acute carditis.
- Digoxin in atrial fibrillation present.

Box 6.3 Morphological findings on echocardiogram in rheumatic valvulitis

Acute mitral valve changes:
- Annular dilation.
- Chordal elongation.
- Chordal rupture resulting in flail leaflet with severe mitral regurgitation.
- Anterior (or less commonly posterior) leaflet tip prolapse.
- Beading/nodularity of leaflet tips.

Chronic mitral valve changes, not seen in acute carditis:
- Leaflet thickening.
- Chordal thickening and fusion.
- Restricted leaflet motion.
- Calcification.

Aortic valve changes in acute or chronic carditis:
- Irregular or focal leaflet thickening.
- Coaptation defect.
- Restricted leaflet motion.
- Leaflet prolapse.

Box 6.4 Investigations for suspected ARF
- White blood cell count.
- ESR (repeat weekly once diagnosis is confirmed).
- CRP.
- Blood culture if febrile.
- ECG.
- CXR.
- Echocardiogram (repeat as necessary every 2–4 weeks if equivocal or if serious carditis).
- Throat swab (preferably before starting antibiotics)—culture for Group A *Streptococcus*.
- Anti-streptococcal serology: both anti streptolysin O and anti-DNase B titres, if available (repeat 10-14 days later if 1st test not confirmed).

- There is little experience with ß-blockers in heart failure due to acute carditis and their use is not recommended.
- Bed rest.

Chorea
- Sydenham's chorea is self-limiting but can run a protracted course resulting in disability and social isolation.
- Anti-inflammatory agents are not effective.
- Carbamazepine can be used initially for severe chorea, and valproic acid may be considered for refractory cases.

- Medication should be continued for 2–4 weeks after chorea has subsided, and then withdrawn.
- Remember that anti-phospholipid syndrome (APS) can cause cardiac valve pathology (including mitral valve) and chorea, and thus may mimic rheumatic fever (see ➔ APS pp. 293–6).

Valve surgery
- Usually deferred until inflammation has subsided.
- Rarely, valve leaflet or chordae tendinae rupture leads to severe regurgitation which require emergency surgery.
- Valve replacement, rather than repair, is usually performed during the acute episode, because of the technical difficulties of repairing friable inflamed tissue.

Prevention
- Primary prophylaxis: prevention of cases of ARF by antibiotic treatment of GAS throat infections.
- Secondary prophylaxis: to prevent recurrent episodes of ARF in patients with a credible history of ARF or RHD, secondary prophylaxis is recommended.
  - Register based co-ordinated control programmes with regular (3 or 4 weekly) IM benzathine penicillin G (1.2 MU or 600,000 U if <20kg) in association with education is effective.
  - Alternatives include long term oral phenoxymethylpenicillin (1m–6y 125mg BD, 6–18y 250mg BD) or erythromycin (1m–2y 125mg bd; 2–18y 250mg bd).
- A vaccine for GAS is in development.

Differentiation from post-streptococcal reactive arthritis (PSRA)
- PSRA is a term coined in the 1980s to differentiate a group of patients from ARF with no/less incidence of carditis where revised Jones Criteria not usually met. The incidence of ARF in the USA and Western Europe is ↓, and PSRA is more prevalent.
- PSRA patients are generally older, have a shorter interval between Group A *Streptococcus* infection and symptom onset and respond less dramatically to salicylates than ARF patients.
- The course of PSRA is characterized by arthritis that, in contrast to ARF, is additive, non-migratory, and is frequently chronic.
- Extra-articular manifestations including renal involvement can be present with PSRA.

Further reading

Gewitz, MH, Baltimore, RS, Tani LY, et al. Revision of the Jones Criteria for the diagnosis of acute rheumatic fever in the era of doppler echocardiography a scientific statement from the American Heart Association. *Circulation.* 2015;**131**:1806–18.

Barash J, Mashiach E, Navon-Elkan P, et al. Differentiation of post-streptococcal reactive arthritis from acute rheumatic fever. *J Pediatr* 2008;**153**:696–9.

WHO Technical Report Series 923; RHEUMATIC FEVER AND RHEUMATIC HEART DISEASE. Report of a WHO Expert Consultation ℘ http://www.who.int/cardiovascular_diseases/publications/trs923/en/

Lyme disease

Lyme disease is caused by infection from the spirochaete *Borrelia burgdorferi*, transmitted by the bite of the *Ixodes* tick, and can affect the skin, joints, nervous system, and heart.

For the rheumatologist the task is to distinguish the arthritis caused by Lyme disease (most commonly a monoarthritis affecting the knee) from that due to other diseases such as JIA, septic arthritis, or TB (Table 6.1). If this distinction is correctly made, and appropriate treatment delivered, Lyme disease in children usually has an excellent prognosis. However, the rheumatologist also needs to be aware of the ongoing controversy surrounding the phenomenon of 'chronic Lyme disease' and the evidence base behind it.

Aetiology and epidemiology

- *Borrelia burgdorferi* is transmitted by a bite from a tick of the *Ixodes* genus, after the tick has been attached for more than 24h. The patient is often unaware of having been bitten.
- The tick is mainly found in temperate regions of Europe, NE USA, and Asia, most commonly in or near densely forested areas. The incidence of Lyme disease is approximately 69 per 100,000 but may be as high as 1:100 in hyperendemic areas.

Clinical presentation

Early localized—erythema chronicum migrans
- First presentation in 89% of children.
- Days to weeks after tick bite.
- Expanding over days to weeks, 8–50cm in diameter.
- May be associated with flu-like symptoms.

Early disseminated
- Weeks after infection.
- Neurological: facial nerve palsy, lymphocytic meningitis, rarely meningoencephalitis.
- Cardiac: conduction defects.
- Articular: arthralgia.

Late disease
- Predominantly articular; chronic cutaneous and neurological features can occur but are uncommon, especially in children, who are more likely to have arthritis as the sole presenting problem.
- Occurs weeks to months after initial infection.
- Arthritis—most commonly single knee with intermittent, relatively painless large effusions lasting days/weeks, remitting and recurring course.
- Small joints not affected.

Diagnosis

Need clinical features *plus* history of exposure *plus* positive serology.

Serology
- Enzyme immunoassay for IgG is sensitive but not specific—if positive, do Western blot (immunoblot is highly specific as well as sensitive). Arthritis is a late stage finding, so by the time this occurs IgG levels are high on Western blot, and serology is therefore reliable.
- If Western-blot negative, then a positive/indeterminate enzyme immunoassay is a false positive.

Joint fluid assessment
- Helpful in excluding septic arthritis.
- PCR for *B. burgdorferi* DNA is very useful in previously untreated patients, with higher positivity on synovial tissue than from fluid. Culture of *B. burgdorferi* rarely successful from joint fluid/synovial biopsy.

Treatment
- If persistent symptoms after 3 months try a second 4-week course of oral or IV antibiotics.
- Thereafter, if persistent symptoms try NSAIDs, IA steroid injections, or DMARD.

Prognosis
- Children treated according to the IDSA guidelines summarized in Box 6.2 have an excellent prognosis, and do not go on to develop chronic arthritis, joint deformities, or recurrence of infection.
- Some patient groups and practitioners advocate that Lyme disease can manifest as a chronic illness, able to evade conventional medical tests and treatments.

Table 6.1 Clinical features of Lyme arthritis compared with septic arthritis and JIA

Lyme arthritis	Septic arthritis	JIA
History of tick bite/travel to forested area exposure to ticks		May be associated with rash, uveitis, autoantibodies
Monoarthritis, large joints Small joints not affected	Monoarthritis, any joint	Any joints may be affected, any number
Intermittent/recurrent symptoms	Persistent symptoms	Persistent symptoms >6 weeks
WBC, ESR, CRP may be normal or raised. Not febrile in late disease	WBC, ESR, CRP raised. May be febrile	WBC, ESR, CRP may be normal or raised. May be febrile
May be relatively painless, not usually stiff	Extremely painful, often unable to weight-bear	May be relatively painless, commonly stiff
High synovial fluid WBC	Very high synovial fluid white blood cell count. Organisms cultured	Moderately raised synovial fluid WBC

NB Always consider TB in cases of monoarthritis (see ➋ TB, pp. 384–90).

Table 6.2 Suggested antimicrobial treatment regimens

Clinical condition	Antimicrobial	Regimen	Duration (d)	Children < 12y	Pregnancy or breastfeeding	Notes
a) Erythema migrans	1st line: doxycycline	100mg bd po	14–21	1st line: amoxicillin	1st line: amoxicillin	Azithromycin requires careful monitoring for treatment failure
b) Early localized Lyme	or amoxicillin	500mg tds po	14–21	2nd line: cefuroxime	2nd line: cefuroxime	
				3rd line: azithromycin	3rd line: azithromycin	
d) Borrelial lymphocytoma	3rd line: azithromycin	500mg od po	10			
e) Asymptomatic Lyme carditis						
Lyme carditis with:						
1st–3rd degree heart block	Cefriaxone	2g od iv	14–21	Cefriaxone	Cefriaxone	IDSA advises cefriaxone to be switched to oral doxycycline or amoxicillin when pacing or iv access no longer required
Neuroborreliosis:						
a) Isolated facial nerve palsy	Doxycycline or Amoxicillin	100mg bd po 500mg tds po	14–21 14–21	Amoxicillin	Amoxicillin	EFNS advises 14d adequate in acute neuroborreliosis

b) Meningitis without encephalitis, myelitis or vasculitis	Doxycycline	100mg bd po	14–21	Ceftriaxone	Ceftriaxone	
c) Meningitis with encephalitis, myelitis or vasculitis	Ceftriaxone	2g od iv	14	Ceftriaxone	Ceftriaxone	
d) Late neuroborreliosis	Ceftriaxone	2g od iv	14–28	Ceftriaxone	Ceftriaxone	
Lyme arthritis	1st line: doxycycline 2nd line: amoxicillin	100mg bd po 500mg tds po	21–28 21–28	Amoxicillin	Amoxicillin	
Refractory Lyme arthritis	Doxycycline or Ceftriaxone	100mg od po 2g od iv	30–60 14–21	Ceftriaxone	Ceftriaxone	Antimicrobial-refractory arthritis should be managed by a rheumatologist
Acrodermatitis chronica atrophicans (ACA)	Doxycycline	100mg bd po	21–28	-		ACA occurs predominantly in older adults.

Source: data from Mygland A, Ljostad U, Fingerle V, Rupprecht T, Schmutzhard E, and Steiner I. EFNS guidelines on the diagnosis and management of European Lyme neuroborreliosis. *European Journal of Neurology*, 2010, Volume 17, Issue 1, pp. 8–14, Copyright © 2009 Mygland A, et al.; Gaubitz M, Dressler F, Huppertz HI, Krause A; Kommission Pharmakotherapie der DGRh; [Diagnosis and treatment of Lyme arthritis. Recommendations of the Pharmacotherapy Commission of the Deutsche Gesellschaft für Rheumatologie (German Society for Rheumatology)]. *Zeitschrift für Rheumatologie*, Volume 73, Issue 5, pp. 469–74, Copyright © 2014 Springer-Verlag Berlin Heidelberg.

Readers are referred to the British National Formulary for information on cautions, contra-indications, side-effects, and drug interactions, including use in pregnancy and breast feeding. Doses given are for adults and will require adjustment for children. The durations for adults and children are the same. Source: data from Mygland A, Ljostad U, Fingerle V, Rupprecht T, Schmutzhard E, and Steiner I. EFNS guidelines on the diagnosis and management of European Lyme neuroborreliosis. *European Journal of Neurology*, 2010, Volume 17, Issue 1, pp. 8–14, Copyright © 2009 Mygland A, et al.; Gaubitz M, Dressler F, Huppertz HI, Krause A; Kommission Pharmakotherapie der DGRh; [Diagnosis and treatment of Lyme arthritis. Recommendations of the Pharmacotherapy Commission of the Deutsche Gesellschaft für Rheumatologie (German Society for Rheumatology)]. *Zeitschrift für Rheumatologie*, Volume 73, Issue 5, pp. 469–74, Copyright © 2014 Springer-Verlag Berlin Heidelberg.

- There is no evidence to support this view, or to show that persistent arthritis is due to continuing or refractory infection, and therefore amenable to prolonged courses of antibiotics.
  - The paediatric rheumatologist needs to be aware that non-accredited laboratories/clinics sometimes incorrectly make a diagnosis of chronic Lyme disease in patients with medically unexplained symptoms based on substandard or inherently unreliable tests.
  - In the UK the Department of Health have provided specific guidance on this difficult subject, found at: ℘ http://www.hpa.org.uk/Topics/InfectiousDiseases/InfectionsAZ/LymeDisease/GeneralInformation/lym020UnorthodoxPractices ℘ https://www.gov.uk/lyme-borreliosis-service
  - HPA is now called the PHE Rare and Imported Pathogen lab/Lyme service. Link: ℘ https://www.gov.uk/lyme-borreliosis-service

Human immunodeficiency virus arthritis

Human immunodeficiency virus (HIV) is highly prevalent in much of the developing world. It is estimated that in 2014 there were 2.6 million children globally living with HIV; 90% of them in Sub-Saharan Africa.

The prevalence of autoimmune disorders in HIV-infected adults is higher than those without HIV for all stages of HIV infection. However, there is very little information with regard to autoimmune disorders in HIV-infected children and adolescents and their true prevalence is unknown. Moreover understanding of the mechanisms or pathogenesis of such autoimmune diseases is lacking. A wide array of rheumatic manifestations have been associated with HIV, including arthralgia, arthritis, myositis, and vasculitis. Features of these rheumatic conditions may be the presenting feature of HIV patients or may occur in patients known to have been infected with HIV, or may be related to the treatment of HIV, either as a direct effect of medication or as part of an immune reconstitution syndrome. The pathogenesis of HIV arthritis is not clear but immune activation secondary to chronic exposure to bacterial lipopolysaccharides, disordered function of regulatory T cells, the formation of auto-reactive CD8 T-cells, the generation of auto-antibodies, and dysregulated B-cell proliferation with hyperglobulinaemia have been postulated. In areas with high HIV prevalence, then HIV should always be excluded before making the diagnosis of another rheumatic disease.

Clinical spectrum of HIV-related arthritis and musculoskeletal disease

Acute infection and sero-conversion

- Arthralgia and non-specific musculoskeletal pain is not an uncommon finding in patients with seroconversion or early HIV infection. Symptoms have been reported to occur in up to a third of patients in prospective studies.
- An acute seroconversion-related arthralgia might be associated with fever, rash, lymphadenopathy, and flu-like illness.
- Intermittent painful articular syndrome, where there is short lived, intensely painful musculoskeletal pain without clinical arthritis has been recognized in adults with HIV infection but has not been described frequently in children.

HIV arthritis

Persistent or chronic HIV arthritis appears to manifest in a range of clinical patterns depending on the number and type of joints and entheseal involvement as well as extra-articular features. The prevalence and profile of children with HIV arthritis has changed since the advent of anti-retroviral therapy (ART).

- Spondylo-arthritis/enthesitis:
  - It has been noted that the prevalence of spondyloarthritis in Africa increased dramatically with the HIV pandemic, despite a low prevalence of HLA-B27 in Africa. Features such as spondylitis, sacroilliitis,

enthesitis, and anterior uveitis are typical of this spondyloarthropa-thy. In a study from Durban these symptoms were found to be more prevalent in a cohort of children with HIV related arthritis than in children with JIA from the same population. Arthritis was the pre-senting feature in 78% of patients with HIV in this cohort of children (Chinniah et al. 2005).
- Polyarthritis:
  - Polyarthritis is well described in adults with HIV. A report on patients South Africa (Webb et al. 2013) found that HIV arthropathy occurred in boys with the following features:
    —Relatively older boys (median age 10 years)
    —Late diagnosis of HIV (WHO Stage 3 infection)
    —Before onset of ART therapy
    —It was the presenting feature of HIV in the majority
    —Lower limb arthritis was common.
  - Oligoarticular arthritis is not uncommon but monoarthritis, especially in the large joints such as hip and knee, should raise suspicion of tuberculous arthritis.
  - Psoriasis is commonly reported to be associated with HIV. Dactylitis and nail dystrophy with asymmetrical large and small joint arthritis is not infrequent in HIV related arthritis.

Musculoskeletal disorders associated with ART
Indinavir and to a lesser extent other protease inhibitors have been associ-ated with arthralgia, monoarthritis, and 'frozen shoulder' in adults but these features have not been reported in children. Avascular necrosis has also been associated with protease inhibitors.

Articular infections associated with HIV arthropathy
- Children infected with HIV are at increased risk for infections.
- The spectrum of organisms associated with osteoarticular infections in children with HIV infection is different to children without HIV; streptococcal infections being more common in the HIV-infected group than staphylococcal infection.
- The choice of empiric antibiotics for osteoarticular infections in areas high HIV prevalence should reflect this difference.
- Infections with *Mycobacterium tuberculosis* (MTB) is much more common in children with HIV; articular MTB is always a consideration when evaluating musculoskeletal complaints in HIV-infected children.

Laboratory investigations
Laboratory infections in HIV are aimed at excluding other infections and confirming the stage of HIV infection.
- Auto-antibodies in HIV:
  - Children infected with HIV tend to have higher rates of autoantibod-ies, the significance of which is often not clear.
  - Rheumatoid factor (RF), anti-citrullinated peptide antibodies (ACPA), anti-nuclear antibody (ANA), and anticardiolipin antibodies (ACL) may often be elevated.

- In the context of HIV infection these tend to be non-specific though they may complicate the process of making an accurate diagnosis.
  - It is postulated that immune dysregulation with polyclonal activation of B-cells and hypergammaglobulinaemia is responsible for this finding.
- Screening for other infections associated with reactive arthritis or joint pathology is critical when evaluating patients with HIV.
  - Organisms associated with viral, enteropathic, or mycobacterial arthritis should be considered based on the preceding or concurrent clinical features (e.g. diarrhoea or rash).
  - Infections known to cause reactive arthritis should be considered if there is urethritis or conjunctivitis.
  - Mycobacterial infections should be considered in virtually all children with HIV who present with musculoskeletal complaints.
- There is a high frequency of HIV and ART associated myositis and measurement of creatine kinase and other muscle enzymes should be done where this is a consideration.
- CD4 counts and HIV viral loads are important in staging HIV and monitoring the effects of ART and immunosuppression.

Imaging in HIV arthritis

- Plain films in are usually used to exclude other causes of musculoskeletal complaints such as avascular necrosis, pathological fractures, and osteoarticular infection. Radiographic features of joint erosions or joint destruction are rare in HIV-related arthritis.
- Joint ultrasound in children with polyarthritis secondary in late HIV infection may reveal exuberant synovial hypertrophy and hyperemia.
- Radioisotope bone scans may be useful in excluding osteoarticular infections and avascular necrosis.

Complications

- Severe untreated HIV arthropathy can lead to joint contractures and disability in some cases.
- Uveitis has been found to be a feature associated with HIV arthritis and also occurs with increased frequency in children with HIV who do not have arthritis. This uveitis can be as devastating as the uveitis associated with JIA.

Treatment

- In the majority of cases HIV arthropathy responds well to treatment with ART. Symptoms resolve within weeks or months of the start of treatment.
- In the majority of cases treatment with NSAIDs will improve the symptoms of arthritis in the initial phase.
- Chloroquine has been shown to have in vitro anti-retroviral effects and is frequently used in the treatment of HIV arthropathy.
- Intra-articular corticosteroids may relieve symptoms during early phases of treatment, as a bridging strategy.

- In cases where arthritis (or uveitis) do not settle with ART, NSAID and chloroquine, then a treatment approach similar to JIA can be followed.
- While methotrexate and sulphasalazine have been used with success, there is insufficient experience with these agents in this setting to make concrete recommendations. Cases of HIV arthritis improving with anti-TNF therapy have been reported but the risk of TB in areas where HIV is prevalent makes this a less attractive option.

Further reading

Muñoz Fernández S et al. Rheumatic manifestations in 556 patients with human immunodeficiency virus infection. *Semin Arthritis Rheum.* 1991 Aug;21(1):30–9.

Marquez J et al. Human immunodeficiency virus-associated rheumatic disorders in the HAART era. *J. Rheumatol.* 31 (4) 741-746

Chinniah K et al. Arthritis in association with human immunodeficiency virus infection in Black African children: causal or coincidental? *Rheumatology.* 2005 Jul;44(7):915-20.

Varicella zoster infections

Infection with varicella zoster virus (VZV) causes varicella (chickenpox), while its reactivation from latency produces zoster (shingles). Cellular immunocompromise dramatically increases the risk of severe and disseminated varicella, including potentially fatal pneumonitis, encephalitis, and hepatitis. In children who have already acquired VZV, immunosuppression increases both the rate and severity of zoster; second episodes of varicella are also well described. VZV disease therefore requires active management in children with present or anticipated immunosuppression. Children may be immunosuppressed due to their underlying diagnosis (e.g. JSLE with lymphopenia) or more commonly due to therapy. Relevant immunosuppressive drugs include systemic corticosteroids (equivalent to prednisolone 1mg/kg/day for 1 month or 2mg/kg/day for 1 week within the previous 3 months), azathioprine, ciclosporin, methotrexate, cyclophosphamide, and biologics, e.g. anti-TNF therapy, anakinra, tocilizumab, etc.

Assessment of VZV immunity

- At diagnosis, assess VZV susceptibility in the patient and family members by eliciting a history of varicella and/or zoster.
- Check VZV serology at diagnosis/prior to commencing immunosuppressive therapy.
- Young children with no history of varicella (or receipt of varicella vaccine—unusual in the UK) are very likely to be seronegative.

Counselling/education

- Families should be warned of the dangers of VZV in immunosuppressed children (see ➲ Biologics, pp. 448–54).
- The need to avoid exposure should be reinforced; varicella vaccination of any other susceptible family members should be advised.
- Families should be advised to contact their medical team immediately in the event of known exposure or suspected VZV disease.

Active vaccination

- The live attenuated varicella vaccine is safe and effective in healthy children above 1yr of age. For optimal protection, 2 doses are advised at least 4 weeks apart.
- Consider vaccinating currently immunocompetent but VZV-susceptible patients who are likely to require immunosuppression later in the disease course (but not for at least 3 weeks). In recently diagnosed oligo-JIA—suggest varicella vaccination at time of joint injection (and can be done at the time of the general anaesthetic). The second dose can be considered 4 weeks later.
- Vaccination is contraindicated in the immunocompromised but not in their healthy varicella-susceptible household contacts—preventing varicella in healthy sibs is an important step towards protecting the immunosuppressed child. *Pre- and post-serology are not required in healthy children; the lack of a history of chicken pox in the young child*

is a good surrogate for being non immune and vaccination is advised. Should vaccine-associated rash develop (<5%), there is a small risk of transmission which should be managed as for wild type exposure of the immunocompromised individual.

Post-exposure prophylaxis

- If significant exposure to VZV is recognized, post-exposure prophylaxis should be given to all immunosuppressed patients who are seronegative. (Significant exposure is defined as any household or nosocomial contact with VZV; any face-to-face contact or 15min in same room as index case of varicella from 48h before rash until all spots crusted over; and contact with exposed dermatomal zoster or any zoster in the immunocompromised.)
- Good evidence supports the use of VZIG as prophylaxis, when administered early (ideally <72h, but may be effective up to 7 days) after exposure; in the UK, stocks are held by HPA laboratories or their equivalent who will advise on its appropriate use. See Fig. 6.4 and 'The Green Book' (see ➔ Further reading, p. 411).
- High-dose oral aciclovir from <7 to 21 days post-exposure is currently used as an alternative or adjunct to VZIG in some UK centres and should be offered if no VZIG has been given within 72h of exposure; however, the evidence base for its use as single agent, post-exposure prophylaxis in the immunocompromised is poor.
- Consider post-exposure prophylaxis using aciclovir in VZV-seropositives who are severely immunosuppressed, e.g. patients on a combination of steroids and biologics or cyclophosphamide.
- Neither VZIG nor aciclovir is completely effective in preventing varicella; clinical infection may follow after a prolonged incubation period (21– 28 days post-exposure) and although usually mild, may occasionally be severe.
- Irrespective of serostatus and prophylaxis after exposure, families should be advised to examine the patient daily for spots and report any suspicion of illness immediately (including non-specific symptoms such as fever, back/abdominal pain as well as rash).

Treatment

- Prompt initiation of antiviral therapy contains viral replication and reduces the risk of dissemination in both varicella and zoster.
- Immunosuppressed children with suspected VZV disease should be admitted without delay to an isolation cubicle for IV aciclovir and general supportive care.
- Suggested laboratory work-up includes FBC, liver and renal function; consider baseline CXR.
- IV aciclovir dose is $500mg/m^2$ 8-hourly (3m–12yr), 10mg/kg 8-hourly (12–18yr). Recommended duration of therapy is at least 7 days; persist with IV therapy until fever and constitutional symptoms have resolved and no new spots have appeared for 48h.
- Remember to consider the possible need for post-exposure prophylaxis among susceptible nosocomial contacts.

Further advice

Paediatric infectious disease specialists, virologists, public health agencies (in the UK see: ℘ http://www.hpa.org.uk/web/HPAweb&HPAwebStandard/HPAweb_C/1287147556958).

Further reading

Chapter 34, Varicella. In Salisbury D, Ramsay M, Noakes K (eds) *Immunisation against infectious disease – 'The Green Book'*. London: The Stationery Office; 2006, 421–42. Available at: ℘ https://www.gov.uk/government/publications/varicella-the-green-book-chapter-34

NICE Clinical Evidence Summary: Chickenpox. Available at: http://cks.nice.org.uk/chickenpox

Fisher J, Bate J, Hambleton S. Preventing varicella in children with cancer; what is the evidence? *Curr Opin Infect Dis* 2011; **24**(3):203–11.

Royal College of Paediatrics and Child Health. *Immunisation of the Immunocompromised Child: Best Practice Statement*. London: Royal College of Paediatrics and Child Health, 2002. Available on BSPAR website: ℘ http://www.bspar.org.uk/pages/clinical_guidelines.asp.

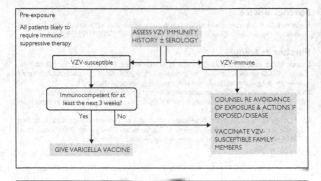

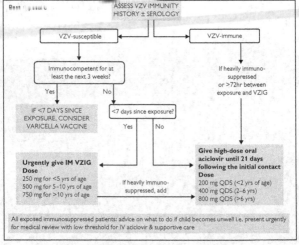

Fig. 6.4 Guidelines for the prevention of severe varicella in the exposed immunocompromised child.

Immunization schedules and the immunocompromised

Immunization of children with paediatric rheumatic diseases raises several issues:

- Risk of disseminated infection with vaccine-strain pathogens after administration of live vaccines to immunocompromised patient.
- Uncertainty regarding induction of adequate immunity.
- The risk of precipitating disease flare by administered vaccine

Since publication in 2011, the European League Against Rheumatism (EULAR) recommendations (Box 6.5) have been supported by higher grade of evidence, in particular accumulation of data regarding the suppressive effect of biologics on immunogenicity of vaccines.

Summary of EULAR recommendations

- Vaccinations do not increase disease activity and do not cause severe adverse events.
- Non-live vaccines are safe and should be given according to national guidelines regardless of disease type or treatment with corticosteroids, disease modifying antirheumatic drugs (DMARDs) or anti-tumour necrosis factor alpha (TNFα) biologics.
  - https://www.gov.uk/government/uploads/system/uploads/attachment_data/file/510450/PHE_2016_Complete_Immunisation_Schedule_A4_17032016.pdf
  - The Green Book online: https://www.gov.uk/government/collections/immunisation-against-infectious-disease-the-green-book
- It is recommended to withhold live-attenuated vaccines in patients on high-dose immunosuppressive drugs and biologics, but booster vaccinations can be considered when essential.
- Immunogenicity of vaccines is good with some exceptions:
  - Responses are reduced in patients on high-dose glucocorticoids and rituximab.
  - Methotrexate reduces responses to pneumococcal polysaccharide vaccines.
  - Anti-TNFα may lower vaccine-induced antibodies and cause accelerated waning of immunity.
- Offering vaccination before commencing immunosuppressive drugs and/or measuring antibody responses after immunization is recommended.

Special warnings

- Following a case report of fatality from disseminated BCG infection in an infant born to a mother taking infliximab during pregnancy, administration of BCG (and other live vaccines, e.g. oral polio, intranasal influenza, VZV, MMR, rotavirus, yellow fever) to infants born to mothers treated with biologics during pregnancy, in particular anti-TNFα monoclonal antibodies, is not recommended during the first 6 months of life.

Box 6.5 Recommendations for vaccinations for children and young people with rheumatic disease

Live-attenuated vaccines
- Adhere to national guidelines[a] *unless* patients on high-dose DMARDs,[b] high-dose glucocorticoids,[b] or biologicals
- Withhold in patients on high-dose DMARDs, high-dose glucocorticoids, or biologicals.
- However, essential booster vaccinations can be considered on a case-by-case basis weighing the risk of infections vs the risk of vaccine-induced adverse events.
- Booster vaccinations against VZV, MMR, and YFV can be administered to patients on methotrexate (<15 mg/m² per week) or low-dose glucocorticoids.
- In case of a negative history (VZV infection or vaccine), especially if anticipating high-dose immunosuppressive therapy or biologicals:
  - VZV vaccine should be considered prior to commencing immuno-suppressive therapy.[c]

Non-live vaccines
- Adhere to national guidelines for vaccination against tetanus, diphtheria, poliovirus, pertussis, Hib, pneumococci, meningococci, HVA, HBV, as well as Japanese encephalitis, typhoid fever, rabies, cholera, or tick-borne encephalitis.
- Adhere to national guidelines for vaccination against HPV.
- If/when not included in national programmes, vaccines against Hib, pneumococci, and meningococci are recommended for patients on high-dose immunosuppressive drugs or biologicals (if possible, prior to commencing therapy).
- Non-live vaccines have been proven safe even when using glucocorticoids, DMARDs, or anti-TNFα therapy.
- Annual inactivated (i.e. non-live) influenza vaccination is recommended for all immunocompromised patients.

Immunosuppressive drugs
- Measure vicinal (pathogen-specific) antibody levels after vaccination in patients on high dose glucocorticoids, rituximab, or other B-cell-depleting therapies, or on anti-TNFα treatment.
- In patients using other biologicals, measuring antibody levels after vaccination should be considered.
- Measure pneumococcal strain-specific antibody levels following pneumococcal polysaccharide vaccination in patients receiving methotrexate at time of vaccination.
- Vaccinate prior to commencing rituximab or other B-cell-depleting therapies whenever possible.

Box 6.5 *Contd.*

- In patients treated with rituximab or other B-cell-depleting therapies in the past 6 months, tetanus immunoglobulin should be administered in case of contaminated (tetanogenic) wound.

Notes: DMARDs—disease-modifying antirheumatic drugs; Hib—*Haemophilus influenzae* type B; HVA—hepatitis A virus; HVB—hepatitis B virus; HPV—human papillomavirus; MMR—measles—mumps—rubella; SLE—systemic lupus erythematosus; TNF—tumour necrosis factor; VZV—varicella zoster virus; YFV—yellow fever virus

[a] National vaccination guidelines worldwide can be found via 🔎 <http://apps.who.int/immunization_monitoring/en/globalsummary/scheduleselect.cfm>

[b] High-dose DMARDs (causing profound immunosuppression) defined as current use or use in the past 3 months of any dose of
  - intravenous (pulse) methylprednisolone, cyclophosphamide, or any biological;
  - mycophenolate mofetil;
  - cyclophosphamide orally (0.5–2.0 mg/kg/day);
  - ciclosporin (2.5–3.0 mg/kg/day);
  - azathioprine (1–3 mg/kg/day);
  - methotrexate (15 mg/m² weekly) (>0.4 mg/kg/day);
  - sulphasalazine (40 mg/kg/day or 2 g/day);
  - leflunomide (0.25–0.5 mg/kg/day);
  - 6-mercaptopurine (1.5 mg/kg/day);
  - high-dose glucocorticoids (≥2 mg/kg or ≥20 mg/day for ≥2 weeks);
  - or combinations of these drugs with other immunosuppressive agents.

[c] Generally, 2–4 weeks is recommended before immunosuppressive therapy is commenced.

Adapted with permission from Heijstek MW, Ott de Bruin LM, Borrow R, et al. EULAR recommendations for vaccination in paediatric patients with rheumatic diseases. *Ann Rheum Dis.*, Volume 70, pp. 1704–1712, Copyright © 2011 BMJ Publishing Group Ltd & European League Against Rheumatism.

- In patients with cryopyrin-associated periodic syndromes (CAPS) unusually severe adverse reactions to pneumococcal vaccination have been reported. Until more data become available, vaccinations should be considered on a case-by-case basis weighing the risk of infections vs the risk of vaccine-induced adverse events.

Further reading

Akikusa JD, Crawford NW. Vaccination in paediatric rheumatology. *Curr Rheumatol Rep.* 2014;**16**:432.

Cheent K, Nolan J, Shariq S, *et al.* Case Report: Fatal case of disseminated BCG infection in an infant born to a mother taking infliximab for Crohn's disease. *J Crohn's Colitis* 2010;**4**:603–5.

Groot N, Heijstek MW, Wulffraat NM. Vaccinations in paediatric rheumatology: an update on current developments. *Curr Rheumatol Rep* 2015;**17**(7):46.

Heijstek MW, Abinun M, Wulffraat NM. Vaccination in immunocompromised children (Chapter 95). In: Watts RA, Conaghan PG, Denton C, *et al.* (Eds.), Oxford Textbook of Rheumatology (4 ed.), Oxford University Press, DOI:10.1093/med/9780199642489.003.0095_update_002.

Heijstek MW *et al.* EULAR recommendations for vaccination in paediatric patients with rheumatic diseases. *Ann Rheum Dis* 2011;**70**:1704–12.

Janow, G, Ilowite NT. Vaccination in pediatric rheumatic disease—risks and benefits. *Nat Rev Rheumatol.* 2012;**8**:188–90.

Ling J, Koren G. Challenges in vaccinating infants born to mothers taking immunoglobulin biologicals during pregnancy. *Expert Rev Vaccines* 2016;**15**(2):239–56.

Silva CA, Aikawa NE, Bonfa E. Vaccinations in juvenile chronic inflammatory diseases: an update. *Nat Rev Rheumatol* 2013;**9**:532–43.

Walker UA et al. brief report: severe inflammation following vaccination against streptococcus pneumoniae in patients with cryopyrin-associated periodic syndromes. *Arthritis Rheumatol* 2016;**68**(2):516–20.

Multi-disciplinary approach to management

The multidisciplinary team

• The experienced MDT is integral to the holistic management of children and young people with rheumatic disease with the patient and family at the centre (See Fig. 3.2) with input from specialist consultant, specialist nurse, paediatric physiotherapist, and paediatric occupational therapist.

• In the context of JIA, the role of the MDT is paramount and emphasized in the BSPAR Standards of Care (see ➔ Chapter 9, pp. 466–8,) and more recently adopted into the NHS England commissioning document for specialized pediatric services. (See ➔ Chapter 8, biologics in JIA pp. 448–54.)

The composition of the paediatric rheumatology MDT may vary from centre to centre and may often involve a managed clinical network with colleagues in primary, community, and hospital care. The roles of the members of the MDT may overlap and are often complementary. The BSPAR position statement outlines the requirements for training and expertise for the MDT. The clinical roles of the nurse specialist, physiotherapist, occupational therapist, and podiatrist are detailed in this chapter. Reference to the important other members of the MDT are given in other chapters role of the clinical psychologist in the context of chronic pain management). The roles of the parent and child/young person in research are also highlighted.

Box 7.1 The paediatric rheumatology MDT

Core members

Access to named member required by every child or young person with JIA:

- Paediatric rheumatologist
- Ophthalmologist
- GP
- Paediatric rheumatology clinical nurse specialist
- Paediatric physiotherapist
- Paediatric clinical psychologist
- Paediatric occupational therapist
- Podiatrist
- Health visitor or school nurse.

The extended team

Access to named member required if clinically indicated:

- Shared care delivery (paediatrician with an interest in rheumatology or adult rheumatologist)
- Adult rheumatologist for transitional care
- Children's community nursing team
- Play therapist/youth worker
- Special educational needs coordinator
- Orthodontist/dentist/maxillofacial surgeon
- Orthopaedic surgeon
- Endocrinologist.

NB The extended team may work in conjunction with a paediatrician with an interest in paediatric rheumatology or an adult rheumatologist with an interest in paediatric rheumatology (operating within a paediatric rheumatology clinical network).

Further reading

Baildam EM, Davidson JE. BSPAR Position Statement on Professional working in Paediatric Rheumatology. *Rheumatology (Oxford)* 2008; **47**(6):743–4. ℘ http://www.bspar.org.uk/downloads/clinical_guidelines/Final_BSPAR_Position_Statement_on_Professionals_working_in_Paediatric_Rheumatology_Teams.pdf.

Davies K, Cleary G, Foster HE, *et al.* on behalf of the British Society of Paediatric and Adolescent Rheumatology: BSPAR Standards of Care for children and young people with Juvenile Idiopathic Arthritis. *Rheumatology* 2010; **49**(7):1406–8. ℘ http://www.bspar.org.uk/downloads/clinical_guidelines/Standards_of_Care.pdf.

'Bringing Networks to Life - An RCPCH guide to implementing Clinical Networks' March 2012

NHS England Specialist Services Commissioning: PAEDIATRIC MEDICINE: RHEUMATOLOGY ℘ https://www.england.nhs.uk/wp-content/uploads/2013/06/e03-paedi-medi-rheum.pdf

The role of the clinical nurse specialist

The clinical nurse specialist (CNS) team is a fundamental component in the care of children and young people with JIA and other rheumatological conditions with a focus on providing the highest quality of clinical care, education, training and patient/carer support. The CNS will be a qualified children's nurse with a diverse training background and broad range of experiences to ensure a holistic approach in achieving safe and effective care.

The role of the CNS is described in the British Society for Paediatric and Adolescent Rheumatology (BSPAR) Position Statement (see ➔ Further reading, p. 422), albeit details of roles and responsibilities may vary between local services.

The role of the CNS has evolved rapidly largely as a result of the era of potent immunosuppression, such as treatment with biologics, and the more pro-active pharmacological approach to management of paediatric rheumatic diseases

Such roles may include:

Clinical coordination

- Holistic care for the child and young person with chronic illness, acting as patient and family advocate in clinical decision-making with care and dignity.
- Clinical care for children with complex illness, often involving other specialist services including social care, education, health and child protection as necessary.
- Clinical networks and regional shared care services with experts knowledge to ensure appropriate support is provided by tertiary centers.
- MDT meetings and their documentation within local/national guidelines that have an agreed purpose, structure, and outcome.
- Day-case administration of infusions, such as intravenous steroids, biologics, cyclophosphamide, and pamidronate with appropriate monitoring and evaluation of care throughout.
- Enhancing standards of clinical care through the support and supervision of nursing colleagues.
- DMARDs and biologic therapy monitoring and liaising with home delivery services.
- Telephone helpline and triage of queries with an agreed response time for all enquiries.
- Coordinating transitional care in conjunction with young people and their carers and transfer to adult services by equipping them with the skills and knowledge to confidently manage their own disease and decision-making.

Other clinical roles

- Nurse-led training and review clinics with proformas to standardize training outcomes of patients, carers, and healthcare professionals.
- Joint injections and delivery of Entonox®.
- Administration and education of subcutaneous and intravenous treatments within a clinical and non-clinical environment.

Clinical governance
- Clinical guideline development and audit to deliver high-quality care.
- Standardized patient information leaflets and educational resources giving consideration to information literacy and possible formats of written information.
- Development of proformas and checklists for use of biologics in accordance with national guidance (see ➲ Approvals for use of biologics therapies, pp. 455–6).
- Nursing dashboard and quality measurements of nursing care, patient experience to be shared nationally.

Training and education
- Disease and treatment education for patients and their families, medical and allied health colleagues involved in shared care (community, general paediatric, and primary care).
- Promoting online resources (e.g. BSPAR, Arthritis Research UK, National Rheumatoid Arthritis Society, Paediatric Rheumatology European Society) for patients and families.
- Promoting online resources (e.g. BSPAR, BSR, Royal College Nursing, RCPCH and Paediatric Musculoskeletal Matters, see Further Reading and References) for continuing professional development and online reading material for health care professionals.
- Disease and treatment education to school and educational services.
- Training and support for patients and families regarding immunosuppressive treatments and home administration where appropriate.
- Education and advice about the unwell patient for families and where to access medical advice out of hours.
- Education around the management of intercurrent infections, fever, infectious diseases, and vaccination schedules for those on immunosuppressive treatments.

Service development
- National guidance on clinical services development through national bodies (such as BSPAR in the UK) and links with other professional bodies (e.g. Royal College of Nursing—see ➲ Further reading, below).
- Development and standardization of training programmes for parenteral methotrexate for nurses to train patients and families.
- Liaising with pharmaceutical companies to develop information packs and devices that are appropriate for use in children and young people, including needle safe devices and solutions to those treatments found to be painful.
- Identify national parent groups for peer support.
- Share positive experiences, outcomes, national awards with other national centres to promote good practice.
- Promote awareness of rheumatological diseases within the public domain, health care planners, and policy makers.

Research
- Contribution to clinical research priority setting within national professional bodies (such as the Clinical Studies Group and BSR).
- Participation in obtaining informed consent and data collection for clinical trials, registries, and clinical research activities.
- Support for children and families taking part in clinical trials.

Further reading

Baildam EM, Davidson, JE. BSPAR Position Statement on Professional working in Paediatric Rheumatology. *Rheumatology (Oxford)* 2008: **47**(6):743–4.

The following documents are available on the BSPAR website (Ͽ http://www.bspar.org.uk).

Department of Health (2004) *National Service Framework for Children, Young People and Maternity Services*. London: DoH.

Royal College of Nursing. *Adolescent transition care – Guidance for nursing staff*. London: RCN, 2004.

Royal College of Nursing. *Administering subcutaneous methotrexate for inflammatory arthritis: Guidance for nurses*. London: RCN, 2007.

Royal College of Nursing. *Assessing, managing and monitoring Biologic therapies for inflammatory arthritis*. London: RCN, 2009.

Royal College of Paediatrics and Child Health. *Bridging the Gaps: Health care for Adolescents*. London: RCPCH, 2003.

Paediatric Musculoskeletal Matters. A free resource for clinicians endorsed by BSPAR and produced by Newcastle University, UK. Ͽ www.pmmonline.org

Paediatric Musculoskeletal Matters for Nurses. Ͽ www.pmmonline.org/nurse

The role of the physiotherapist

Generic roles of the physiotherapist

- Assessment of musculoskeletal system:
  - Joints—active disease, range of movement, abnormal biomechanics.
  - Muscles—strength, stamina, length, and biomechanics and normal patterns of movement.
  - Generalized stamina and fitness.
  - Balance, proprioception, and gait.
- Physiotherapy treatment can:
  - Reduce pain, reduce fatigue, and ↑ energy.
  - Improve or maintain joint range of movement, minimize joint deformity.
  - ↑ or maximize muscle strength and function, ↑ generalized fitness.
  - Improve balance and proprioception, restore normal gait patterns.
- Family and patient education:
  - Pain management, disease management, goal setting and pacing.
  - Ensure full participation with school, family and friends, advice re sport and physical activity.

Condition-specific focus

Juvenile idiopathic arthritis

- Combined with medical management aim to maintain full range of movement in all joints.
- Maintain full muscle strength for all muscle groups.
- Re-education balance and proprioception, re-educate gait.
- Regain full fitness to ensure full participation with all sport and physical activities.

Juvenile dermatomyositis

- Physiotherapy combined with medical management and ideally started at the time of diagnosis:
  - Muscle function assessments (see ➲ JDM, pp. 280–7).
  - Maintenance of full muscle length/joint range (splinting, stretching, active movement).
  - Encouraging muscle function immediately; advice on safe handling and mobility.
- Graduated and progressive, resisted specific muscle strengthening programme with re-education balance, proprioception, and gait with aim to regain to full fitness to ensure optimal participation.

Juvenile systemic lupus erythematosus

- ↑ general fitness to reduce fatigue.

Juvenile scleroderma

- Assessment and monitoring of progression combined with medical management:
  - Stretches to maintain joint range, muscle length, skin mobility.
  - Deep tissue massage, wax treatment, and specific muscle strength training.

Non-inflammatory musculoskeletal pain syndromes
- Hypermobility/anterior knee pain/back pain:
  - Assessment of biomechanical changes, specifically muscle function.
  - Explanation for young person and family about pain and treatment goals and objectives—regain full specific muscle strength/stamina with progressive/resisted specific muscle training, high reps and low weights emphasized.
  - Pain management techniques, restore balance and proprioception, re-educate gait.
- Complex regional pain syndrome:
  - Family education about disease and treatment; function despite pain approach.
  - Regain normal movement of affected limb immediately to reduce pain—desensitization is most effective through regaining normal movement and muscle strength.
  - Regain all physical, social, and psychological function.
- Chronic fatigue:
  - Education about paced approach to life, specific strength training, global fitness training.
  - Training to be 'fit for life'.

The role of the occupational therapist (OT)

Overview of the role of the OT

- The OT works as part of an MDT approach.
- The role of the OT is to assess, identify occupational performance goals, plan patient led intervention, and evaluate outcomes.
- The OT approach is based on encouraging, educating, offering support, and facilitating the patient and their parent/carer from referral to transition/discharge.
- The OT adopts a functional approach to disease management using a range of interventions. This requires a holistic approach to meet the physical, emotional, psychosocial, and cognitive needs of the patient and their family.

Clinical role

The OT clinical role is diverse and may include a number of the following:

- To encourage, empower, and support the patient and their family, especially at the point of referral or transition to enable independence and self-advocacy.
- Provide specific age appropriate disease education for the patient and their family.
- To carry out a range of standardized assessment (such as that defined by BSPAR ℘ http://www.bspar.org.uk/pages/bspar_home.asp) with regular monitoring of the patient's function appropriate to their developmental stage.
- To help the patient manage pain, fatigue, anxiety, and psychosocial difficulties through educative coping strategies. This may include energy conservation, relaxation, pacing/grading.
- To support the development of self-esteem and self confidence in activities of daily living (self-care, productivity, and leisure).
- To provide advice to schools and other educational establishments, in order to promote inclusion, participation, and fulfilment of the patients' potential.
- To promote joint protection strategies during activities of daily living.
- To encourage physical functioning during periods of acute and chronic disease activity, utilizing pacing and energy conservation techniques.
- To assess and provide splints for the upper limb; to preserve range of movement, increase function, joint protection, comfort/pain relief, using a variety of splinting materials thermoplastic, neoprene, etc.

Training and development

- Increase awareness of current standards of care, approaches, treatment with JIA to the clinical network and under shared care arrangements.
- Promote evidence-based practice.
- Audit current practice standards of care and BSPAR guidelines.
- Patient specific information leaflets and educational resources.

- Facilitate the development of a family support network.
- Promote the role of occupational therapy within paediatric rheumatology.
- Raise the profile of paediatric rheumatology within student education.

Further reading

Melvin J, Jensen G. *Rheumatologic Rehabilitation Series Volume 1: Assessment and Management.* Bethesda, MD: The American Occupational Therapy Association, 1998; p. P08.

The role of the podiatrist

- The podiatrist has a specialized role to diagnose and treat all types of foot pathology including structural and functional problems.
- There is some overlap in this role with physiotherapists who might also diagnose and treat mechanical problems, and with orthotists who may be asked to provide orthoses.
- In paediatric rheumatology, the podiatrist's 1° role is to improve the child's functional foot position so that soft tissue strain is reduced and gait efficiency can be improved.
- The podiatrist can also advise on and treat skin and nail pathologies that may occur with many of the rheumatological conditions.
- A child should be referred to the podiatrist if the foot is considered to be in a poor position. This can be identified in standing or by an inefficient gait, or if the child is reporting discomfort in the foot or ankle that is exacerbated by activity.
- As it is considered that a poor mechanical foot position can add to the persistence of local joint or tendon synovitis, a referral should be considered for any child with ongoing ankle or foot disease.

Podiatry therapeutic approaches

- Functional orthosis, footwear advice, footwear adaptations
  - Orthoses modify the foot position and alter the timing of the foot joint motions during gait. Both prefabricated (ready-made yet individualized) orthoses and customized orthoses can be used and have been shown to be effective in randomized controlled trials in JIA.
- Gait re-education, exercises, shoe raises, and orthodigital splinting.

The healthy paediatric foot (see ➲ Normal variants, p 9)

The healthy child (<6yr) will typically have a low-arch profile involving some bulging of the talonavicular joint medially, and a valgus heel position. This is called the *pronated, pes planus*, or *valgus foot*. The healthy foot is mobile, efficient in gait, and pain-free.

Changes in the foot caused by JIA

- Although possessing individual joint capsules, many of the joints appear to interconnect and synovitis affecting a single foot joint is the exception rather than the rule. Synovitis and stiffness in one joint is often accompanied by either reduced movement or a compensatory movement in a neighbouring joint and thus a good overview of foot anatomy, mechanics, and function is essential when treating the foot in inflammatory joint disease.
- When the foot joints are sore due to local joint disease, the child may adopt new foot positions or changes in gait to off-load the painful areas. Typically the double support phase of stance lengthens, the propulsive phase shortens, and ankle power in plantarflexion at toe-off is reduced. With rearfoot and midfoot synovitis in JIA, the bony integrity of the subtalar and midtarsal joints may be lost. This frequently leads to collapse of the medial longitudinal arch with excessive foot pronation

being seen. This change in position results in an increase in soft tissue strain locally, including the anti-pronatory muscles which are overused in an effort to stabilize the foot. The affected joints have a reduced range of motion and fixed deformities may develop.
- Although the pronated foot type is common when rearfoot and midfoot synovitis is present, many other foot deformities are seen and may be related to the combination of joints affected, to local tenosynovitis, to muscle weakness, or be related to the impact of the more proximal joints on the foot (such as genu valgum and fixed flexion deformities at the hip or knee which influence the foot position).
- Inflammatory joint disease can affect other synovial structures in the foot:
  - Tenosynovitis often occurs in conditions such as JIA.
  - Swelling in the rearfoot needs careful examination to differentiate ankle or subtalar synovitis from tenosynovitis of tibialis anterior, tibialis posterior, long flexor or extensor tendons, or peroneal involvement, especially if local treatment with joint injections are being planned. Clinically, differentiation of individual tendons is difficult and MRI scans would be appropriate when planning injections.
  - Although not common, bursitis can occur in the forefoot with RF+ve JIA.
  - Enthesitis of the Achilles and plantar fascia insertions are frequently seen in enthesitis-related arthritis and respond well to shock absorbing, custom orthoses.

Leg-length discrepancy in JIA
- This is much less observed with prompt access to appropriate care but needs to be considered when asymmetrical knee joint involvement has featured.
- The asymmetry created by the leg-length discrepancy can have a large impact on the musculoskeletal system with initial compensation mechanisms occurring in the feet and impacting on the knee, pelvis, and spinal positions.
- As a rule of thumb, when a leg-length discrepancy is seen to create asymmetry in gait or joint positions, it should be treated by a full-length raise within or placed externally on the sole of the shoe. Such asymmetry is usually observed when a leg-length difference exceeds 1cm. The leg-length discrepancy should be reviewed six monthly for adjustment of any raise.

Compensatory gait change from pain
- Changes in gait occur as the child attempts to reduce the pain and discomfort of walking. These changes may become habitual and remain even when the joint disease has improved.
- It is the role of the podiatrist to assess the child's gait and use re-education, orthoses, or shoe adaptations to improve gait efficiency.

The foot in other rheumatological conditions

- Conditions such as JDM and SLE can affect the feet and require assessment and treatment by a podiatrist when a change in the feet or gait is noted.
- Although the muscle weakness with JDM is considered to be a proximal weakness, distal changes are seen. The muscle weakness associated with JDM may affect the feet by causing an increase in subtalar joint pronation as the muscle weakness reduces control of the foot position. Contracture of the tendoachilles is frequently seen and causes toe-walking to develop or excessive foot pronation, as the subtalar joint compensates for the tightness in an attempt to allow the heel to weightbear.

Choice of footwear for children with inflammatory foot disease

- A podiatrist will not prescribe orthoses until the child is wearing suitable footwear that will support the foot and accommodate the orthoses.
- It is important for all children to wear good footwear, particularly in the presence of joint inflammation or where the foot position requires support to reduce soft tissue strain.
- Good footwear means a supportive shoe, with a deep heel counter so that the shoe fits snugly up to the malleoli. The heel counter should be strong enough to control some of the varus/valgus movement of the heel. A fastening mechanism is needed to hold the foot into the strong heel counter and the sole should have some shock-absorbing properties.
- There is no single make of shoe that can be recommended for children, therefore it is important to direct the child and parents towards local shoe shops where the staff have a good knowledge of fitting 'difficult' feet, are familiar with fitting a shoe with or without orthoses, and have a range of shoes that they can be tried.
- A boot is sometimes recommended when extra support is needed as they often have stronger support, higher into the heel counter, although this does have to be balanced against some potential loss in ankle range of movement.

Transitional care

Definition of transitional care

- Transition is a multifaceted active process that attends to the medical, psychosocial, and educational/vocational needs of adolescents as they move from child into adult care.
- Transfer to adult services is a single event within this process, requiring close liaison between paediatric and adult services and primary care.

Key principles of transitional care

- Is an active, future-focused process with the aim to maximize life-long functioning and potential of young people.
- Is young-person-centred and inclusive of parents/care-givers.
- Involves paediatric and adult hospital services as well as primary care, education, social and youth services, and voluntary agencies.
- Is age and developmentally appropriate, recognizing the three phases of adolescent development: early (11–13yrs), mid (14–16yrs) and late (17–19yrs) as well as emerging adulthood (20–25yrs).
- Includes knowledge and skills training for the young person in health and disease education, communication, decision-making, assertiveness, self-care, and self-management.
- Is based on a resilience framework to enhance sense of control and interdependence in health care.

Interdependence of adolescent health care and transitional care

Transitional care is only one part of adolescent and young adult rheumatology care and there is no 'one-size-fits-all' process for transition. Local solutions and core principles of adolescent medicine should underpin transitional care including:

- Acknowledgement of the reciprocal influences of adolescent development and the rheumatic condition in question.
- Acknowledgement that adolescents and young adults (AYA) development (including brain development) continues into the mid-twenties.
- The importance of routine psychosocial screening of all adolescents (e.g. the HEEADSSSS screening tool—Home, Exercise, Education, Activities, Drugs, Sexual health, Suicide, Sleep, Safety).
- Giving young people the opportunity to be seen independently.
- Respecting and assuring their rights to confidentiality.
- Effective use of strategies including motivational interviewing (see ℛ http://motivationalinterviewing.org).
- AYA rheumatology services should meet the 'You're Welcome' quality criteria of accessibility, publicity, confidentiality and consent, environment, staff training, joined-up working, monitoring/evaluation involving young people, and adolescent health issues for young person-friendly health services (see ℛ https://www.gov.uk/government/publications/quality-criteria-for-young-people-friendly-health-services).

Core components of transitional care in rheumatology

- Written departmental/local transition policy agreed with all key stakeholders including young people and parents/care-givers.
- Transition lead professional.
- Transition care coordinator.
- Multidisciplinary team.
- Assessment of transition readiness with regular documented review during transition planning process.
- Education, skills training, and informational resources for young people, parents, and professionals.
- Informed adult rheumatology/ophthalmology/orthopaedic/renal services, and primary health care.
- Links with education/vocational/youth/social services and voluntary agencies.
- Administrative support including transfer summaries, tracking mechanisms to confirm attendance at first two adult clinic appointments.
- Monitoring, evaluation, and audit of services involving young people.

Transition planning for young people

Transition planning should consider the following issues (pertinent also to young people seen de novo in adult rheumatology services). These issues should be considered in a developmentally appropriate context and through education, assessment of understanding, skills-training, and sign-posting to young people (the HEEADSSSS screening interview is useful in this regard):

- Health issues:
  - Specific to rheumatic disease: disease knowledge, treatment, out-come, pain and fatigue management, independent health care utiliza-tion, self-medication and adherence, procedural pain management, shared decision-making skills, etc.
  - Generic health: exercise, healthy eating, sleep, sexual health, smok-ing, alcohol, recreational/illegal drug use, emotional well-being, safety.
- Psychosocial issues—household chores, independence, self-care, mobility, benefits, driving, leisure activities, social and peer support, self-esteem, body image, bullying, coping strategies.
- Educational/vocational issues:
  - Impact of condition, disclosure, rights, Equality Act (2010).
  - Career plan, work experience, career counselling.
- Family issues—concept of transition, knowledge of condition and impact on adolescent development, transitional care needs, understanding of confidentiality.

Transition planning should also include preparation for the event of transfer and specifically address the differences between the paediatric and adult services, the need to engage with primary care as well as the particular skills young people will need to negotiate these services.

Transition models

- Different models of transition exist depending on the local health services and resources:
  - A developmental transition model includes an adolescent clinic (11–16yrs) and young adult clinic (16–25yrs).
  - Evidence suggests an early start, ideally in early adolescence.
- The timing of transfer should be flexible, acknowledging disease status, readiness and maturity of the young person, and completion of growth and development.
- An evidence-based transitional care programme showed short-term benefits in rheumatology. Young adult clinics have been reported to be associated with successful transition. Further research is needed to determine the impact of such models on long-term outcomes.

Further reading

Foster HE, Minden K et al. EULAR/PReS Recommendations for Transition in Rheumatology. *Ann Rheum Dis* 2017:76:639–646 doi:10.1136/.

Campbell F, Biggs K, Aldiss SK, O'Neill PM, Clowes M, McDonagh J, While A, Gibson F. Transition of care for adolescents from paediatric services to adult health services. *Cochrane Database Syst Rev.* 2016 Apr 29;4:CD009794. Review.

Clemente D, Leon L, Foster H, Carmona L, Minden K. Transitional care for rheumatic conditions in Europe: current clinical practice and available resources. *Pediatr Rheumatol Online J.* 2017 Jun 9;15(1):49.

Clemente D et al. Systematic review and critical appraisal of transitional care programmes in rheumatolog. *Seminars in Arthritis and Rheumatism* 2016 ℗ http://dx.doi.org/10.1016/j.semarthrit.2016.06.003.

Barbara Ansell National Network for Adolescent Rheumatology ℗ www.bannar.org.uk

Department of Health. *You're welcome quality criteria. Making health services young people friendly.* London: DoH, 2011 ℗ http://www.gov.uk.

e-Learning for Healthcare website: ℗ http://www.e-lfh.org.uk.

Doukrou M, Segal TY. Fifteen-minute consultation: communicating with young people -how to use HEEADSSS, a psychosocial interview for adolescents. *Arch Dis Child Educ Pract Ed.* 2017 Jun 14. [Epub ahead of print].

McDonagh JE. Young people first, juvenile idiopathic arthritis second: Transitional care in rheumatology. *Arthritis Rheum* 2008: 59(8):1162–70.

Tattersall R, McDonagh JE. Transition: a rheumatology perspective. *Br J Hosp Med (Lond).* 2010 Jun;71(6):315–9.

Youth health Talk ℗ http://www.healthtalk.org/young-peoples-experiences.

Transition from children's to adults' services for young people using health or social care services. NICE guidance 2016. ℗ http://www.nice.org.uk/guidance/ng43

Pregnancy and rheumatic disease in adolescents and young adults

Pregnancy and JIA

Many children with JIA continue to have active disease throughout adolescence and young adulthood. Adult forms of arthritis, such as RA, can present in young adults around the time that they are considering starting families and therefore the management of adolescents and young adults with JIA or other inflammatory arthritides is an important topic and one which is routinely discussed in transition and young adult clinics. Patients should ideally be managed in a specialist unit with an MDT with interest in CTD and pregnancy and include an obstetrician, rheumatologist, and allied health professional. Safeguarding concerns will need to be addressed with younger adolescents who become pregnant.

Active inflammatory disease is associated with adverse pregnancy outcomes and an overarching principle in maternal medicine is that maintaining health in the mother plays a key role in both fertility and a positive pregnancy outcome. Prescribing in pregnancy is complicated by a lack of clinical trials and knowledge that may lead to patient misinformation or withdrawal of appropriate medication. Fortunately there have been recent guidelines published by both the British Society of Rheumatology and the European League Against Rheumatism (Table 7.1).

Biologics and their use in pregnancy

There is data available from registries about the use of some biologic therapies in the perinatal period. Anti-TNF therapies (Infliximab, Etanercept, Adalimumab, Certolizumab) are not teratogenic and are considered safe in the perinatal period and in the first trimester. If possible, it is recommended that Infliximab, Etanercept and Adalimumab should be stopped in the second or third trimester due to placental transfer of these drugs and the theoretical risk of immunosuppression in the neonate (although the placental transfer of Etanercept is much lower that of Infliximab and Adalimumab). However, any potential deleterious effects on stopping these drugs to maternal health and subsequently foetal health must be considered. There is minimal transfer of Certolizumab across the placenta due to the fact that it is a pegylated molecule and therefore can be continued throughout pregnancy. If any anti-TNF therapy is continued throughout pregnancy then live vaccines should be avoided for the first 7 months of the neonate's life.

Pregnancy and SLE

Patients with SLE are at increased risk of adverse pregnancy outcomes that include pre-eclampsia, eclampsia, preterm delivery and foetal growth restriction. Obstetric outcomes can be improved with pre-pregnancy planning and disease quiescence for at least 6 months prior to conception. Appropriate counselling is an essential part of the care of any adolescent or young adult with SLE. The combined oral contraceptive pill is not recommended for patients with a history of thrombosis, LAC or aPL antibodies. Low oestrogen formulations can be considered in non-smokers in stable disease without renal involvement. Although condom use should be encouraged, it is not adequate alone to prevent pregnancy in this high-risk population.

Special considerations in connective tissue disease (CTD) pregnancies

- Patients should ideally be managed in a specialist unit with an MDT including an obstetrician and rheumatologist with an interest in CTD and pregnancy.
- Disease activity (including dsDNA, complement, urine dip and BP) should be measured at baseline and at regular intervals throughout pregnancy.
- Maternal Ro/La should be checked due to the 1-2% risk of foetal congenital heart block. If positive, a foetal cardiac scan should be performed at 16-20 and 28 weeks gestation.
- Antiphospholipid syndrome confers a risk of increased pregnancy morbidity. Antibody testing should be performed in early pregnancy. LAC confers the strongest predictor of adverse pregnancy outcome in SLE. Patients should be assessed for the need for therapeutic dose Low molecular weight heparin (LMWH), e.g. tinzaparin. All those previously taking warfarin should be changed to this form of LMWH.
- Low-dose aspirin therapy should be considered in all pregnant patients with lupus, especially those with aPL antibodies.
- Flares of disease should be treated promptly with the lowest effective dose of prednisolone.
- Women with pulmonary hypertension, stage 4/5 chronic kidney disease, and active disease should be strongly advised against pregnancy.

Disease modifying anti-rheumatic drugs (DMARDS)

- Mycophenolate (MMF), methotrexate, and cyclophosphamide are known teratogens and should be withdrawn before planned pregnancy (Table 7.1). In the case of unplanned pregnancy when on any of these agents, the decision to terminate or continue the pregnancy should be made with counselling, individual risk assessment, and detailed foetal ultrasound available. Sexually active men (including those post vasectomy) are recommended to use condoms during and for a period after cessation of treatment with MMF due to the risk of transfer of the drug in seminal fluid.
- Hydroxychloroquine should be continued in all SLE pregnancies.
- In severe refractory maternal disease, pulsed intravenous methylprednisolone, IVIG or second or third trimester cyclophosphamide should be considered.
- Rituximab has not been shown to be teratogenic and only second or third trimester exposure is associated with neonatal B cell depletion.

Table 7.1 Drug compatibility in pregnancy and breast-feeding for commonly used traditional DMARDs

	Peri-conception	Compatible with 1st trimester	Compatible with 2nd/3rd trimester	Compatible with breast-feeding	Compatible with paternal exposure
Corticosteroids (prednisolone & methyl-prednisolone)	Yes	Yes	Yes	Yes	Yes
Hydroxy-chloroquine	Yes	Yes	Yes	No	Yes (limited data)
Azathioprine <2mg/kg/day	Yes	Yes	Yes	Yes	Yes
Sulphasalazine (with folic acid)	Yes	Yes	Yes	Yes	Yes (although oligo-spermia has been reported)
Leflunomide	No (requires choles-tyramine washout)	No	No	No data	Yes (limited data)
Methotrexate	Stop at least 3/12 in advance	No	No	No	Yes (limited data)
Ciclosporin	Yes	Yes	Yes	*Yes (limited data)	Yes (limited data)
Tacrolimus	Yes	Yes	Yes	Yes (limited data)	Yes (limited data)
Mycophenolate mofetil	Stop 6/52 in advance	No	No	No	No
Cyclo-phosphamide	No	No	No	No	No
IVIG	Yes	Yes	Yes	Yes	Yes (limited data)
Rituximab	Stop 6/12 in advance	No	No	No data	Yes (limited data)

* Manufacturer recommends avoiding ciclosporin when breastfeeding.

References

Ostensen M, Andreoli L, Brucato et al. State of the art: reproduction and pregnancy in rheumatic diseases. *Autoimm Rev* 2015;14:376–86

Skorpen CG, Hoeltzenbein M, Tincani A et al. The EULAR points to consider for use of antirheumatic drugs before pregnancy, and during pregnancy and lactation. *Ann Rheum Dis* 2016;0:1–16. Doi10.1136/annrheumdis-2015-208840

Flint J, Panchal S, Hurrell A et al. BSR and BHPR guidelines on prescribing drugs in pregnancy and breastfeeding – Part I; standard and biologic disease modifying anti-rheumatic drugs and corticosteroids. *Rheumatology* 2016;doi:10.1093/rheumatology/kev404

Soh MC, Nelson-Piercy. High-risk pregnancy and the rheumatologist. *Rheumatology* 2015;54(4): 572–587. doi: 10.1093/rheumatology/keu394

Tesher MS, Whitaker A, Gilliam M et al. *Paediatric Rheumatology*. 2010;8:10 doi: 10.1186/1546-0096-8-10

CELLCEPT® (MYCOPHENOLATE MOFETIL) GUIDE FOR HEALTHCARE PROVIDERS: Risk of miscarriage and birth defects. British Generic Manufacturers Association March 2016.

Chapter 8

Specialized therapeutic approaches

Corticosteroid intra-articular injections

Intra-articular corticosteroid injections are increasingly used as they allow rapid symptom control and allow time for other therapies, such as methotrexate (MTX) to have their effect. They often remove the need for the use of oral or IV corticosteroids and avoidance of side-effects. There is no limit to the number of joints that can be injected at any one time or the total dose of corticosteroid.

Anaesthesia and analgesia

Various modalities are available:
- General anaesthetic is needed for multiple joints or in younger children.
- Inhaled nitrous oxide (Entonox®) is useful in older children and for 1–4 joints.
- 'Wide awake' is feasible in older children and adolescents—ethyl chloride topical spray gives local skin anaesthesia.
- Sedation is not recommended and difficult to achieve adequately— general anaesthetic is a much safer option.

Choice and dose of intra-articular corticosteroid

- Triamcinolone hexacetonide (TH) is the drug of choice with longer duration of remission, less systemic absorption, and without ↑ in local side-effects compared to other more soluble corticosteroid preparations. TH is available from specialist suppliers (check with your pharmacy). Triamcinolone acetonide (TA; Kenolog®), is an acceptable alternative but produces many more systemic side-effects due to ↑ systemic absorption. Other corticosteroid preparations are not recommended.
- Corticosteroid doses (given assuming TH is used) depends on body weight and the joint injected:
  - Large joints (knees, shoulders, hips): 1mg per kg per joint (max. 40mg/joint)—larger doses may be used in older larger patients albeit expert advice is recommended.
  - Medium joints (ankles, subtalars, elbows, wrists,) 0.5mg per kg per joint (max. 30mg/joint).
  - Temporomandibular joint 0.25mg per kg per joint.
  - Small joints (fingers and toes) 0.04–1mg total dose per joint.

These dosages can be safely rounded up or down and should be doubled when using TA—there is no maximum total dose that can be used at one time, but if TA is used, then there is a significant likelihood of systemic side-effects with larger total doses.

Side-effects of intra-articular corticosteroids

- Systemic:
  - Transient increases in BP, appetite and weight gain are described and more likely with TA. Striae from weight gain are uncommon.

- Local:
  - Subcutaneous atrophy—most likely with joints with a small intra-articular volume such as fingers, wrists, and subtalar joints.
  - Sepsis—very small risk (<1 in 10,000 with good aseptic technique).
  - Periarticular calcification—observed on x-ray but unlikely to cause clinical symptoms.
  - Cartilage growth disturbance—may occur if corticosteroids are incorrectly placed into growing cartilage.
  - Correct needle placement and appropriate dosage will reduce but not eradicate local side-effects.

Procedure
- Informed consent/assent must be recorded in the patient's case notes and irrespective of the type of anaesthesia used.
- Aseptic technique—operator should have clean hands and wear sterile gloves. Gowns and masks are not necessary. Steroid preparation should be drawn up in a 2mL syringe (or 1mL syringe for PIPJs, MCPJs, and MTPJs).
- Needle size:
  - 21-gauge for shoulders, knees, ankles, and subtalars; 23-gauge for wrists and TMJs; 25-gauge for PIPJs, MCPJs, and MTPJs.
  - Spinal needle should be used for the hips.
  - The needle should be placed into the joint capsule and attempts to aspirate the joint should be made—drawing back synovial fluid confirms needle placement, but the lack of fluid does not necessarily mean that the needle is not in the correct place. Once the operator is happy with the placement of the needle, 50% of the corticosteroid should be injected; the remaining corticosteroid should be injected after waiting a few seconds. The operator should then wait for a further 30sec before removing the needle and then pressing lightly on the injection site.
  - Never force an injection: if there is a need to use force then it is likely that the needle is incorrectly placed and the procedure should be abandoned and then restarted.
  - The use of an image intensifier or US can be used to aid correct needle placement.

Post-injection management
- Injected joints should be rested for 24h postoperatively—there is no need for bed rest but patients should defer from taking part in vigorous exercise for 48h postoperatively.
- Patients and carers should have clear instructions on who to call in the event of any postoperative complications developing.

Site of injection

- It is important to learn under the guidance of an experienced clinician with opportunities initially to observe and then perform under supervision.

  Knee: the needle is inserted approximately 1cm medial (or lateral) to the patella, at the level of the junction of the upper 2/3 and lower 1/3. The needle is directed slightly caudally and at an angle to go under the patella (see Fig 8.1).
- Ankle: the needle is inserted anteriorly just lateral to the extensor hallucis longus tendon see Fig 8.2.
- Subtalar: the needle is inserted perpendicularly into the space just distal to the lateral malleolus see Fig 8.3.

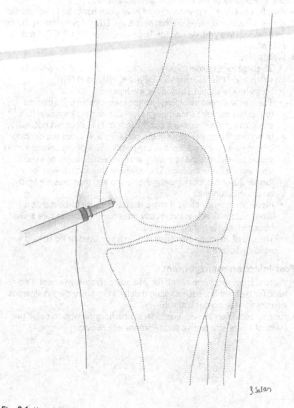

Fig. 8.1 Knee joint
Reproduced by kind permission of Barbara Salas, Copyright © 2016 Barbara Salas.

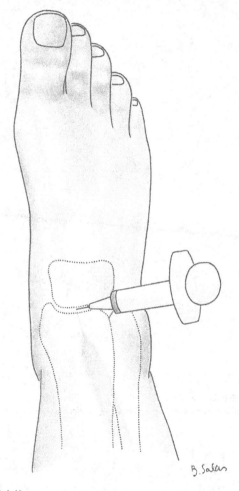

Fig. 8.2 Ankle

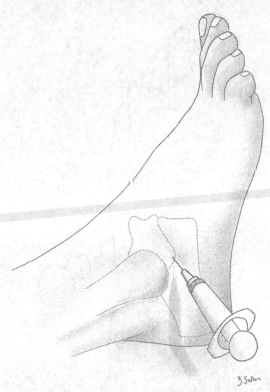

Fig. 8.3 Subtalar joint

Reproduced by kind permission of Barbara Salas, Copyright © 2016 Barbara Salas.

- Hip: a line should be drawn between the anterior superior iliac crest (ASIC) and the pubic tubercle. A 2nd line should be drawn from the ASIC towards the medial border of the patella. A 3rd line should be drawn perpendicularly from the mid-point of the 1st line until it bisects the 2nd line. That bisection point is the site of needle entry. The needle is then directed towards the mid-point of the original line and at an angle of 60° to the skin Fig 8.4. The needle should be slowly inserted until it hits bone. The needle should then be lying against the neck of the femur. The needle placement should be checked with fluoroscopy prior to injection of the drug.
- TMJ: the needle is placed a few millimetres anterior to the tragus and advanced until it hits the joint just distal to the head of the mandible.
- Shoulder: the needle is inserted anteriorly just lateral to the coracoid process and superior to the head of the humerus Fig 8.5.

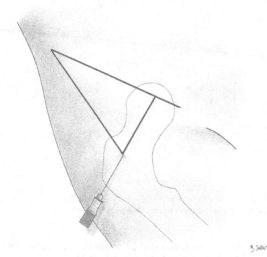

Fig. 8.4 Hip joint
Reproduced by kind permission of Barbara Salas, Copyright © 2016 Barbara Salas.

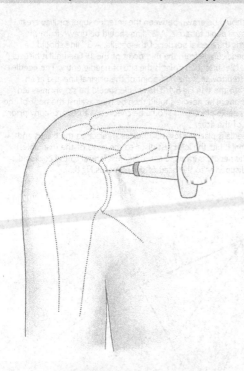

Fig. 8.5 Glenohumeral shoulder joint
Reproduced by kind permission of Barbara Salas, Copyright © 2016 Barbara Salas.

- Elbow: with the elbow flexed to 90° the needle is inserted between the epicondyles and above the olecranon process Fig 8.6.
- Wrist: the needle is inserted just distal to the end of the radius angled at 60° to the dorsal forearm with the wrist slightly palmar flexed Figs 8.7 and 8.8.
- Small joints of fingers and toes: these joints should only be injected by experienced clinicians see Figs 8.9–11. Needle placement should be confirmed by image intensifier or US.

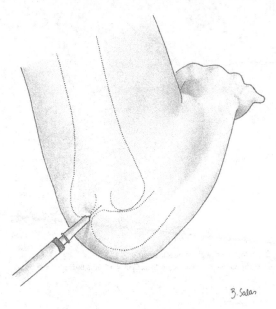

Fig. 8.6 Elbow joint
Reproduced by kind permission of Barbara Salas, Copyright © 2016 Barbara Salas.

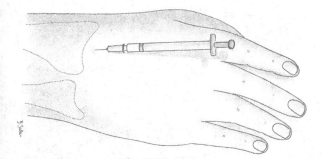

Fig. 8.7 Wrist joint
Reproduced by kind permission of Barbara Salas, Copyright © 2016 Barbara Salas.

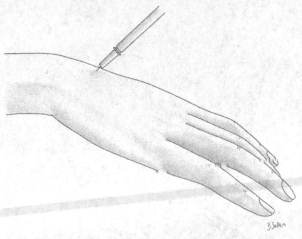

Fig. 8.8 Wrist joint; angle of needle insertion
Reproduced by kind permission of Barbara Salas, Copyright © 2016 Barbara Salas.

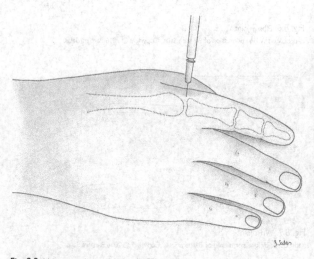

Fig. 8.9 Metacarpophalangeal joint (MCP)
Reproduced by kind permission of Barbara Salas, Copyright © 2016 Barbara Salas.

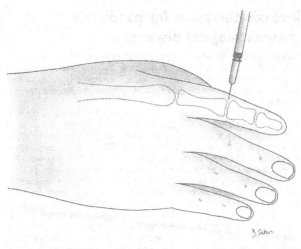

Fig. 8.10 Proximal Interphalangeal Joint (PIP)
Reproduced by kind permission of Barbara Salas, Copyright © 2016 Barbara Salas.

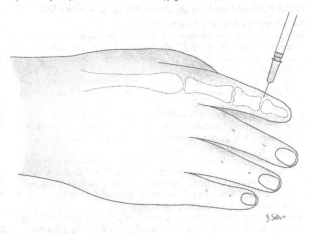

Fig. 8.11 Distal Interphalangeal joint (DIP)
Reproduced by kind permission of Barbara Salas, Copyright © 2016 Barbara Salas.

Further reading

Ryder CAJ, Southwood TR, Malleson PN. Intra-articular corticosteroid injections. In Szer I, Kimura Y, Malleson PN, et al. (eds.) *Arthritis in Children and Adolescents*. Oxford: Oxford University Press, 2006; pp. 442–7.

Biologic therapies for paediatric rheumatological diseases

Biologic agents are genetically engineered drugs designed to target specific areas of the immune system which are implicated in disease aetiology by selectively blocking inflammatory pathways. They include monoclonal antibodies, soluble cytokine receptors and recombinant receptor antagonists (Table 8.1).

It is recognized that early aggressive management of paediatric rheumatological disease is needed to improve short-term and long-term outcomes and this has been much aided by the advent of biologics, particularly in patients who fail conventional treatment with DMARDs. However, a proportion of children do not respond to initial biologic, flare after period of quiescence, or suffer adverse events necessitating cessation of drug.

In JIA the efficacy of biologics has been shown in landmark clinical trials made possible by international multicentre collaboration. There are many reports of efficacy and safety in off-label use of biologics for a range of paediatric rheumatological diseases. There is concern about rare adverse events and long-term safety of biologics with emerging cases of infection, autoimmune disease, malignancy, and demyelination, which highlights the important role of registries to document efficacy and long-term safety as adverse events may not be identified in short-term clinical trials.

NICE guidance on biologic therapies for JIA in the UK

Biologic agents approved by NICE for use in JIA:

- Etanercept was first approved in 2002 for children aged 4–17yr with active polyarticular-course JIA who failed to respond adequately to, or who proved intolerant of, MTX (see ℘ http://www.nice.org.uk/nicemedia/pdf/JIA-PDF.pdf).
  - This 2002 NICE guidance has now been updated: ℘ https://www.nice.org.uk/guidance/ta373; etanercept is now approved from the age of 2yr.
- Initiation of treatment should be in accordance with BSPAR recommendations (see Appendix D in NICE guidelines), undertaken by an experienced consultant together with a nurse specialist who is able to teach families injection techniques.
- Use of tocilizumab in children with systemic JIA aged 2 years and older whose disease has responded inadequately to NSAIDs, systemic corticosteroids and methotrexate (see ℘ https://www.nice.org.uk/guidance/ta238/resources/guidance-tocilizumab-for-the-treatment-of-systemic-juvenile-idiopathic-arthritis-pdf)
- NHS England Interim Clinical Commissioning Policy Statement: Biologic therapies for JIA was published in January 2015 providing guidance on the use of biologic therapies in all subgroups of JIA. This policy is pending any future guidance from NICE ℘ www.engage.england.nhs.uk/consultation/specialised-services-policies/user_uploads/biolgcs-juvenl-idiop-arthrs-pol.pdf

Table 8.1. Use of biologics in paediatric rheumatological diseases

Biologic Agent	Mode of action	Administration	Commonly used doses	Current indications	Licensed
Abatacept	Humanized selective T cell costimulatory modulator	IV infusion (subcutaneous only licensed in adults)	10mg/kg at 0, 2, 4 weeks then 4 weekly afterwards	#Polyarticular JIA (excluding ERA and PsA; not included in RCT). †JIA-associated uveitis	In USA and EU for refractory polyarticular JIA >6yrs
Adalimumab	Humanized soluble anti-TNF monoclonal antibody	Subcutaneous injection (use 40mg in 0.8mL paediatric vials for small doses)	24mg/m² up to 40mg fortnightly Maximum of 20mg in patients 2–<4yrs of age	#Polyarticular JIA. †JIA-associated uveitis. †Systemic vasculitis. †CRMO/SAPHO	Licensed EU for refractory polyarticular JIA in ≥2yrs age and in USA from >4yrs
Anakinra	Humanized anti-IL1 receptor antagonist	Subcutaneous injection	2mg/kg daily (max 100mg) Dose for CAPS depends on response to 2mg/kg; but higher doses have been used	#Systemic JIA,† Cryopyrin-associated periodic syndromes (CAPS).* †CRMO/SAPHO.	Off label for sJIA. Licensed for CAPs in children over 8 months in EU (not USA)
Belimumab	B lymphocyte stimulator (BLyS)-specific inhibitor	Intravenous	10mg/kg 4 weekly	#[in progress]SLE	Adult SLE
Canakinumab	Human anti–IL-1β monoclonal antibody	Subcutaneous	Dose in CAPS dependent on age/weight, increased in line with response up to maximum of 8mg/kg or 300mg 8 weekly 4mg/kg (max 300mg) every 4 week for SJIA	# CAPS #SJIA	In adults and children with CAPS in EU older than 2yrs. In EU licensed for sJIA in patients older than 2yrs but not approved by NICE

Table 8.1 Contd.

Biologic Agent	Mode of action	Administration	Commonly used doses	Current indications	Licensed
Certolizumab	Pegylated anti-TNFα inhibitor	Subcutaneous	200mg every 2 weeks or 400mg every 4 weeks in adults	#in progress JIA (Safety and efficacy in children yet to be established)	In adults with axial spondylo-arthritis or RA
Etanercept	Soluble TNF p75 receptor fusion protein	Subcutaneous	0.4mg/kg twice weekly (max 25mg per dose); 0.8mg/kg once weekly (max 50mg per dose)	#Polyarticular JIA (reduced efficacy in sJIA) †ERA. †PsA †JIA <4yrs of age. †Systemic vasculitis †CRMO/Sz-PHO	EU licence for refractory polyarticular JIA in age 2–17 yrs NICE approval. Licensed >2yrs in USA
Golimumab	Fully humanized monoclonal antibody to soluble and trans-membranous TNFα	Subcutaneous or intravenous infusion	50mg SC for adults or 2mg/kg 8-weekly infusion	#In progress: Polyarticular JIA	In adults with axial spondylo-arthritis or RA.
Infliximab	Chimeric human murine anti-TNF monoclonal antibody	2 hours IV infusion	6mg/kg Initially at 0, 2 & 6 weeks; then at intervals of 4–8 weekly depending on clinical response	# Refractory polyarticular JIA. †JIA-associated uveitis. JSLE † Refractory JDM; Sarcoid †Systemic vasculitis †PSA, ERA #Behcets #Refractory Kawasaki's disease †CRMO/SAPHO	Off label

Rilonacept	Soluble fusion protein of IL-1 receptor and IgG Fc	Subcutaneous	Initial dose 4.4 mg/kg (max 320mg) then once-weekly at 2.2 mg/kg (max 160mg)	#CAPS †SJIA	In adults and children with CAPS in EU & USA (≥12yrs age)
Rituximab	Anti-CD20 antibody (B cell depletor)	IV infusion (often used synergistically with cyclophosphamide & methylprednisolone	750mg/m² (max 1g) on day 0 and day 14	†JSLE; †SJIA †Refractory polyarticular JIA †Refractory JDM †Systemic vasculitis (particularly AAV)	Off label
Tocilizumab	Humanizad anti-IL-6 receptor monoclonal antibody	1 hour IV infusion (SC dosing study in JIA in progress)	8–12mg/kg 2–4 weekly depending on weight and indication	#SJIA #Poly JIA	NICE approval for SJIA Licensed in EU & USA for poly JIA from age 2yrs upwards

* Cryopyrin associated periodic syndromes (CAPS) includes familial cold-induced autoinflammatory syndrome, Muckle-Wells syndrome, and chronic infantile neurologic, cutaneous, articular [CINCA] syndrome (also known as neonatal-onset multisystem inflammatory disease (NOMID).

Level of evidence for efficacy and safety: # indicated clinical trial performed, †indicates case series or observational studies, no symbol indicates clinical use but no paediatric data published.

N.B. Within clinical trials polyarticular refers to any subtype of JIA that involves ≥5 joints, including EOJIA, SJIA, ERA, as well as RhF positive and negative polyarthritis.

- Abatacept, adalimumab, etanercept, tocilizumab for treating JIA [TA373; December 2015) replaces guidance TA35
  - ℘ http://www.nice.org.uk/guidance/TA373
- Adalimumab for children with severe refractory uveitis (November 2015)
  - ℘ https://www.england.nhs.uk/commissioning/wp-content/uploads/sites/12/2015/11/d12x02-paediatric-uveitis-anti-tnf.pdf
- Infliximab not currently licensed for JIA in the UK and NICE have withdrawn infliximab from appraisal at this time.
- Use of biologics for treatment of JDM, JSLE, juvenile scleroderma, and vasculitis (in children) is currently off-label and not under NICE guidance: see relevant chapters.

Assessment checklist prior to commencing biologic therapy

- *Education (verbal and written; ideally provided by rheumatology CNS):*
  - Age appropriate, in format that family understand, with time for reflection to make informed decision.
  - Include knowledge of medication/side-effects, dose needed (mg/mL), appropriate storage of medication (if keeping at home), and safe disposal of medication/equipment.
  - A frank and honest discussion is required to maintain trust between child and healthcare workers (e.g. adalimumab and anakinra injections may hurt).
- *Blood screen:*
  - FBC, ESR, U&E, LFT, CRP, antibody screen (ANA, anti dsDNA, anti ENA), immunity status (measles, varicella IgG), and hepatitis serology where applicable.
- *Measurements:*
  - Accurate height, weight, and surface area to calculate dose of medication.
  - Plot growth chart.
- *Risk assessment for tuberculosis (see ⇒ TB, pp. 384–90):*
  - History—recent visits or previous residence in high-risk countries/close family/friend contact/past history of TB.
  - Baseline CXR for all patients; Mantoux (if not on immunosuppressant/steroid therapy).
  - Consider immunological testing (T spot or QuantiFERON), particularly if high index of suspicion. If positive, treat TB before starting biologic therapy—seek expert advice.
- *Sexual health and contraception:*
  - Effects of biologic therapy on developing foetus unknown and pregnancy should be avoided. Education needed for all young people with potential of being sexually active (best provided by rheumatology CNS).
  - Meaning of confidentiality should be explained to young person and practiced by health professionals.
- *Training on SC injections if applicable:*
  - The CNS/nurse teaching the patient/family must have experience and training in giving SC injections and be confident in ability to teach the patient/family, ensuring competence and safety.

- Important to review injection technique especially if apparent waning of clinical response.
- *Dealing with needle phobia where applicable:*
  - Suitable environment, allowing element of control with help of play specialist / psychologist.
- *Arrange delivery/pick up of medication/equipment:*
  - Homecare delivery services are available to regularly supply medication direct to the patient's home and collect waste/sharps bins.
  - Some companies provide a teaching/assessing service for home administration.
- *Safety checks:*
  - Families must understand the importance of safe handling and disposal of medication and equipment.
- *Vaccinations:*
  - Consider varicella vaccination for non-immune patients if able to delay start of biologic treatment and vaccination not contra-indicated by other immunosuppressive therapy (see ➔ Varicella, pp. 409–11).
  - Families need explicit and written instruction if child is non-immune (e.g. varicella or measles).
  - Live vaccinations (including MMR, varicella, BCG, yellow fever) should *not* be given to patients on biologic therapy or for 6 months after treatment has finished (see ➔ Immunizations, pp. 413–15).
  - Killed vaccinations can be administered safely and are recommended (annual flu vaccine, 5-yearly pneumococcal vaccine, human papillomavirus vaccine).
- *Counselling regarding infection:*
  - Essential that patient and family understand importance of seeking medical advice quickly in event of infection. Biologic treatment may predispose to serious manifestations of common bacterial infections and a low threshold for antibiotics is prudent. Consider opportunistic and atypical infections (see ➔ Infection and the immunocompromised, pp. 69–73).
  - Withhold biologic treatment if child has an infection with raised temperature, but remember that serious infection may be present in the absence of pyrexia in a child receiving immunosuppression.
  - Varicella infection and varicella exposure in the non-immune (see ➔ Varicella, pp. 409–11). In the event of infection, biologic therapy should be stopped until the child is well and the chicken pox lesions have crusted over. If the patient is varicella non-immune and there has been close (family) contacts with chicken pox, give prophylactic VZIG or aciclovir (see ➔ Varicella, pp. 409–11) but the biologic therapy can be continued if the child does not develop lesions beyond the incubation period. It is advisable for a child's school/nursery to inform the family if there is a chicken pox outbreak. Consider vaccination of healthy siblings.
  - Exclude TB prior to starting biologic treatment and have low threshold for investigating for TB if symptomatic on treatment. See ➔ TB, pp. 384–90.

- Counsel regarding increased risk of skin / soft tissue infections, particularly if young people considering piercings / tattoos (regular cleaning advised after piercings).
- *Baseline 'core set criteria'* (see ➜ *Outcome measures, pp. 43–9*)
  - Clearly documented before starting biologic treatment and monitor regularly throughout (recommended 3-monthly for first year).
- *Supply contact details:*
  - Patient/family should have contact details for the hospital/local services including who to contact at weekends/bank holidays if necessary.
- *Follow-up appointments and blood monitoring:*
  - Recommended to be at least every 3 months for the first year.
  - Families to be aware of clinic dates and plans for blood monitoring before discharge.
  - Families to have CNS helpline number.
  - Families to have written instructions when to seek healthcare if child unwell (e.g. febrile) and have open access to day units as necessary.
- *Monitoring and reporting treatment response adverse events:*
  - For etanercept the BSPAR Etanercept cohort study: ℳ https://www.aruk.manchester.ac.uk/bspar/
  - Other agents used in JIA (and in the future, other diseases) the Biologics for Children with Rheumatic Diseases Registry: ℳ http://www.bcrdstudy.org/
  - In the UK suspected adverse reactions are reported through the 'Yellow card scheme': ℳ http://yellowcard.mhra.gov.uk.

Further reading

Beresford MW, Baildam EM. New advances in the management of juvenile idiopathic arthritis – 2: The era of biologicals. *Arch Dis Child Educ Pract Ed* 2009; **94**:151–6.

Gartlehner G, Hansen RA, Jonas BL, et al. Biologics for the treatment of juvenile idiopathic arthritis: A systematic review and critical analysis of the evidence. *Clin Rheumatol* 2008; **27**:67–76.

Ungar W, Costa V, Burnett HF, et al. The use of biologic response modifiers in polyarticular course juvenile idiopathic arthriits: a systematic review. *Sem Arth Rheum* 2013;**42**:597–618.

Woo P. Theoretical and practical basis for early aggressive therapy in paediatric autoimmune disorders. *Curr Opin Rheumatol* 2009; **21**:552–7.

Approvals for the use of biologic therapies

Abatacept (Orencia®), adalimumab (Humira®), canakinumab (Ilaris®), etanercept (Enbrel®) and tocilizumab (RoActemera®) in paediatric rheumatology

- National Institute for Health Care Excellence (NICE) is funded by the Department of Health (UK) to provide independent appraisal of licensed therapies based on efficacy and cost effectiveness.
- NICE guidance (2015) abatacept, adalimumab, etanercept, tocilizumab for treating JIA ℘ http://www.nice.org.uk/guidance/ta373)
- European Medicines Agency (EMA) issues the licenses for drugs used in the UK ℘ www.ema.europa.eu/ema/
- NHS England policy (2015) on biologics describes the use of biologics in JIA including their sequential use based on consensus opinion, emphasizes the need to enroll eligible patients in clinical trials where possible and national registries. (℘ https://www.engage.england.nhs.uk/consultation/specialised-services-policies/user_uploads/biolgcs-juvenl-idiop-arthrs-pol.pdf
- There is currently no NICE guidance for the use of biosimilars in JIA. (℘ https://www.nice.org.uk/guidance/ktt15/resources/biosimilar-medicines-58757954414533)

Licensed and/or NICE approved

- Etanercept is approved by NICE for poly-articular juvenile idiopathic arthritis (JIA).
- Tocilizumab is approved by NICE for systemic-onset JIA.
- Etanercept (2002) NICE technology appraisal guidance [TA35].
- ℘ http://guidance.nice.org/TA35/Guidance/pdf/English.
- Tocilizumab (2011) NICE technology appraisal guidance [TA238].
- ℘ http://guidance.nice.org/TA238/Guidance/pdf/English.
- Abatacept, adalimumab, etanercept, tocilizumab NICE technology appraisal ℘ http://www.nice.org.uk/guidance/TA373)—this replaces TA35.
- NHS England policy (2015) on adalimumab and infliximab as anti TNF treatment options for paediatric patients with severe refractory uveitis. ℘ https://www.engage.england.nhs.uk/consultation/specialised-services-consultation/user_uploads/uveitis-paediatrics-policy.pdf

Licensed but not NICE approved

- Anakinra gained licence for use in CAPS in April 2014.
- Canakinumab gained licence for use in October 2009.

NICE advocates that patients on these biologics undergo long-term monitoring and surveillance (see ➲ Biologics and Guidelines pp. 493–4).

- Patients on etanercept are invited to be recruited to the BSPAR Biologics and New Drug Registry ℘ https://www.aruk.manchester.ac.uk/bspar/
- For all other biologics patients are invited to be recruited to The Extended Biologics Study ℘ http://bcrdstudy.org/.

Emerging information at time of publication

Nov 2015: NHS England have stated they will routinely commission Adalimumab for paediatric patients (aged 2–18yrs) with severe refractory uveitis (JIA and non-JIA-related uveitis). This is on an interim basis pending a full policy following publication of a major UK clinical trial (SYCAMORE).

Further reading

Royal College of Nursing. Assessing, managing and monitoring biologic therapies for inflammatory arthritis: guidance for rheumatology practitioners. London: RCN, 2015. ℘ http://www.rcn.org.uk.

NHS England: Interim Clinical Commissioning Policy Statement: Biologic Therapies for the treatment of Juvenile Idiopathic Arthritis (JIA) January 2015 (NHS England (E03/PS/a) ℘ https://www.engage.england.nhs.uk/consultation/specialised-services-policies/user_uploads/biolgcs-juvenl-idiop-arthrs-pol.pdf.

NHS England: Clinical Commissioning Policy: Adalimumab (Humira) and Infliximab (Remicade) as Anti-TNF Alpha Treatment Options for Patients with Severe Refractory Uveitis. July 2015 (NHS England D12/P/b)

NHS England: Interim Clinical Commissioning Policy Statement: Adalimumab for the treatment of severe uveitis in children. November 2015. (NHS England D12x02) ℘ https://www.england.nhs.uk/commissioning/wp-content/uploads/sites/12/2015/11/d12x02-paediatric-uveitis-anti-tnf.pdf.

Medicines for children and paediatric rheumatology

- Many drugs prescribed for children are used outside the terms of their product licence ('off-label') or are not licensed for any use in the applicable country.
- It is the responsibility of the prescriber to ensure an appropriate evidence base for safety and efficacy exists for an unlicensed use and specific guidance is provided by the General Medical Council 'Good practice in prescribing and managing medicines and devices (2013)' (ℬ http://www.gmc-uk.org/guidance/ethical_guidance/14316.asp).
- The Summary of Product Characteristics (SmPC) for the drug product in question (ℬ http://www.medicines.org.uk/emc) should be consulted to ascertain the licensed indications, dosages, precautions, and possible side effects.

Paediatric pharmacokinetics

Growth and development influence the absorption, distribution, metabolism, and excretion (ADME) of drugs requiring constant adjustment of dosage regimens from birth to adolescence. In addition, it should be noted that:

- Absorption and bioavailability are influenced by the choice of formulation, route, fed/fasted state and concomitant medication for the oral route, and by the need for manipulation of the dosage form, which will additionally affect dose accuracy.
- Metabolism and excretion can be affected by the complexity of some multi-system auto-immune, auto-inflammatory disorders where renal and hepatic involvement may be part of the underlying disease process (e.g. SLE, sJIA, systemic vasculitides) and by concomitant medications that induce or inhibit drug metabolizing enzymes or affect renal function, thus impacting upon efficacy and toxicity which may necessitate dose adjustment or monitoring.
- Drugs with a narrow therapeutic index require close monitoring and dose adjustment (e.g. methotrexate, ciclosporin). Conditions such as nephrotic syndrome can affect drug excretion.

Safety issues

- Manual handling and inadvertent exposure to cytotoxic drugs (methotrexate, azathioprine, cyclophosphamide) must be avoided. Cytotoxic injectables should be prepared in the pharmacy in accordance with national guidance and local management policy on safe preparation and administration.
  - If manipulation (e.g. opening capsules or breaking tablets) is required, it should be referred to the pharmacy; detailed guidelines were developed as independent research commissioned by the National Institute for Health Research (MODRIC—Manipulation Of Drugs Required In Children) available online at (ℬ http://www. alderhey.nhs.uk/wp-content/uploads/MODRIC_Guideline_FULL-DOCUMENT.pdf)

- Be aware of different product strengths available (e.g. methotrexate tablets and unlicensed methotrexate oral liquids) that can lead to dosing errors. Patients and carers should be educated to check every new prescription, dispensed product, and dosing instructions. Recommendations in safety alerts issued for methotrexate should be complied with. For primary care transfer, discharge letters should specify the strength to prescribe (plus manufacturer if difficult to source) and relevant monitoring.
- Monoclonal antibody (mAb) products should be treated as biohazardous—insufficient data exists on low-level long-term exposure to mAbs. Safe preparation and handling guidelines should be followed to minimize staff contamination and patient cross-contamination.

Dose calculation

Children's doses are usually calculated based on body weight (mg/kg) or body surface area (BSA) (mg/m^2) and should be obtained from appropriate paediatric formularies (e.g. BNFC). Several formulae of variable accuracy for estimation of BSA are available. The 2 commonly used equations are the Mosteller equation that provides a simple calculation for BSA based on height and weight and the Boyd equation (used in the BNFC tables) based on weight alone. Points to note:

- For overweight patients (e.g. those exposed to high doses/long-term corticosteroids): consider whether actual body weight or ideal body weight is appropriate to use.
- For NSAIDS, use body weight. Round doses if appropriate to avoid manipulation of dosage forms which leads to dose inaccuracies.
- For drugs with a narrow therapeutic index (NTI) (e.g. cytotoxics), use BSA.
- Consider when dose capping is required—the total daily dose should not exceed the maximum adult daily dose.
- When both body weight and BSA are used for dose calculation, ensure consistency. Check local guidelines on which measure is to be used.
- Methotrexate often causes nausea and vomiting when given orally at higher doses. Consider switching from the oral to SC route to improve tolerability and bioavailability. Currently, the corresponding oral dose is used for the SC route.
- Due to differences in bioavailability between brands, certain oral drug products are not interchangeable (e.g. ciclosporin). Where brand switching is necessary blood levels should be monitored. Such status is usually stated in the BNFC. In general, switching oral formulations, e.g. tablets to liquid (even within the same brand), can affect bioavailability. Check for information on bioequivalence of different formulations of a specific brand in its SmPC.

Considerations for the drug classes used: see ⊇ Guidelines, pp. 465–524

- NSAIDs—the choice of NSAID depends on its side-effect profile, individual efficacy, and tolerance, and availability of age-appropriate formulations.

- Analgesics—step-up protocols from paracetamol, codeine, co-codamol to opioid analgesics must be followed and used as an adjunct to NSAIDs. (𝒮 https://www.gov.uk/drug-safety-update/codeine-for-analgesia-restricted-use-in-children-because-of-reports-of-morphine-toxicity)
- Steroids—for oral therapy the minimum effective dose should be used. Long-term steroid use has osteoporotic side-effects; calcium and vitamin D supplementation and the use of bisphosphonates for prevention and treatment should be considered.
- Mycophenolate mofetil (MMF)—oral treatment for short or long term, FBC must be monitored pre-treatment and regularly thereafter due to high risk of neutropenia development.
- Cytotoxic immunosuppressants:
  - Cyclophosphamide: toxic effects such as malignancy and infertility are related to cumulative doses therefore update the cumulative dose sheet in patient notes after each dose and dose cap as appropriate; consider fluid tolerance issues.
  - Methotrexate: always prescribe the same strength formulation (i.e. 2.5mg tablets) and pay attention to the dosing interval (weekly doses). Homecare providers can greatly improve patient and parent convenience by reducing hospital visits. However, training must be provided and the suitability and competence of the patient/carer to administer medication must be assessed in advance.
- Immunoglobulin: for IgG replacement therapy, be aware that infusion rates vary for the different brands available. Access to immunoglobulin is restricted due to availability/supply issues. Refer to the local/national guidance on clinical prioritization and managing supplies.
- Biologics: biosimilars (similar biological medicinal products) must not be treated as generics since they are not proven to have identical clinical characteristics to the 'reference' biological medicine due to (differences in starting materials, manufacturing processes, and immunogenic reactions). Thus, all biologics and biosimilars should be prescribed by brand name in line with existing recommendations from the Medicines and Healthcare Products Regulatory Agency (MHRA) and the British Society for Rheumatology. Biosimilars are not interchangeable and must not be substituted without appropriate patient monitoring.
- Subcutaneous treatments are preferable to intravenous administration as it enables the child not to miss school.

Issues to consider when selecting oral dosage forms
See Table 8.2.

Table 8.2 Advantages and disadvantages of different dosage forms

Dosage form	Advantages	Disadvantages
Tablets and capsules	Portable, more palatable than liquids especially for drugs where taste is an issue Lower contamination risks (cytotoxics) than liquids (spills/breakages)	Fixed dose Swallowing difficulty Unavailability of higher strength products may require several to be taken or a single unit to be manipulated for lower doses
Dispersible tablets	Overcomes swallowing difficulty More portable than liquids	Fixed dose Limited strengths available Taking proportion of liquid leads to poor dose uniformity & reproducibility
Sustained release tablets & capsules	Reduces number of daily doses, avoids school time doses, interference with activities or sleep May improve compliance	Fixed dose, lack of paediatric PK data in most cases Dosage forms cannot be manipulated Lack of efficacy may complicate dose escalation and add-on therapy (e.g. pain management)
Oral liquids	Dose flexibility, usually flavoured, can be administered via feeding tubes Overcomes swallowing difficulty May provide better/more consistent absorption than solids for patients with GI problems	Palatability, may contain unsuitable excipients such as alcohol, preservatives, colours, sugars (impact on oral health) Inconvenient/bulky for travel
Effervescent products	More convenient to carry than liquids Forms a liquid: overcomes swallowing difficulty	Palatability Need to be fully dissolved in large volume of liquid Compliance with ingesting large volume Usually have high Na^+/K^+—unsuitable for certain groups (e.g. renal patients)

Haematopoietic stem cell transplantation

- In a small proportion of affected children, autoimmune/ autoinflammatory rheumatic disease is severe and/or resistant to conventional treatments, including the biologic DMARDs.
- These children often develop significant side-effects from the long-term treatment with multiple and often combined disease modifying agents.
- This small group of children may benefit from haematopoietic stem cell transplantation (HSCT), and UK national guidance is available for autologous HSCT; whilst allogeneic HSCT is 'generally not recommended'. However, results of rarely performed allogeneic HSCT are surprisingly good.

Autologous T cell depleted (TCD) HSCT for autoimmune disease (AID)

The hypothesis
- Deletion of presumed auto-aggressive lymphocyte clones:
  - Immunosuppressive conditioning (usually anti-T lymphocyte globulin-ATG, cyclophosphamide and fludarabine).
  - T cell depletion (TCD) (usually by CD34+cell selection).
- Newly developing lymphocyte population lead to 're-setting' of the immune system, i.e. self-tolerance.

The evidence
- TCD auto-HSCT for JIA can induce complete remission (CR):
  - Immediate improvement of acute inflammation, due to the immuno-suppressive conditioning regimen.
  - Subsequent improvement in disease activity (CR> 50%), due to 'immunomodulation' (re-establishment of immune tolerance).
  - Albeit may be a transient effect.
  - Significant transplant-related mortality (TRM).

Potential weakness of the hypothesis for sJIA
  - Disease recurrence following long-term remission (7–9 yrs) post autologous HSCT for sJIA.
  - Many now regard sJIA as an autoinflammatory disease rather than an autoimmune disease.
  - Some patients with sJIA have genetic predisposition to haemophago-cytic lymphohistiocytosis (HLH) and there may be some overlap between sJIA/severe macrophage activation syndrome (MAS) with typical primary HLH patients.
  - Induction of self-tolerance by autologous HSCT may thus only provide partial or temporary improvement in those patients.
  - Allogeneic HSCT may arguably be a more logical approach in this subgroup – still an area of ongoing debate, but with emerging sup-porting new evidence.

Inclusion criteria for autologous T cell depleted HSCT for JIA

Severity of disease and persistent disease activity

- Any JIA subtype with a polyarticular course, with persisting active inflammatory disease, total disease duration > 1yr, active disease > 6mo.
- The persistence of active disease should be despite immunosuppressive medication or only controlled with unacceptable drug toxicity (see below).
- The patient must be in a satisfactory general condition—significant end organ disease (e.g. from amyloidosis, hypertension, other major organ involvement or immunosuppression related or other pathology) may or may not preclude autologous HSCT.
- Patients with sJIA should not have uncontrolled active systemic features due to increased risk of MAS at conditioning (see ➲ MAS, pp. 321–4).
- There should be no evidence of active ongoing infection, including with opportunistic organisms.
- Consideration should be given to the potential for improvement in functional disability (previously established joint/bone damage cannot be restored).
- Psychosocial factors need to be considered by the referring team who are likely to know the child and family well, and are best placed to judge how they would cope with autologous HSCT.

Failure of immunosuppressive and anti-inflammatory therapy

- It is difficult to define 'failure of treatment' as treatment options are ever increasing. The key point is to think ahead for severe and 'refractory' cases as the process of auto-HSCT takes time.
- Conventional treatment for JIA is methotrexate, and in the era of emerging novel therapies most patients, prior to consideration of auto-HSCT, will have failed >1 biological therapy and a trial of parenteral methotrexate, each for at least 3–6 months before being deemed 'failure'.
- The use of combination therapy, changing from one to another biological (anti-TNF, anti-IL-1, anti-IL6, etc.) should be considered before auto-HSCT. The downside is that if these approaches fail disease and therapy-related damage may accrue.
- An informal discussion with the transplant team and potential referral for independent assessment may be helpful when dealing with a child with severe, persistently active JIA who has failed immunosuppressive and anti-inflammatory therapy—i.e. disease uncontrolled on:
  - Systemic corticosteroids (>0.3 mg/kg/day) and/or repeated iv pulses of methylprednisolone (30 mg/kg/day) and,
  - High dose methotrexate (≥15 mg/m2/week) given parenterally for >3 months with biologic (failed >2 biologics), given at appropriate doses for > 3–6 months.

Drug toxicity or intolerance to medication as defined by any of the following
- Evidence of corticosteroid toxicity.
- Intolerance of methotrexate (e.g. unacceptable nausea / vomiting despite anti-emetic medication, psychological intervention, and trial of parenteral route; alopecia; severe mucosal ulceration).
- Unacceptable elevation in liver enzymes related to methotrexate or drug induced cytopenia or other toxicity e.g. renal toxicity or hypertension related to ciclosporin.

Allogeneic HSCT for severe childhood autoimmune/autoinflammatory disorders
- Benefit—potentially curative procedure (immune replacement), based on very few case reports:
  - Initially procedures were intended for treatment of coincidental malignancy;
  - Subsequently, procedures undertaken for intentional treatment of severe and recalcitrant autoimmune or autoinflammatory disorders.
- Retrospective survey (35 patients with miscellaneous severe autoimmune diseases (AID); EBMT Working Party/AID, 1984–2007):
  - Complete response in 55%; partial response in further 24%.
  - TRM ~20%
  - Risk of acute/ chronic graft-versus-host disease (GvHD) ~40%.
- Retrospective survey (15 patients with miscellaneous severe autoimmune disease (such as cytopenias, vasculitides) British Society of Blood and Marrow Transplantation 1997–2009)
  - Overall survival at 1 and 5yrs–87% and 65%, resp.
  - Progression free survival at 1 and 5yrs—80% and 65%, resp.
  - Non-relapse mortality at 1yr—13% (infection, pulmonary toxicity/ respiratory failure).
- The risk : benefit ratio—may be further improved
  - Reduced intensity conditioning (immunosuppressive, less myelo-ablative), and
  - Better GvHD prophylaxis (ciclsporin, mycophenolate mofetil).

Notes on HSCT for AID/rheumatic disorders and clinical outcomes
- TRM associated with autologous TCD HSCT is higher (~10–15%) than of non-TCD (~3–5%), almost comparable to that of allogeneic HSCT.
  - The most likely reason for this is the combined effect of conditioning immunosuppression and T cell depletion, leading to severe and prolonged T cell immunodeficiency state (6–12 months).
- HSCT should not be regarded any longer as 'experimental treatment' and should be offered earlier in the course of the disease:
  - If the approach with autologous TCD HSCT is still considered a valid treatment option, it should be brought forward to avoid increased risks of TRM from infectious complications (occurring as a cumulative result of long-term and combined immunosuppression).
  - Experience with allogeneic HSCT for AID/rheumatic disorders is encouraging and this treatment should be offered to selective patients in specialized centres.

Further reading

Abinun M. Haematopoietic stem cell transplantation for rheumatological conditions. *Paediatric Child Health* 2011; 21(12):558–62.

Foster HE, Davidson J, Baildam E, Abinun M, Wedderburn LR; British Society for Paediatric and Adolescent Rheumatology (BSPAR). Autologous haematopoeitic stem cell rescue (AHSCR) for severe rheumatic disease in children: guidance for BSPAR members-Executive summary. *Rheumatology* . 2006:45:1570–1.

Silva J, Glanville J, Ladomenou F, et al. Allogeneic Haematopoietic Stem Cell Transplantation for Systemic Onset Juvenile Idiopathic Arthritis. *Biol Blood Marrow Transplant* 2015; 21:S46.

Snowden JA, Pearce RM, Lee J, et al. Haematopoietic stem cell transplantation (HSCT) in severe autoimmune diseases: analysis of UK outcomes from the British Society of Blood and Marrow Transplantation (BSBMT) data registry 1997–2009. *Br J Haematol* 2012:157(6):742–6.

Clinical guidelines and protocols

ARMA/BSPAR standards of care for children and young people with JIA

- The ARMA (ARthritis and Musculoskeletal Alliance)/BSPAR Standards of Care (SOC) were developed by a working group comprising patients with JIA, their families, and professionals from health and education, and published in 2010. They build on and supersede the previously published BSPAR Standards of Care for JIA.
- The SOC are based on the fundamental principle that all children and young people with JIA have the right to equitable access to the highest quality of integrated services.
- The SOC are primarily aimed at professionals working in paediatric rheumatology, designed to support clinical service development, and delivery in conjunction with colleagues and funding bodies and by being in the public domain, promote awareness of good clinical practice to parents and families affected by JIA. Key standards include:

Standards to improve access, early diagnosis, and treatment

- All healthcare practitioners likely to come into contact with a child with JIA should acquire the necessary clinical skills and knowledge to recognize the condition early.
- Musculoskeletal clinical examination should be included in education and training of medical students and hospital trainees.
- All children and young people with suspected JIA should be referred to a paediatric rheumatology team (PRT) ≤6 weeks of the onset of symptoms and should be seen by the PRT ≤4 weeks of referral, with 45 minutes allocated for the first appointment.
- On diagnosis all children and young people with JIA should have prompt access to a multidisciplinary PRT who must have appropriate experience and training as defined by their relevant professional bodies.
- On diagnosis all children/young people with JIA should have a full assessment of their disease, general health, psychosocial, educational, and pain management needs.
- On confirmation of the diagnosis:
  - Within 6 weeks all patients should have a slit lamp examination performed by an experienced paediatric ophthalmologist or optometrist.
  - Where required, IA corticosteroid injections should be performed by a member of the PRT in ≤6 weeks and SC MTX should be available within ≤4 weeks.

Standards to empower patients and their families by improving information, access to support, and knowledge

- Children and young people with JIA and their families will be encouraged to participate in disease management.

- Information for patients and families must be provided to inform decision-making, and optimize their physical, psychosocial, and emotional development. Information should be provided:
  - In a variety of formats, be developmentally appropriate, and presented in clear simple language avoiding jargon.
  - About JIA, treatment options, and general health issues.
  - About the members of the PRT and how to access them.

Standards to improve access to ongoing and responsive treatment and support

- Patients with active disease should be assessed at intervals not greater than 4 months apart.
- Patients should have regular ophthalmology reviews in accordance with BSPAR/Royal College Guidelines (see Chapter 9 and ➔ Uveitis screening in JIA, pp. 148–51).
- Each patient should have an individualized care plan (pathways for treatment, information on what to do in the event of worsening symptoms), details of national or local support groups, and provision of information for schools and employers.
- Patients and families should have:
  - Access to their named MDT members with direct and easy access during flares of disease.
  - A dedicated telephone helpline managed by the PR clinical nurse specialist.
  - The opportunity to participate in clinical research and clinical trials.
- Paediatric rheumatology clinical networks should have referral pathways, guidelines, and framework for clinical governance.
- Drugs used for the treatment of JIA must be prescribed and monitored in accordance with BSPAR/NICE guidelines (see ➔ Biologics, pp. 448–54) and should be available without undue delay.
- Specialist surgery should be performed by a surgeon with training in the management of JIA and communicating with children and adolescents and who is linked to the paediatric rheumatology clinical network.

Standards to maximize independence, inclusion, and quality of life

- The psychosocial well-being of the child/young person with JIA and their family should be addressed by all professionals (health, education, and community).
- The PRT should encourage and facilitate age-appropriate participation in interests, sport, and community life.
- The educational setting (school and college) should ensure full inclusion of the child/young person with JIA.
- Young people with JIA should be supported to develop the skills to move into employment.
- The child/young person with JIA and their families should be provided with support/strategies to manage distressing aspects of their treatment.

- The child/young person with JIA should be given the skills to disclose their arthritis to others, should they choose to do so.
- Age and developmentally appropriate individualized transitional care for the child/young person with JIA, should take place reflecting early, mid, and late phases of adolescent development (see ➔ Transitional care, pp. 430–2).

Further reading

*** BSPAR/ARMA Standards of Care for Children and Young People with Juvenile Idiopathic Arthritis (hard copy (booklet) published by ARMA 2010. Available online at ℞ http://arma.uk.net/wp-content/uploads/pdfs/Juvenile%20Idiopathic%20Arthritis.pdf

Davies K, Cleary G, Foster H, et al. on behalf of the British Society of Paediatric and Adolescent Rheumatology: BSPAR standards of care for children and young people with juvenile idiopathic arthritis. Rheumatology 2010; 49(7):1406–8.

BSPAR drug information leaflets for parents and families

Medication is a major component in the treatment of rheumatic diseases. It is estimated that half to a third of all medications are not taken as recommended (NICE 2009). Non adherence to medicines is one issue and has a huge impact on the National Health Service not only in the form of wasted medications, admissions to hospital due to flares of disease but on patient's health outcomes. A market research survey in 2009 (℘ http://www.ipsosmori.com/default.aspx) found that patients want more medicines information than they get and that they want it from a variety of sources.

The clinical nurse specialist (CNS) plays a major role in patient and family education about medicines. By providing unbiased evidence-based information the CNS helps patients and carers to participate fully in decision-making about the medication prescribed for them by health professionals. Working as a partner with patients and carers and providing sufficient high quality information on which to base their decisions will help achieve self care, a key government objective. It is important that both patients and carers understand why a drug is being prescribed, the risks and benefits, and the importance of any monitoring required. The CNS needs to have a good understanding of the medicine that is being prescribed including:
- Pre-screening that may be required prior to commencement of drug.
- How to report adverse events (e.g. yellow card system) and awareness of drug alerts (℘ http://www.mhra.gov.uk).
- How to access psychological support/counselling for non-adherence.
- Shared care guidelines with local and tertiary services.

Drug information should initially be given verbally and key messages reinforced with patient information leaflets (PILs) and where appropriate 'signposting' to relevant websites. Guidance for PILs is available (℘ http://www.mhra.gov.uk) and should be:
- Fit for purpose, i.e. appropriate for the intended target group.
- Proof read by a pharmacist for content accuracy.
- Assessed for readability (℘ http://www.plainenglish.co.uk).
- Inclusive of public and patient involvement (℘ http://www.dh.gov.uk).

The following aspects should be included:
- Formulary and generic names of the drug.
- Drug interactions, contraindications, side-effects, monitoring required (blood tests).
- Counselling as appropriate; sexual health, contraception and pregnancy (℘ http://www.brook.org.uk; http://www.fpa.org.uk), alcohol (℘ https://drinkaware.co.uk) and smoking.
- Potential risk of infection. 'Do's and do not's, when to seek medical attention, and travel information (taking medication abroad, insurance, and contact if become unwell).
- Immunizations and impact on live vaccines and avoidance of live vaccines where applicable.
- Formulations available, e.g. liquid, tablet, melt, and its suitability for the patient and family.
- Dose intervals of drug and how they fit around daily activities.

Points relevant to paediatric rheumatology practice
(see ➔ Medicines for children, pp. 457–9)

NSAIDs

- Gastric protection—NSAIDs should be administered with or after food. Gastro protective drugs may be required, especially if symptoms occur or prophylactically if on combination therapies such as prednisolone.
- Sun protection against pseudoporphyria, especially with naproxen.

Corticosteroid

- Gastric protection (as for NSAIDs).
- Weight gain—dietary advice for the whole family.
- Body image and risk of bullying—psychology/counselling support (🕸 http://www.bullying.co.uk).
- Changes in mood and behaviour.
- Acne—seek dermatology opinion for latest treatment.
- Osteoporosis—activity levels, calcium and vitamin D intake.

Second line drugs

- Blood monitoring (see ➔ specific guidance for individual drugs, p. 472).
- Sexual health and pregnancy (consult latest product literature).
- Infection risks.
- Potential hair loss.
- Safe handling and disposal as per local guidelines.

Methotrexate (MTX)

- Use 2.5mg tablets to minimize confusion and medication errors.
- Parenteral administration—RCN document: 🕸 http://www.rcn.org.uk.
- Nausea—the use of antiemetic, change time of dosing and/or split the dose over 24h.
- Liver toxicity—alcohol advice and counselling: 🕸 http://www.nidirect. gov.uk/young-people-and-alcohol-what-are-risks.

Biologics

(🕸 http://www.rcn.org.uk: assessing, managing, and monitoring biologic therapies).

- Need for pre-treatment screening, e.g. TB.
- Long-term unknown side-effects.
- Potential risks of malignancy (see BSPAR statement).
- Risk of serious infections—when to seek medical advice.
- When to stop or omit—i.e. surgery, active infection—temperature >38°C.
- Injection site reactions for SC drugs—apply cold packs pre- and post injection, antihistamine cream/oral.
- IV infusion reactions including potential anaphylaxis.

This section covers some of the issues that should be considered when giving information about treatments. It is important that patients and families feel empowered about their treatment and it is their right to be given a balanced view of all the information available so that they can make informed choices.

Box 9.1 Issues to consider for all DMARDs and biologic therapies (see ➲ Biologics, pp. 448–54)

Blood monitoring
- Age of child.
- Difficulty with venous access.
- Capabilities of local services.
- Distance from home.
- Play therapy/psychology input.
- As infrequent as possible.
- Local anaesthetic cream, cold spray, buzzy bee, cold packs.
- Establish a monitoring agreement with GP.

Travel
- Vaccinations required.
- Letter re: medications.
- Adequate supply of drug.
- Travel insurance.
- Clinic letter.
- Carriage of medicines.

Further reading

PReS Information on Paediatric Rheumatic Diseases—information for families on a wide range of conditions and available in many languages (2016) ✍ http://www.printo.it/pediatric-rheumatology/

BSPAR treatments used in paediatric rheumatology

A current list of available classes of treatments is given below: readers are directed to recommended drug formularies (℘ http//:www.bnf.org. uk) for more details and current guidelines. Patient information leaflets are available on the BSPAR website (℘ http//:www.bspar.org.uk).

- NSAIDs.
- Corticosteroids—oral, IV, intra-articular, and IM.
- Conventional DMARDs: MTX, sulphasalazine, hydroxychloroquine. mycophenolate mofetil.
- Biologic agents (see ➔ pp. 448–54)
  - Anti-tumour necrosis factor α: etanercept, infliximab, adalimumab.
  - T-Cell co-stimulatory inhibitors: abatacept
  - Interleukin-1 inhibitors: anakinra, rilonacept, canakinumab.
  - Interleukin-6 inhibitors: tocilizumab.
  - Anti-B-cell therapy: rituximab.
- Autologous or allogeneic haemopoeitic stem cell transplant—see ➔ p. 461.
- Cyclophosphamide—see ➔, pp. 485–9.

Non-steroidal anti-inflammatory drugs (NSAIDs)

The choice of NSAIDs is based on taste, formulation, convenience of dosing regimen, and side-effect profile (Table 9.1). No Cox-2 inhibitors are licensed for use in children.

Slow-release preparations given in the evening may be helpful for early morning stiffness.

High dose ibuprofen is helpful for symptomatic relief of pericarditis.

Drug interactions

See cBNF for full details, but in general:

- ACE inhibitors: Increased risk of hyperkalemia and renal damage with NSAIDS.
- Warfarin: effect enhanced by NSAIDs.
- MTX: elimination can be reduced by NSAIDs; however, in clinical practice this is not a problem and NSAIDs and MTX are regularly co-prescribed.

Contraindications

Absolute (rare)

- Active or previous peptic ulceration or GI bleeding.
- Severe heart failure.
- Moderate to severe renal impairment.

Relative

- Asthma.
- Coagulation defects.
- Renal, cardiac, or hepatic impairment.

Side-effects

- Gastrointestinal—nausea, abdominal pain, rarely bleeding, ulceration.
  - Ibuprofen has the lowest risk. Apparent intolerance of NSAIDS should raise concern of GI pathology (e.g. *Helicobacter pylori* infection, inflammatory bowel disease).
- Oral health—risk of caries with sugared liquid preparations: use sugar free or tablets where possible.
- Central nervous system—headache, hyperactivity, dizziness, vertigo, anxiety, depression, and tinnitus may occur.
- Haematologic—blood disorders are rare, albeit bleeding times may be prolonged.
- Renal—may provoke renal failure, hypertension in pre-existing renal impairment. Rarely papillary necrosis or tubulointerstitial nephritis (later interstitial fibrosis) leading to renal impairment.
- Skin—NSAIDs may cause pseudoporphyria (photosensitive blistering rash leaving scars—most common with naproxen and in fair-skinned individuals).
- Other rare side-effects—hepatic damage, alveolitis, pulmonary eosinophilia, pancreatitis, eye changes, Stevens Johnson Syndrome, toxic epidermal necrolysis.

Table 9.1 Dosage, administration, formulations of NSAIDs

Drug	Age	Dose	Formulations	Comments
Ibuprofen	>3 months	5–10mg/kg/dose 3–4 doses/day Max.total 2.4g/day	Tablet Suspension/Syrup	Weakest NSAID, but least side-effects May be used up to 6 doses/day in systemic JIA only Associated with aseptic meningitis in SLE Use sugar-free syrups where possible
Naproxen	>2 years	5–7.5 mg/kg/dose 2 doses/day Max.total 1g daily	Tablets Suspension may be available a special order	Good efficacy Generally low incidence of side effects but associated with pseudoporphyria in JIA
Diclofenac	>6 months	1.5–2.5mg/kg/dose 2–3 doses/day Max.total 150mg/day	Tablets Dispersible tablets Suppositories	Similar actions and side effects to naproxen May trigger hepatic porphyria
Piroxicam	See 'dose'	Dose depends on patients weight: <15kg: 5mg 16–25kg: 10mg 26–45kg: 15mg >46kg: 20mg One dose/day Max.total 20mg/day	Tablets Dispersible tabs Also available as 'melts'	More GI side-effects, more serious skin reactions Should not be used 1st line and should only be initiated by physicians experienced in treating rheumatic disease Treatment should be reviewed after 2 weeks and periodically thereafter
Indomethacin	>1 month	0.5–1mg/kg/dose(2mg/kg under specialist supervision) 2 doses/day Max. total 200mg/day	Capsules Suppositories Suspension	Mostly used to treat enthesitis-related arthritis and systemic JIA High incidence of side-effects

Disease-modifying anti-rheumatic drugs (DMARDs): hydroxychloroquine (HCQ)

Hydroxychloroquine is an anti-malarial quinolone with some immuno-modulatory effects.

There is evidence of benefit in SLE, including modifying cardiovascular risk, and in juvenile dermatomyositis (see ➔ separate chapters).

Pre-treatment considerations
- HCQ: 5–6.5mg/kg/day—beneficial for skin and joint disease, may reduce fatigue, and is helpful for long-term cardiovascular protection.
- Baseline bloods including FBC, U+Es, LFTs.

Contraindications
- Absolute:
  - Severe renal impairment- creatinine clearance <10ml/min/1.73m^2.
  - Pre existing maculopathy.
- Relative:
  - Mild/ moderate renal impairment—reduce dose on prolonged use.
  - Neurological disorders (especially a history of epilepsy).
  - Liver disease—avoid concurrent use of hepatotoxic drugs.
  - Severe gastrointestinal disorders.
  - Porphyria conditions.
  - G6PD deficiency.
  - Quinine sensitivity.
  - May exacerbate psoriasis and aggravate myasthenia gravis.

Drug interactions
- Major:
  - Increased risk of ventricular arrhythmias with: amiodarone, moxifloxacin.
  - Increased risk of seizures with: antiepileptics, mefloquine.
  - May increase plasma concentrations of: digoxin, ciclosporin.
  - Avoid other antimalarials: artemether/ luefantrine.
- Minor:
  - Inhibits the effects of: agalsidase beta (used in Fabry's disease), laronidase (used in mucopolysaccaridosis), neostigmine, pyridostigmine.
  - Effect reduced by: kaolin, antacids.
  - Plasma concentrations increased by cimetidine.

Side-effects
- GI disturbance—nausea, diarrhoea, anorexia, abdominal cramps.
- Headache, skin reactions—rash, pruritis. Rarely pigmentary changes, bleaching of hair and hair loss. Visual changes—see above.
- Other: ECG changes, convulsions, ototoxicity.
- Rarely: blood disorders, psychological disturbance, myopathy, Steven Johnson syndrome, acute generalized exanthematous pustulosis, exfoliative dermatitis, photosensitivity, hepatic damage.

Dosage and administration
- Child 1 month–18yrs: 5–6.5mg/kg o.d. Maximum dose: 400mg once daily.

Monitoring
- Blood monitoring—not routinely required.
- Assessment and monitoring of vision: The incidence of HCQ-induced retinopathy is very low and dependent on the maximum dose and duration of treatment. In the UK, the Royal College of Ophthalmologists recommend baseline assessment of renal and liver function, inquiry about visual symptoms, and recording of near visual acuity at each visit and measurement of visual acuity annually. A yearly sight test including colour vision (local optician) is recommended.

Fertility/pregnancy/breast-feeding
- Pregnancy: Not necessary to withdraw antimalarial drug during pregnancy if rheumatological disease is well controlled. However manufacturer advises to avoid- possibly increased risk of cochlear damage.
- Breastfeeding: *Avoid*—risk of toxicity to infant.

Disease-modifying anti-rheumatic drugs: sulfasalazine (SSZ)

The mechanism of action of SSZ is unclear. Despite being licensed for use in JIA, it is not widely used.

Pre-treatment investigations

FBC, U&E, creatinine, LFTs.

Contraindications

- Absolute:
  - Hypersensitivity to sulphonamides, co-trimoxazole or aspirin.
  - Children < 2 years, severe renal failure.

Relative

- Systemic JIA: use has been associated with macrophage activation syndrome.
- G6PD deficiency: risk of haemolysis.
- Moderate renal impairment: crystalluria may develop—ensure high fluid intake.
- Slow acetylators (especially if predisposing haplotypes present): potential risk of drug-induced lupus—withdraw treatment if clinically suspected.

Side-effects

Up to 20% of children experience dose-related side-effects:

- GI disturbance (most common)—nausea, anorexia, dyspepsia, diarrhoea.
- Dermatological—photosensitive rash, hypersensitivity reactions, oral ulcers.
- Haematological—neutropenia, thrombocytopenia, macrocytic anaemia.
- Drug-induced SLE, Raynaud's, interstitial pneumonitis, fibrosing alveolitis, hepatitis.
- Staining of soft contact lenses and orange discolouration of urine.
- Others: fever, headache, dizziness.

Dosage and administration

- 1st week: 5 mg / kg twice-daily.
- 2nd week: 10 mg / kg twice-daily
- 3rd week: 20 mg / kg twice-daily
- Maintenance dose: 20-25 mg / kg twice daily.
  - Max. Dose 2g/day (2–12yrs) or 3g/day (12–18yrs).
  - Time to response: minimum of 3 months.

Monitoring

- Check for G6PD before starting.
- After checking FBC and LFTs monthly for 3 months the same monitoring regime as for methotrexate is recommended.

Fertility/pregnancy/breast-feeding

- Fertility: reversible oligospermia has been reported.
- Pregnancy: theoretical risk of foetal haemolysis in 3rd trimester. Folic acid should be offered to all pregnant women taking SSZ and total dose should not exceed 2g/day.
- Breast-feeding: Theoretical risk of neonatal haemolysis—especially in G6PD-deficient infants.

Disease-modifying anti-rheumatic drugs (DMARDs): mycophenolate Mofetil (MMF)

MMF works by inhibiting monophosphate dehydrogenase—an important enzyme in T- and B-lymphocytes mitosis. It is licensed in the UK for children >2yrs for the prophylaxis of acute rejection in renal transplantation. In rheumatology it is most widely used 'off-licence' in the treatment of systemic vasculitides including SLE.

Pre-treatment investigations

- Advise adequate contraception in sexually active females of child-bearing age.
- FBC, liver transaminase levels, serum creatinine.
- Varicella immunity status (consider also checking measles status). Consider immunization *before treatment* starts if child is non-immune.
- Consider testing for TB in high risk individuals.
- Important aspects of patient education:
  - Patients taking MMF are immunosuppressed during and for ≥3 months after stopping treatment.
  - Live vaccines are all contraindicated; inactivated vaccines are safe, but may have reduced efficacy. Annual flu vaccine and 5 yearly pneumovax advised. (See ➔ Vaccines, pp. 413–15).

Contra-indications

Absolute
- Known hypersensitivity to MMF.
- Pregnancy—this applies to both females and male partners who are taking MMF (See ➔ Pregnancy, pp. 433–6).
- Chronic/active infection.

Relative
- Reduce dose in renal impairment.
- Gastric/ duodenal ulceration.

Drug interactions

- Absorption of MMF reduced by antacids, oral iron salts, and cholestyramine.
- Plasma concentration of active metabolite of MMF reduced by rifampicin.
- For full list see BNF.

Side-effects

- GI disturbances—including ulceration and bleeding.
- Hepatitis.
- Renal failure.
- Malignancy—particularly skin.
- Blood disorders.
- Foetal abnormalities.

Dosage and administration
- Child 1month—18yrs: 10–20mg/kg bd. Usual maximum dose 1g bd.

Monitoring
- FBC, U&E, creatinine, LFTs weekly for 4 weeks, then 2-weekly for 2 months, then monthly.
- If recurrent infections develop check immunoglobulin levels.

Fertility/pregnancy/breast-feeding
- Pregnancy—contraindicated. MMF is a known teratogen and effective contraception is needed in sexually active patients during treatment and for at least 6 weeks after treatment is discontinued.
- Breastfeeding—manufacturer advises avoid.

Disease-modifying anti-rheumatic drugs (DMARDs): Methotrexate (MTX)

MTX is first line DMARD for JIA and used in many other rheumatic conditions (see ➲ JIA p. 162). MTX is an antagonist of Folic acid but its exact mechanism of action as a DMARD is unclear.

Before commencing MTX the following should be checked:

- FBC, liver transaminase levels, serum creatinine.
- Varicella immunity status (consider also checking measles status). Consider immunization *before treatment* starts if child is non-immune and seek specialist advice from paediatric infectious diseases when planning treatment. (See ➲ Vaccines pp. 413–15.)
- Consider testing for TB in high risk individuals.
- Important aspects of patient education:
  - Patients taking MTX are immunosuppressed during and for ≥3 months after stopping treatment.
  - Live vaccines are all contraindicated; inactivated vaccines are safe, but may have reduced efficacy. Annual flu vaccine and 5 yearly pneumovax advised. (See ➲ Vaccines pp. 413–15.)
  - Alcohol: there is no safe proven intake limit in children. In older adolescents (>14 years), a maximum of 5 units/week is widely regarded as safe.
  - MTX is a teratogen; pregnancy must be avoided and reliable contraception is needed in sexually active females. Male patients should not father a child whilst on MTX although evidence for this advice is lacking.
- Trimethoprim-containing antibiotics are avoided (risk of toxicity increased).
- Folic acid supplementation may reduce side-effects. Widely used regimens include: 5mg given weekly, 3 days after MTX; or 1mg given daily, except on day MTX is given.

Side-effects

- Nausea, vomiting, and anorexia. These are very common and are the most common reason for stopping treatment with MTX. It may be helped by:
  - Ondansetron given orally 1 hour before MTX, and 8hrs afterwards as needed.
  - Dividing the weekly dose and giving 12 hours apart.
  - Giving subcutaneously rather than orally.
  - Daily folic acid (except MTX dosing day).
  - Clinical psychology may help anticipatory nausea.
- Hepatotoxicity: Irreversible liver damage extremely rare in children. Transient elevation of liver enzymes is common (often during/after intercurrent viral infection).
- Headaches, hair loss, mood changes. Less common.
- Bone marrow suppression: Extremely rare, but potentially fatal. More likely after the first year MTX.
- Pulmonary fibrosis & renal toxicity: extremely rare in children.

Dosage and administration

- Usual starting dose 10–15mg/m^2 / once weekly SC or oral.
  - IV route may be used in patients attending for regular IV biologic infusions.
  - Doses up to 25mg/m^2/dose are used but efficacy unclear and side-effects common at higher doses.
- SC route gives optimal bioavailability.
- Intramuscular administration is more painful and confers no advantage over SC.
- Auto-injector pens are available at various doses and may optimize tolerance.

Monitoring

- FBC, and either aspartate (AST) or alanine (ALT) aminotransferase levels at 2–4 monthly intervals. Serum creatinine at 6-monthly intervals.
- The recommendations given in Table 9.2 are from BSPAR and are consensus based.

Table 9.2 BSPAR recommendations for monitoring MTX

Monitoring Parameter	Action
AST or ALT >3 times upper limit of normal reference range	Consider omitting MTX for 1–2 weeks and repeating blood test.
WCC <3.0×10^9/l (or steadily falling).	May necessitate dose reduction, or rarely discontinuation. Avoid abrupt cessation as may result in disease flare.
Neutrophils <1.5×10^9/l (or steadily falling).	
Lymphocytes <0.5×10^9/l (or steadily falling).	Consider other more common causes for abnormal blood test results.
Platelets <150×10^9/l (or steadily falling).	
New or worsening unexplained dyspnoea or cough.	Consider omitting MTX whilst investigating cause.
Rising creatinine (falling creatinine clearance).	Seek renal opinion.
Rash or unexplained bruising, temperature above 38.5°C or chicken pox contact in non-immune patients.	Patient must be reviewed by medical team prior to continuing with MTX.

Reproduced with permission from British Society for Paediatric and Adolescent Rheumatology, *Methotrexate use in Paediatric Rheumatology: Information for health professionals*, Copyright © 2013, available from http://80.87.12.43/includes/documents/cm_docs/2016/b/bspar_guideline_for_methotrexate_2013.pdf

Azathioprine

Azathioprine is mainly used primarily to treat patients with vasculitis or inflammatory bowel disease. It takes approximately 2–4 months to achieve its effect.

Pre-treatment consideration/testing

- FBC, U&Es, creatinine, LFTs, urinalysis, zoster immune status, thiopurine methyltransferase (TPMT) activity.
- In renal or hepatic impairment dose should be reduced and frequency of blood monitoring for toxicity ↑.
- Severe myelosuppression may occur due to TPMT deficiency, an enzyme necessary in the catabolic pathway for azathioprine. Pre treatment testing of TPMT activity identifies those with TPMT deficiency (azathioprine contraindicated), low activity (azathioprine recommended to be started at a lower dose and ↑ with careful monitoring) and normal activity (full azathioprine dose can be commenced). Myelosuppression can also occur in individuals with normal TPMT activity and therefore ongoing monitoring in all patients is recommended.
- Theoretical ↑ risk of malignancy.

Contraindications

Absolute

- Hypersensitivity to azathioprine or mercaptopurine (as per BNF contraindications).
- TPMT deficiency.

Relative

- TPMT low activity (prescribe at lower dose; see above). See ➲ Pre-treatment considerations/ testing, p. 481)
- Pregnancy.

Drug interactions

Major

- Allopurinol—enhanced effects and ↑ toxicity of azathioprine when given with allopurinol (reduce dose of azathioprine to 1/4 of the usual dose).
- ↑ haematological toxicity seen with trimethoprim and co-trimoxazole.
- Avoid concurrent use of other drugs that suppress the bone marrow.

Minor

- For a full list of drug interactions please refer to the BNFC.

Side effects

- Nausea/vomiting/diarrhoea—usually dose-related, responds to reducing the dose. Occasional patients show an idiosyncratic reaction with abdominal pain and severe vomiting; in these patients azathioprine must be discontinued permanently.
- Haematological—bone marrow suppression usually dose related. Sore throat, bruising, severe mouth ulcers, or fever necessitates an urgent

FBC. Stop treatment and discuss with rheumatologist caring for the patient if:
- White cell count <3.5 × 10⁹ /L.
- Neutrophil count <1.5 ×10⁹ /L.
- Platelet count <150 × 10⁹ /L.
- Rashes/mouth ulcers—usually mild but severe rash or mucosal ulceration is an indication to stop treatment.
- Hair loss—this is usually insignificant and reversible on stopping.
- Liver toxicity his is an occasional problem. If liver transaminases are > 2× levels then azathioprine should be stopped.
- Flu-like illness—this may be 2° to azathioprine immune-mediated reaction and the drug should be stopped.

Dosage and administration
- *Starting dose:* 1mg/kg/day (max. 50mg) taken with/after food. Total daily dose may be given in 2 divided doses.
- *Increments:* 0.5–1mg/kg/day every 2–4 weeks if no side effects, depending on clinical condition and response.
- *Maximum:* 3mg/kg/day (doses of > 200mg/day in adults are seldom necessary).

Monitoring
All patients on azathioprine should carry monitoring cards in which the results of each blood test are recorded.
- FBC and LFTs should be checked fortnightly for the first 8 weeks and for 4 weeks after an ↑ in the dose. FBC should be checked monthly once the dose is stable.
- LFTs should be checked 3-monthly once the dose is stable except in hepatic impairment when LFTs should be checked monthly.

Fertility/pregnancy/breastfeeding
- There have been reports of premature birth and low birth-weight following exposure to azathioprine, particularly in combination with corticosteroids. Spontaneous abortion has been reported following maternal or paternal exposure.
- Azathioprine is teratogenic in *animal* studies.
- Breastfeeding—teratogenic metabolite present in milk in low concentration but no evidence of harm in small studies—consider if potential benefit outweighs risk.

Intravenous cyclophosphamide

Cytotoxic drugs such as cyclophosphamide act predominantly on rapidly dividing cells, such as T and B lymphocytes, and are therefore immuno-suppressive and anti-inflammatory, as well as having anti-cancer properties. Pulse IV cyclophosphamide may be used for the treatment of some vascu-litic disorders (e.g. PAN, AAV, TA), systemic lupus erythematous (SLE), and dermatomyositis.

Potential adverse effects

- Includes bone marrow suppression, GI symptoms, haemorrhagic cystitis, and hair loss. Males may be rendered azoospermic. Amenorrhoea and female infertility can occur with an increase in risk with increasing age over 25 years.
- Cyclophosphamide is contraindicated in pregnancy.
- Contact with infectious diseases should be avoided as far as possible during the period of cyclophosphamide therapy and infections should be treated vigorously.

Dose

- Cyclophosphamide IV 500–1000mg/m² per dose (based on National Institutes of Health (NIH) protocol, usual starting dose 500mg/m²; maximum dose 1.2g).
- The NIH protocol is often used but alternative regimens exist including the Birmingham Vasculitis protocol of which there are several modified versions. One example is as follows:
  - Dose: 15mg/kg (maximum 1g) of cyclophosphamide given by IV bolus over 15mins every 2 weeks for 3 doses, then every 3 weeks for 3 doses, then every 4 weeks for 3 doses.
  - After each dose of cyclophosphamide the patient may also receive 30mg/kg of methylprednisolone (maximum 1g) over 6hrs in their post-hydration fluid.
  - The use of ondansetron and sodium 2-mercapto-ethanesulphonate (MESNA) is the same as for the NIH protocol.
  - Another increasingly referred to protocol is the 'EUROLUPUS' protocol used in a trial involving adults with lupus nephritis: 6 fort-nightly pulses at a fixed dose of 500 mg IV every 2 weeks (again with MESNA as per above)

Investigations

Each dose is preceded by a FBC, U&Es, LFTs, and creatinine. Dosage should be reduced or delayed if there is evidence of bone marrow suppression, particularly if neutrophils are less than 1.5×10^9L; and/or total WCC is < 4×10^9L. Bone marrow suppression is most likely to occur 7–10 days fol-lowing administration of the dose so the full blood count should be checked at this time. Urine should be monitored for haematuria and proteinuria throughout the treatment period.

Suggested guidance for dosing based on total WCC is provided in Table 9.3.

Table 9.3 IV cyclophosphamide dosing

WCC (total) level on day of pulse or day before pulse	CYC dose	Adjustment for next doses
≥4 × 10⁹/L	500mg/m² for first dose Then increase to 750mg/ m² thereafter. (Maximum 1.2g per dose)	750mg/m² or previous adjusted dose* If hepatic impairment or GFR <30ml/min/1.73m² dose reduced to 80%
<4x10⁹/L	Cancel pulse Recheck FBC weekly until leukocyte >4	Once >4, reduce previous dose by 25%
Nadir total WCC (**10–14 days after a pulse)– even if total WCC >4 immediately prior to next dose		
Total WCC 1–2 × 10⁹/L		Reduce dose of last pulse by 40%
Total WCC 2×3 × 10⁹/L		Reduce dose of last pulse by 20%

* Previous dose is the last dose actually administered to the patient.

** For the second and third doses, the nadir blood test will be performed at day 13–14 which coincides with the dose immediately prior to the infusion.

NB: for GFR <30 mls/min/1.73 m² and/or significant hepatic impairment the CYC dose will be reduced to 80% dosing e.g. 750 mg/m² would be reduced to 600 mg/m².

Administration

- The dose is given with MESNA cover (120% of cyclophosphamide dose) with IV hydration, to reduce the incidence of haemorrhagic cystitis, and with ondansetron to reduce nausea.
- MESNA is a sulphydryl-containing compound that is excreted in the urine. Co-administration with alkylating agents, such as cyclophosphamide significantly reduces their urotoxic effects by reacting with the metabolites in the urinary system.
- For patients with a history of haemorrhagic cystitis the total MESNA dose may be increased in 20% increments up to 180%. Administration time for the cyclophosphamide is increased, and the hydration time may also be increased to 16–20h.
- For those patients who have an allergic reaction to MESNA a revised protocol is used: give IV cyclophosphamide over 1h. Omit MESNA, but ensure patient is adequately hydrated and increase hydration fluids to 125mL/m²/h for 12h.

Sequence of administration

See cyclophosphamide infusion chart, Fig. 9.1.

- 15min before cyclophosphamide slow IV bolus of ondansetron 5mg/m^2 (max 8mg), *and*
- MESNA (20% cyclophosphamide dose) IV bolus over 15min.
- Cyclophosphamide (20mg/mL concentration) given over at least 10min via 3-way tap into hydration fluids, with the patient supine.
- *Hydration with:* MESNA (100% cyclophosphamide dose) in 2.5% glucose/0.45% NaCl run over 12h at 85mL/m^2/h.
- Ondansetron 4mg (4–12 years) or 8mg (over 12 years) orally twice a day for 2 days if required.
- If emesis is still a problem despite ondansetron an IV dose of dexamethasone 100microgram/kg (maximum 4mg) may also be given.

Take care to ensure that the IV cannula is correctly sited and that saline flushes in easily before administering cyclophosphamide. If extravasation occurs, the duty plastic surgery team is contacted.

Personal protective equipment

Personal protective equipment (PPE) is necessary when preparing, handling, and administering cytotoxic drugs, to minimize the risk of accidental contamination.

Infection and the patient on cyclophosphamide

Patients receiving cyclophosphamide are highly vulnerable to all infections, and the manifestations of infection may be less clinically obvious. This is particularly important in those patients with indwelling venous catheters.

INTRAVENOUS PRESCRIPTION CHART

CHEMOTHERAPY

WARD

SURNAME	FIRST NAME	HOSP NUMBER	D.O.B	WEIGHT:	DATE:	HEIGHT	SURF AREA	ALLERGIES?
			AGE	WEIGHT:	DATE:			

DATE	IV FLUID	VOLUME	ADDITIVES	RATE	DURATION	DRS SIG	DATE & TIME	NURSE UNIT	NOTES
–0:15	*CYCLOPHOSPHAMIDE*		Ondansetron_____mg	Slow IV bolus					5mg/m^2 (max 8mg)
–0:15			Mesna___________mg	Slow IV bolus	Over 15 mins				20% Cyclophosphamide dose
0:00			Cyclophosphamide__mg	Slow IV bolus	Over at least 10 mins				Give via 3-way tap into hydration fluids
0:00	Glucose 2.5%/ Sodium Chloride 0.45%	ml	Mesna___________mg (_______mg per 500ml bag or_______mg per 1000ml bag)	ml/hr	12hr				Hydration rate = 85ml/m^2/hr Mesna dose =100% Cyclophosphamide dose

Fig. 9.1 Cyclophosphamide infusion chart.

Prophylaxis

Should be commenced at the start of therapy and should only be discontinued after discussion with the consultant paediatric rheumatologist/nephrologist, and not within 2 months of finishing treatment:

- **Bacteria and *Pneumocystis jirovecii*:** Co-trimoxazole (Septrin®): 450 mg/m^2 twice daily (max. 960 mg twice daily) for 3 days a week (either consecutively or alternate days; dose regimens may vary locally). Alternatively, children under 5yrs could receive 240mg od, and those over 5yrs 480mg od. Patients unable to take co-trimoxazole may be offered once-daily azithromycin 10mg/kg (max 500 mg) as an alternative; this is usually taken 3 days per week (e.g. Monday/Wednesday/Friday)
- **Fungal:** Patients with JSLE and those with significant immunosuppression, especially if neutropenic (total neutrophil count <1.0) should receive once-daily itraconazole prophylaxis 5mg/kg/day. To protect against Aspergillus a trough level of >0.5mg/L is needed so the level should be checked after 1–2 weeks of treatment and the dose altered accordingly.
- **Viral:** Prophylaxis against herpes viruses with acyclovir is not routinely needed but non-immune children with complex immunosuppression, especially if lymphopaenic (<1) may benefit. Children in contact (same room for >15mins, or face to face contact) with varicella or measles should be dealt with as follows:

Known immunity

No treatment but child must be fully undressed and examined by parent/carer twice a day and if spots develop admitted to hospital. For children who are very heavily immunosuppressed with a Varicella contact consider giving prophylactic oral aciclovir 10mg/kg/dose qds for 7 days (discuss with consultant first).

Unknown/non-immune

Within 72 hrs of exposure these children may be given either of the following:

Exposure to varicella:

- Zoster immunoglobulin (ZIG): consider IVIG if child is thrombocytopaenic as IM ZIG may cause excessive bruising:
  - <5yrs of age: 250mg.
  - 5–10yrs: 500mg.
  - >10yrs: 750mg.
- Oral acyclovir: 10mg/kg/dose QDS for 7 days.

Exposure to measles:

Children are infectious from 3 days before onset of rash until desquamation (usually ~4days). Children within 6 days (most effective if within 3 days) of contact should receive normal human immunoglobulin (HI):

- Normal HI
  - <1yr: 250mg IM.
  - 1-2yr: 500mg IM.
  - >2yr: 750mg IM.
- Standard immunoglobulin may be used only if normal HI not available. Dose is 0.2mg/kg given IV.

Patients taking cyclophosphamide should have access to urgent paediatric assessment with:

- Single episode of fever >38.5C.
- Two episodes of fever > 38C within 24h.
- Close contact with infectious disease (e.g. varicella). This normally refers to 'kissing contacts' such as close family members rather than schoolfriends, but patients are also at risk if they have been in the same room as an infectious person for longer than 15mins. If in doubt parents should seek advice (see ➲ Varicella zoster infections, pp. 409–11).
- Parental/patient concern. Especially in the presence of symptoms that may indicate infection (even without documented pyrexia) such as nausea, vomiting, diarrhoea, cough, coryza.
- Any evidence (even 1 spot) of chickenpox, zoster (shingles), or herpes simplex (cold sore).

In all circumstances where an acute infection is suspected the patient MUST be reviewed on the paediatric ward as soon as possible (ideally within the hour) and the following checked:

- FBC (note however that, although profoundly immunosuppressed, the WCC may be: normal; low due to previous cyclophosphamide; or raised due to steroid therapy).
- ESR and CRP.
- U+E, creatinine, LFTs.
- Blood cultures.
- Urine cultures.

Other investigations such as throat swabs, cough swabs, viral PCR, lumbar puncture, etc. should be done if clinically indicated but are not routine; however, if respiratory signs are present (e.g. hypoxia, tachypnoea) then pneumocystis infection must be considered. These patients will almost always need admission and IV antibiotics. They must be discussed with the consultant paediatric rheumatologist/nephrologist if admitted during normal working hours. Antibiotic regimes may vary according to individual circumstances but in general the following regimes are applicable in patients with normal renal function (for patients with impaired renal function this *must* be discussed with the nephrologist on-call before starting treatment):

- Central line in situ: teicoplanin 6mg/kg 12hourly for 3 doses then once-daily and meropenem 20mg/kg tds (max 2g).
- No central line: ceftazidime 50mg/kg tds (max. 2g) and gentamicin 5mg/kg od, or meropenem 20mg/kg tds (max 1g) and gentamicin 5mg/kg od.
- Varicella (chickenpox or shingles): IV aciclovir 500mg/m^2/dose 8-hourly for at least 5 days, and then prophylaxis with oral acyclovir 10mg/kg/dose twice a day until at least 2 months after finishing cyclophosphamide.

Further reading

Boumpas I., Austin HA, 3rd, Vaughan EM, et al. Risk for sustained amenorrhea in patients with systemic lupus erythematosus receiving intermittent pulse cyclophosphamide therapy. *Ann Intern Med* 1993;119: 366–9.

Brogan PA, and Dillon MJ The use of immunosuppressive and cytotoxic drugs in non-malignant disease. *Arch Dis Child* 2000;83: 259–64.

Pamidronate

Pamidronate is one of bisphosphonate family of drugs. It works by inhibiting the action of osteoclasts and thus promoting ↑ in bone density. In children it has a long-standing role in the treatment of children with osteogenesis imperfecta (but has also been used to treat congenital or steroid-induced osteoporosis, bone pain due to osteoporotic vertebral or sacral insufficiency fractures (see ➔ Metabolic bone disease, pp. 358–61), chronic recurrent multifocal osteomyelitis (CRMO), and synovitis acne pustulosis hyperostosis osteitis syndrome (SAPHO) (see ➔ CRMO pp. 313–15).

Contraindications

Absolute

Patient must not be hypocalcaemic and should be taking regular calcium and vitamin D3 supplements.

Relative

Caution must be used in renal impairment. Patients should be well hydrated and pamidronate should not be given if creatinine clearance is <30mL/min/1.73m².

Drug interactions

↑ risk of hypocalcaemia when given with aminoglycoside antibiotics.

Side-effects

(See BNFC for full listing.)

- Hypocalcaemia—maximum effect occurs a few days post administration.
- Hypophosphataemia.
- Fever and flu-like reactions.
- Transient bone pain—this can be quite severe.
- Nausea, vomiting, headaches, arthralgias, myalgias, diarrhoea, and rash.
- Acute renal failure has been reported, especially in pre-existing renal impairment.

Dosage and administration

- Usual dose is 1mg/kg given once a day for 3 days every 3 months. However, because of the risk of fever and flu-like reactions the dose on the 1st day of the first ever infusion given is often reduced to 0.5mg/kg. All subsequent doses are 1mg/kg.
- Pamidronate is dissolved in a 250mL bag of 0.9% saline and given by IV infusion over 2h. In patients requiring lower fluid volumes the maximum stated concentration is 60mg/250mL for Aredia® and 90mg/250mL for Medac® and longer infusion times may be needed accordingly.

Monitoring

- Patients with osteoporosis or osteogenesis imperfecta should all have a DEXA scan done before starting pamidronate and yearly whilst receiving ongoing treatment. Children with CRMO or SAPHO syndromes do not need this checking.

- Before commencing infusion—check FBC, ESR, U&Es, LFTs, Ca, Mg, CRP.
- During infusion—monitor temperature, pulse, and BP:
  - At baseline.
  - After 15 min, 30min, 1h, 90min, and at completion.
  - Children should remain for 1h after completion of pamidronate infusion.

Epoprostenol/iloprost

Epoprostenol (prostacyclin), and its synthetic analogue iloprost may be used to treat severe Raynaud's syndrome where digital infarction is likely. Both are given by IV infusion via a syringe driver to ensure accurate and consistent dosing (see **➜** Overlap syndromes pp. 288–92).

Contraindications

- *Absolute*: severe coronary heart disease, pulmonary veno-occlusive disease where there is risk of haemorrhage.
- *Relative*: half the dose of iloprost in liver disease.

Side effects

- Hypotension.
- Facial flushing.
- Bradycardia.
- Nausea.
- Sweating.
- Abdominal discomfort.
- Headaches.

Dosage

Epoprostenol

Between 1 and 5 nanogrammes (ng) per kg bodyweight per minute (1–5ng/kg/min).

- The rate is started at 1ng/kg/min.
- ↑ rate every 20min as tolerated up to 5ng/kg/min.
- Once the maximum rate is achieved this is continued for a further 5–7h (depending on tolerance and patient convenience). This is given daily, for 1–5 days. Doses of 1–20ng/kg/min (or higher) continuously for many days have been used to treat peripheral ischaemia due to vasculitis, under expert supervision only.

Iloprost

Between 0.5 and 2ng/kg/min. Start at 0.5ng/kg/min and increase as for epoprostenol to maximum of 2ng/kg/min. Run for 6h/day for 3–5 days.

Monitoring

Postural hypotension may be marked and patients should be nursed lying down.

BP and pulse should be measured:

- Every 20min for the first hour.
- Every 30min thereafter until finished.

Fertility/pregnancy/breastfeeding

Toxic in animal studies during pregnancy so manufacturers advise to avoid, no information available for breastfeeding.

Etanercept (Enbrel®)

(See ➲ Biologics pp. 448–54)

Clinical/drug information summary

Etanercept blocks the action of the pro-inflammatory cytokine tumour-necrosis factor-α (TNF-α). It is licensed for use in JIA and approved by NICE for children whose disease is not well controlled by, or who are intolerant of SC MTX. Etanercept may take between 2 and 12 weeks to become effective.

Pre-treatment investigations

Before starting etanercept the following should be checked:
- FBC, urea, creatinine & electrolytes, LFT.
- Auto-antibody screen including anti-nuclear antibody (ANA) and anti-dsDNA.
- TB screening: this may take several forms but most include a combination from CXR, Mantoux test, and/or QuantiFERON-Gold or similar immunological test.
- Varicella zoster immune status—as for methotrexate.

Before starting etanercept the patient / carer must be informed of the following:
- Pregnancy and breast-feeding—there is insufficient data to suggest either are safe.
- Tattoos and body piercing—there is an increased risk of soft-tissue infections described in children taking anti-TNF treatment so counselling advised.

Contra-indications

- Chronic active infection or recent severe infection.
- Known / suspected TB.
- Previous history of demyelinating disease.
- Previous history of, or susceptibility to, malignancy.

Drug interactions

There are no specific drug interactions reported for this drug but combining its use alongside other 'biologic' treatments is not recommended.

Side-effects

- Immunosuppression—particularly soft-tissue infections, and re-activation of latent TB.
  - Good skin / nail care important (ingrowing toenails can become infected).
- Injection site inflammation is common, but usually improves with continued use.
- Generally well tolerated. Reports of exacerbation of eczema, headache, dizziness, rash, abdominal pain, or indigestion.
- Neutropenia.
- Demyelinating diseases—case reports but causal relationship with etanercept is unclear.

- Malignancy—theoretical concern but no evidence to date in paediatric use.
- Anecdotal reports of worsening of pre-existing uveitis, or de-novo uveitis so caution is advised, especially if used as monotherapy.

Dosage and administration
- Dose: Usual starting dose 0.4mg/kg given SC twice a week—may be increased up to 0.8mg/kg if necessary in refractory disease.
- Maximum dose: Usually 25mg twice a week, but doses up to 50mg twice-weekly have been used.
- Often given in combination with MTX or can be used as monotherapy. The dose of MTX can be reduced to optimize tolerance.

Formulation
There are several different formulations of etanercept available from the manufacturer. All are injected subcutaneously. Many patients report that the 'Vial and Diluent' preparations cause less injection-site pain on injection and are often therefore preferred.
- 10mg vial of dry powder with accompanying water for home reconstitution.
- 25mg vial of dry powder with accompanying water for home reconstitution.
- 25mg / 50mg pre-filled syringes and 50mg auto-injector pen—not yet licensed for children.

Monitoring
- FBC, ESR, U+E, LFTs, & CRP, should be checked every 3 months for the first year on etanercept. Thereafter this may be reduced to 6–12 monthly.
- ANA and anti-dsDNA should be checked yearly.
  - Patients who do develop anti-dsDNA antibodies without clinical features of SLE should continue to receive treatment but should be monitored more closely.
  - Patients developing any features of SLE should stop taking the drug. The same response to abnormal results/side-effects as with MTX should be used.

Adalimumab (Humira®)

(see ➲ biologics pp. 448–54)

Clinical/drug information summary

Adalimumab is a fully humanized monoclonal antibody which works by binding to the receptor for TNF-α and thus preventing its action. Adalimumab is licensed for use in children over the age of 2 with JIA whose disease is not well controlled by, or who are intolerant of subcutaneous MTX.

It may take between 2 and 12 weeks to become effective after commencing treatment or a dose increase

Pre-treatment investigations / contra-indication / drug interaction

As for etanercept; see ➲ pp. 493–4.

Side-effects

- As for etanercept except it is not associated with an increased risk of flares of uveitis. Indeed it has good evidence to support its use to treat uveitis that complicates JIA.
- The formation of Human Anti-Chimeric Antibodies (HACA) may prevent long-term use of Infliximab but the risk of this may be lessened if MTX is co-administered.

Dosage and administration

- Adalimumab dose—usual starting dose is $24mg/m^2$ subcutaneously every 14 days. However in practice most patients receive either 20 or 40mg / dose.
  - Age 2–4yrs maximum dose 20mg.
  - Age >4yrs maximum dose 40mg.
- Co-treatment with MTX recommended.

Formulation

Adalimumab is produced as a pre-filled pen or syringe. A paediatric pack to allow easier use of lower doses is also available.

Monitoring

As for etanercept.

Infliximab (Remicade®)

(see biologics, → pp. 448–54)

Clinical/drug information summary

Infliximab is a chimeric monoclonal antibody which works by binding to the receptor for TNF-α and thus preventing its action. Infliximab is not licensed for use in JIA but in practice is widely used for children with JIA whose arthritis justifies treatment with an anti-TNF drug but for whom the risk of a flare of their uveitis would exclude the use of etanercept, and for whom home-treatment with adalimumab is inappropriate or adherence to therapy is suspected to be sub-optimal.

It may take between 2 and 12 weeks to become effective after commencing treatment or a dose increase

Pre-treatment investigations / contra indication / drug interaction

As for etanercept; see → pp. 493–4.

Side-effects

- As for etanercept, except that it is not associated with an increased risk of flares of uveitis. Indeed, it is most often used to treat uveitis that complicates JIA.
- The formation of human anti-chimeric antibodies (HACA) may prevent long-term use of infliximab but the risk of this may be lessened if MTX is co-administered.
- The risk of hypersensitivity reactions is greater with infliximab, than with other TNF-inhibitors.

Dosage and administration

- Usual starting dose is 6mg/kg given intravenously
- Second dose is usually given 2 weeks after the first. Thereafter doses may be given at 3–8 week intervals depending on severity of symptoms and therapeutic response. Most children require 4–6 weekly dose intervals.
- Dose range 3–10mg/kg.
- Co-treatment with MTX recommended.

Formulation

Infliximab—100mg dry powder for reconstitution.

Monitoring

As for etanercept; see → pp. 493–4.

Note: Golimumab and certolizumab are other anti-TNF treatments, but are not yet available in the UK for children and are therefore not dealt with in this chapter.

Anti-IL-1 treatments: anakinra (Kineret®), rilonacept (Regeneron®), and canakinumab (Ilaris®)

(see ➲ biologics pp. 448–54)

Anakinra, rilonacept, and canakinumab all act on IL-1β to inhibit its activity.

Canakinumab, but not the others, is licensed in the UK for use in systemic-JIA (sJIA) and cryopyrin-associated periodic syndrome (CAPS) but high cost has resulted in this drug not being currently approved by NICE.

Anakinra is also now licensed for CAPS, and there is some evidence to support its use in sJIA, particularly when complicated by macrophage-activation syndrome.

Pre-treatment investigations

As for etanercept.

Contra-indications / drug interactions

As for etanercept except:
• No documented dietary restrictions.
• For anakinra:
  • Patients with known hypersensitivity to *E coli*-derived proteins.
  • Latex allergy—needle cover (natural rubber) may induce allergic reactions.

Side-effects

• Most common is injection site reaction (redness, swelling, and pain). The incidence of this appears to be much lower with canakinumab. Other mild side effects reported include coryza, headache, nausea, diarrhoea, sinusitis, arthralgia, flu-like symptoms, and abdominal pain.
• All can cause serious side effects including:
  • Infections—cellulitis, pneumonia (especially in asthmatics), and bone and joint infections.
  • Neutropenia.
  • hepato-toxicity.
  • Hypersensitivity reactions—hypersensitivity reactions including anaphylactic reactions, angioedema, urticaria, rash, and pruritis have been reported rarely.
  • Malignancies—the role of IL-1 blockers in the possible development of malignancy is unknown.

Dosage and administration

Anakinra
• Dose: Usual starting dose is 1–2mg/kg or 60mg/m^2 given daily SC, maximum dose 100mg daily.
  • Moderate—severe renal failure may need a lower dose or alternate-day dosing.
  • Can be used alongside MTX, but not recommended for use with other 'biologics'.

Canakinumab

The recommended starting dose for CAPS patients is:

Adults, adolescents and children ≥4 years of age
- 150 mg every 8 weeks for patients with bodyweight >40 kg.
- 2 mg per kilogram for patients with bodyweight ≥ 15 kg and ≤ 40 kg.
- 4 mg per kilogram for patients with bodyweight ≥ 7.5 kg and <15 kg.

Children 2–4 years of age
- 4 mg per kilogram for patients with bodyweight ≥ 7.5 kg.

The recommended dose for systemic JIA is:

Child 2–17 years (bodyweight 7.5 kg and above)
- 4 mg per kilogram every 4 weeks (maximum dose 300 mg).

Rilonacept
- First dose 4.4 mg/kg injected SC, maximum 320 mg.
- Subsequent doses 2.2 mg/kg (maximum of 160 mg).

Formulation
- Anakinra—100mg in 0.67mls pre-filled syringes.
- Canakinumab—150mg dry powder for reconstitution with 1ml water for injections.
- Rilonacept—80mg dry powder for reconstitution in 1ml water for injections.

Monitoring

As for etanercept; see ➔ pp. 493–4.

Abatacept (Orencia®)

(see ➔ biologics pp. 448–54)

Clinical / drug information summary

Abatacept (Orencia®) blocks the co-stimulatory pathway between T-cells and antigen-presenting cells. It is licensed for use in children with JIA over the age of 6yrs whose disease is not well controlled by, or who are intolerant of SC MTX. It can be used as monotherapy, or in combination with MTX. Time to respond is approximately 3 months.

Pre-treatment investigations / contra-indications

- As for etanercept, except demyelinating disorders not reported with abatacept.

Drug interactions

Patients receiving both abatacept, and another biologic therapy such as anti-TNF had a much higher risk of serious infection. Thus combination of abatacept with other biologic agents is *not* recommended.

Side-effects

- Most common headache, URTI, sore throat, and nausea.
- Serious infections: pneumonia, infections caused by viruses, bacteria, or fungi.
- Allergic reactions: can occur at the time of infusion or can be delayed (even next day)—pre-dosing with hydrocortisone may reduce this risk.
- Respiratory problems have been reported in adults with chronic obstructive lung disease.
- Other side-effects may include diarrhoea, cough, fever, and abdominal pain.

Dosage and administration

- Dose: Usual starting dose is *10mg/kg given intravenously*. Maximum dose 1g
- Second dose is usually given 2 weeks after the first, thereafter at 4-weekly intervals.

Monitoring

As for etanercept; see ➔ pp. 493–4.

Ciclosporin

Ciclosporin is a DMARD used occasionally in the treatment of JIA, JIA-associated uveitis, JDM, and macrophage activation syndrome. Its use is most limited by renal toxicity and cosmetic problems with hirsutism.

Pre-treatment consideration / testing
- FBC and differential WCC, U&Es, creatinine, magnesium, LFTs, fasting lipids.
- Calculated GFR.
- Urinalysis.
- BP.

Contraindications
Absolute
- Renal failure
- Liver failure.
- Uncontrolled hypertension.
- Uncontrolled infection.
- Malignancy.
- Severe electrolyte imbalance.
- Concomitant use of tacrolimus or rosuvastatin.

Drug interactions
There are multiple drug interactions. See BNFC for full listing.
- Always halve the dose of diclofenac if ciclosporin is co-prescribed.
- Care is also needed with other potentially nephrotoxic drugs, e.g. aciclovir, aminoglycosides, amphotericin, ciprofloxacin, trimethoprim, vancomycin.
- Ciclosporin levels can be increased by erythromycin, clarithromycin, ketoconazole, fluconazole, oral contraceptives, methylprednisolone (high dose), hydroxychloroquine.
- Ciclosporin levels can be decreased by carbamazepine, phenytoin, rifampicin, St John's wort.

Side-effects
Common
- Hypertension.
- Renal dysfunction.
- Hyperlipidaemia, hypercholesterolaemia.
- Tremor, headache, convulsions.
- Paraesthesia.
- Nausea, vomiting, abdominal pain, diarrhoea, anorexia, gingival hyperplasia.
- Hepatic dysfunction.
- Hyperuricaemia, hyperkalaemia, hypomagnesaemia.
- Hypertrichosis, hirsutism.
- Muscle cramps, myalgia, fatigue.
- Immunosuppression and infections—viral, bacterial, fungal, and parasitic.

Other less common side-effects listed in BNFC but may include a possible increased risk of secondary neoplasia, and the posterior reversible encephalopathy syndrome (PRES).

Dosage and administration

Switching between formulations without close monitoring may lead to clinically important changes in blood-ciclosporin concentration. Therefore prescribing and dispensing of ciclosporin should be by brand name to avoid inadvertent switching. If it is necessary to switch a patient to a different brand or formulation of ciclosporin, the patient should be monitored closely for changes in blood-ciclosporin concentration, serum creatinine, and BP.

Dose

2–4mg/kg/day in 2 divided doses gradually increased over 6 weeks according to response, tolerance, and blood level to a maximum dose 6mg/kg daily.

If *no* clinical response at maximum tolerated dose for 3 months, then withdraw treatment.

- The total daily dose is given in 2 doses 12h apart, taken with food or drink.
- Grapefruit juice should be avoided for 1h prior to administration. Do not mix with grapefruit juice.
  - Grapefruit juice is a potent inhibitor of the intestinal cytochrome P-450 3A4 system which is responsible for the first-pass metabolism of many medications. This interaction can lead to increases in bioavailability and corresponding increases in serum ciclosporin levels.
- Mix the oral solution with orange/apple juice (to improve taste) or with water immediately before administration.
- Do not administer via a nasogastric tube (interaction with plastic).
- Do not keep oral liquid in the fridge. Keep at room temperature (15–25°C).

Monitoring

- Routine monitoring of ciclosporin levels not usually necessary once desired level and steady state achieved unless concerns regarding adherence to therapy.
- U&Es, creatinine—every 2 weeks until dose and trend stable, then monthly.
  - Creatinine rise >30% from baseline, or fall in calculated GFR of >10%—withhold and discuss with specialist team.
  - Potassium rises above reference range—withhold and discuss with specialist team.
- LFTs—once a month until dose and trend stable for 3 months, then 3 monthly.
- FBC—once a month until dose and trend stable for 3 months, then 3 monthly. If platelets <150 × 10^9/L or abnormal bruising withhold and discuss with specialist team.
- Fasting lipids—no clear guideline in children but suggested every 6 months.

- BP should be checked at every clinic visit. Treat BP if >95th centile for age on 2 consecutive readings 2 weeks apart. If BP cannot be controlled, stop ciclosporin.

Fertility / pregnancy / breastfeeding

- Ciclosporin does cross the placenta but limited data available from organ transplant recipients indicate that, compared with other immunosuppressive agents, ciclosporin treatment imposes no increased risk of adverse effects on the course and outcome of pregnancy.
- However, in the absence of adequate studies, avoid in pregnancy unless potential benefit to mother outweighs the potential risk to the fetus.
- Ciclosporin is excreted in breast milk and breast-feeding should be avoided.
- There is limited data of the effect of ciclosporin on fertility.

References

British National Formulary for Children (BNFC), 2015

Electronic Medicines Compendium, Summary of Product Characteristics for Neoral Oral Solution, updated 09/01/2015. Accessed at: Ⓝ www.medicines.org.uk

Chakravarty K, et al. BSR/BHPR guideline for disease-modifying anti-rheumatic drug (DMARD) therapy in consultation with the British Association of Dermatologists. *Rheumatology (Oxford)* 2008;47:924–5.

Anti-IL-6 treatment: tocilizumab (RoActemra®)

(see ➲ biologics pp. 448–54)

Tocilizumab is a recombinant humanized anti-human interleukin-6 (IL-6) receptor monoclonal antibody which binds specifically to both soluble and membrane-bound IL-6 receptors to inhibit the action of IL-6. It is licensed in the UK for the treatment of sJIA and poly-articular course JIA, and approved by NICE for the treatment of sJIA.

Pre-treatment investigations / contra-indications / drug interactions / monitoring

As for etanercept.

Side-effects

Most common are infusion reactions and pre-dosing with hydrocortisone is advised. Tocilizumab has also been reported to cause severe infections (pneumonia, varicella), deranged LFTs (ALT / AST, and bilirubin) and neutropenia.

Dosage and administration for sJIA

<30kg body weight
- Dose: 12mg/kg given by intravenous infusion over 1hr.
- Frequency: every 2 weeks.

≥30kg body weight
- Dose: 8mg/kg/dose given by intravenous infusion over 1 hr.
- Frequency: every 2 weeks.

Dosage for poly JIA

Child 2 to 17 years (<30kg)
- Dose: 10mg/kg every 4 weeks.

Child ≥30kg
- Dose: 8mg/kg every 4 weeks.

Anti-B-cell therapies: rituximab (Mabthera®) (also, see chapter on anti-B cell therapy in SLE)

(see ➲ biologics pp. 448–54)

Clinical/drug information summary

Rituximab is a chimeric monoclonal antibody directed against B cells. It binds to CD20 antigen located on pre-B and mature B lymphocytes, thus caus-ing B-cell lysis. Rituximab spares B cell progenitors (and antibody secreting plasma cells), and B cells reappear 4–12 months after therapy. However memory B-cells can remain suppressed for 2 years. Rituximab is licensed for use in adults with RA and AAV, but not in children. Reports of good effect in adolescents with poly-articular IIA (RF positive), treatment resistant (JOLE), JDM, and some forms of vasculitis (particularly AAV). Rituximab may take approximately 3 months to be effective.

Pre-treatment investigations/contraindications/cautions

As for etanercept plus:
- Check BP before, during, and after treatment.
- Pregnancy is contraindicated and recommended that breast-feeding is avoided.
- Patients with a history of cardiovascular or renal impairment may require dose reduction.
- Live vaccines are currently contraindicated post rituximab whilst B cells are depleted.
- Anti-CD 19 and immunoglobulins should also be measured, see 'monitoring' below, and see ➲ anti B cell therapy in SLE, pp. 256–61.

Drug interactions:

- Renal toxicity has been reported in combination with cisplatin in clinical trials.

Side-effects

- Infusion reactions (fever, rigor, dyspnoea and bronchospasm, pruritis and rashes, angioedema, and transient hypotension) usually present ≤ 12 hours.
  - Pre-medication with chlorphenamine, paracetamol, and methylpred-nisolone may reduce the incidence of infusion reactions.
- A decline in immunoglobulin levels may make children more susceptible to infections, especially varicella.

Dosage and administration

- Dose: 2 doses of 750 mg/m² given by intravenous infusion 2 weeks apart. Maximum dose per infusion is 1g.
- Other regimens, e.g. 375 mg/m² weekly for 4 weeks have been described.
  - Dilute the required dose with sodium chloride 0.9% or glucose 5% to a final concentration of 1–4mg/mL.

- The initial infusion rate is 25mg/hour, which can be increased by increments of 25mg/hour every 30 minutes up to a maximum of 200mg/hour as tolerated.
- In SLE each rituximab may be followed the next day by 375mg/m^2 of IV cyclophosphamide: see ➲ anti B cell therapy in SLE, pp. 256–61.
- In JIA concomitant use of MTX is recommended.

Monitoring

As a minimum, the following immune monitoring is recommended:

- Lymphocyte subsets requesting CD19 (or CD20 if available) on day 7–10 after infusion, then monthly from 4 months after first dose until peripheral B cells return (repopulation may occur earlier than 4 months, particularly in SLE).
- Immunoglobulins (GAM): Day 7–10; 2 months after first dose; then monthly from 4 months after first dose until B cells return.

Systemic corticosteroid therapy (oral, intra-muscular, and intravenous)

Systemic corticosteroid therapy is often needed at 'induction' or to treat flares of disease (e.g polyarticular JIA, sJIA, JSLE, scleroderma, JDM or vasculitis—see ➔ relevant chapters).

Pre-treatment consideration / testing

- Consider need for prevention and treatment of steroid induced osteoporosis with daily vitamin D and calcium supplementation. Use of activated vitamin D (such as 1-alpha calcidol, or calcitriol) or bisphosphonates to prevent corticosteroid induced osteoporosis not routinely recommended.
- Give steroid card and advice re chicken pox and measles.
- FBC, ESR, CRP U&Es creatinine, glucose, and LFTs (if not done already as part of disease monitoring). Varicella zoster serology prior to the first dose.
- Avoid live virus vaccines during, and for 3 months after, administration of oral, IM, or IV steroids (live vaccines may be given if patients have received IA steroids only and > 6 weeks before systemic immunosuppression (e.g. MTX) started.

Contraindications / cautions

Major

- Active peptic ulceration, acute infections.

Minor

- Diabetes, benign intracranial hypertension, previous peptic ulcer disease, hepatic impairment.
- Reduce the dose or the rate of IV infusion in patients more at risk of hypertension/renal crisis such as those with SLE nephritis or systemic sclerosis patients.
- Some advise avoiding high dose IV methylprednisolone in those with systemic sclerosis because of the risk of renal hypertensive crisis. This recommendation is made for adults with this disease in particular, with little or no data to support this recommendation in paediatric patients with systemic sclerosis. If in doubt SEEK EXPERT ADVICE.

Drug interactions

Major

- NSAIDS (including aspirin)—increased risk of GI bleeding. Gastro-protection should be given, usually with a proton pump inhibitor.
- Anti-coagulants—corticosteroids may enhance effect of warfarin.
- Ciclosporin—corticosteroids may increase plasma levels of ciclosporin.

Minor

- All anti-hypertensive treatments are physiologically counteracted by corticosteroids.

Side-effects

- Mild—facial flushing, metallic taste, hyperactivity, mood changes, blurred vision, tiredness.
- Rare—hypertension (even with IV infusions) and often responds to slowing infusion rate and only occasionally requires treatment (e.g. nifedipine).
- Extremely rare—altered conscious state or psychosis, seizures.

Dosage and administration

Intravenous

- Usual dose is 30mg / kg / day IV methylprednisolone (maximum of 1000 mg/day).
- Each dose is normally given over 30–60mins in 30–250ml of 0.9% sodium chloride—and usually given once per day for 3 days.
- This may need to be repeated in subsequent weeks depending on the nature and severity of the condition being treated.
- Oral steroids are stopped on days that methylprednisolone is given, and restarted with a weaning regimen appropriate for the individual and disease being treated.

Intra-muscular

- Usual dose is 1mg/kg, max.80mg, of triamcinolone acetonide (Kenolog®)
- Must be given by deep IM injection to the gluteal muscles to try and avoid causing subcutaneous atrophy.
- In larger doses consider splitting the dose and giving half the dose to each buttock.
- Pain of administration limits its use in children but is often tolerated better by older adolescents.

Oral

- The starting dose is entirely dependent on the disease (and its severity) being treated, but usually is in the range of 1–2mg/kg.
- Aim to wean as quickly as possible thereafter (dependent on clinical response and toxicity in individual patients).

Monitoring—for intravenous route only

- Temperature, pulse, respiratory rate (RR), BP—before, during and after infusion.
- Urinalysis for glycosuria prior to first dose. If patient is known to have diabetes hyperglycaemia should be expected, insulin requirements will rise and can be unpredictable; blood glucose (BM stix) must be monitored regularly.
- If the patient feels unwell, check TPR, BP, and blood glucose; consider slowing rate of infusion.

Suggested treatment pathway for oligo-articular jia and joint injections

See Figure 9.2.

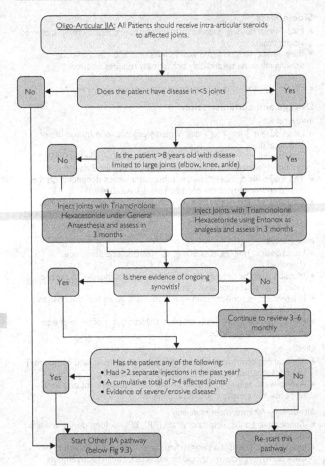

Fig. 9.2 Suggested treatment pathway for oligo-articular JIA and joint injections.

Suggested treatment flow chart for non-oligo JIA

Fig. 9.3 Suggested treatment pathway for polyarticular or systemic JIA. This is based on the NHS England Interim Statement for the use of Biologics in JIA (2015)—see chapter 8—Approvals for the use of biologics in JIA page 446.

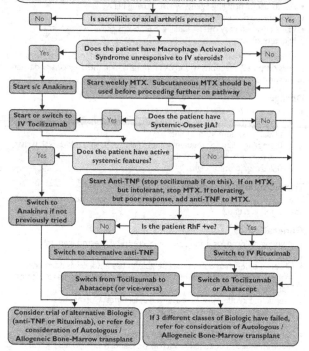

Oligo-Articular JIA: See previous pathway
Other JIA: At diagnosis all patients should receive either intra-articular corticosteroids to <u>all</u> affected joints, or systemic (preferably IV) corticosteroids.
- Apart from the 2 specific circumstances of Macrophage Activation Syndrome or Sacroiliitis, all patients should start treatment with Methotrexate (MTX) as their first line DMARD and be re-assessed at least every 3/12.
- Patients should only proceed to the next step of the pathway if treatment has failed (active systemic features, >2 joints with active arthritis, or intolerant of the treatment). 'Flares' of arthritis may be treated with steroids as above.
- Consider access to research studies at all treatment decision points.

Is sacroiliitis or axial arthritis present? — No / Yes

Does the patient have Macrophage Activation Syndrome unresponsive to IV steroids? — Yes / No

Start s/c Anakinra

Start weekly MTX. Subcutaneous MTX should be used before proceeding further on pathway

Start or switch to IV Tocilizumab — Yes — Does the patient have Systemic-Onset JIA? — No

Does the patient have active systemic features? — No

Yes

Switch to Anakinra if not previously tried

Start Anti-TNF (stop tocilizumab if on this). If on MTX, but intolerant, stop MTX. If tolerating, but poor response, add anti-TNF to MTX.

Is the patient RhF +ve? — No / Yes

Switch to alternative anti-TNF

Switch to IV Rituximab

Switch from Tocilizumab to Abatacept (or vice-versa)

Switch to Tocilizumab or Abatacept

Consider trial of alternative Biologic (anti-TNF or Rituximab), or refer for consideration of Autologous / Allogeneic Bone-Marrow transplant

If 3 different classes of Biologic have failed, refer for consideration of Autologous / Allogeneic Bone-Marrow transplant

Fig. 9.3 Suggested treatment flow chart for JIA. This flow chart is based on the NHS England Interim Clinical Commissioning Policy Statement: Biologic therapies.

Reproduced with permission from NHS England, *Interim Clinical Commissioning Policy Statement: Biologic therapies for the treatment of Juvenile Idiopathic Arthritis (JIA)*, ℘ https://www. engage.england.nhs.uk/consultation/specialised-services-policies/user_uploads/biolgcs-juvenl-idiop-arthrs-pol.pdf, accessed 01 May 2016, Copyright © NHS England.

Intra-articular (IA) corticosteroid use in JIA

See ➔ JIA, p. 162 see Corticosteroid Intra-articular injections, p. 438.

Intra-articular corticosteroid injections

- Result in minimal systemic steroid absorption.
- Are the treatment of choice for oligo-articular JIA.
- Act as useful bridging agents whilst starting MTX.
- Minimize exposure to systemic corticosteroids.
- Have good efficacy often inducing ≥ 6months of remission in the injected joint.

Re-injection is advised if synovitis recurs. However if recurrent synovitis occurs despite 2 injections within 6–12 months then the diagnosis and treatment should be reviewed.

Dosage

- Triamcinolone hexacetonide:
  - 1mg/kg/joint for large joints (knees, ankles, elbows, shoulders). Usual maximum 40mg/joint.
  - 0.5mg/kg/joint for medium joints (hips, sub-talars, mid-tarsal, wrists, and temporo-mandibular joints).
  - 0.2–2mg/joint for digits.

Triamcinolone acetonide

The dose is double that of triamcinolone hexacetonide, but systemic absorption is greater.

General notes

- In young children, or if multiple joints are to be injected, general anaesthesia is needed.
- Children older than 6–8yrs may be able to use entonox as adequate analgesia. Older teenagers may be able to use local anaesthesia such as EMLA cream.
- Aseptic technique must be observed at all times. Correct needle placement should reduce risk of SC atrophy and injection of corticosteroid into the cartilage that can cause growth disturbance.
- X-ray or ultrasound imaging may aid accuracy, and is strongly recommended in deep joints such as hips, and in small joints such as fingers.
- Joint injection followed by casting may help to reduce contractures if combined with intensive physiotherapy.

Side-effects

- Septic arthritis is a potential risk but with good technique, almost never observed.
- Facial flushing and Cushingoid appearance are transient. Cushing syndrome and adreno-suppression are very rare.
- Periarticular calcification may occur (≤5% of injections).

- Diabetic patients may notice increased insulin requirements transiently after injections.
- SC atrophy can occur, mainly smaller joints; skin changes may fade but unlikely to resolve completely.
- Chemical synovitis may cause increased pain and swelling 12–24 hours post injection (albeit rarely observed in practice).
- Post injection pain is uncommon; simple analgesia (with paracetamol) usually suffices. Post-injection rest is impossible to achieve and should not be enforced.

The CARRA consensus treatment plans for polyarticular JIA

Purpose

- There is wide variation in current treatment practices for polyarticular forms of JIA.
- The consensus treatment plans (CTPs) were developed by the Childhood Arthritis and Rheumatology Research Alliance (CARRA) JIA Research Committee to facilitate observational research evaluating the effectiveness, safety, and tolerability of the most commonly used treatment approaches for polyarticular JIA.

Development

- The CTPs were designed using a combination of surveys and in-person meetings from May 2011 to June 2013.
- First, an electronic survey was conducted in May 2011 of the entire CARRA voting membership. Participants were presented with scenarios and asked which medications they use as initial and subsequent therapy. This survey identified 3 main treatment strategies varying in the timing of when non-biologic and biologic DMARDs were started in new-onset polyarticular JIA.
- At the June 2011 CARRA Annual Scientific Meeting, the process of converting the survey results into CTPs began and continued through the next 2 years. This process included a literature review, breakout groups that used modified nominal group technique to discuss and achieve consensus at face-to-face meetings, and an expert workgroup that continued to meet by conference calls to refine the CTPs.
- The CTPs were finalized at the June 2013 CARRA meeting: 96% of voters agreed that they would be willing to implement these CTPs in their practice.

Inclusion and exclusion criteria, endpoints, reasons to change approach (all CTPs)

- Inclusion criteria: rheumatoid factor positive or negative polyarticular JIA, extended oligoarticular JIA, enthesitis-related arthritis, psoriatic JIA, undifferentiated JIA, with arthritis in > 4 joints during the disease course, age at baseline less than 19 years.
- Exclusions:
  - Systemic JIA, inflammatory bowel disease, coeliac disease, trisomy 21, current or past history of malignancy, recurrent infection.
  - Prior treatment with non-biologic or biologic disease modifying anti-rheumatic agents or oral steroids.
  - Live vaccine within a month of entry.
- Treatment response is assessed at 3, 6, and 12 months following initiation of therapy.
- Reasons to modify treatment approach: 1) if 'the patient was not much better', 2) the physician global assessment was greater than or equal to 2 (on a scale of 0–10), or 3) the patient is still on oral prednisone.
- Primary end point: paediatric ACR90 score at 12 months.

- Secondary end points: clinically inactive disease, radiographic evaluation of at least one involved joint at 12 months.

The CTPs

Three treatment strategies were created: Step Up, Early Combination and Biologic First Treatment Plans.

Step Up Treatment Plan

- Patients start on a non-biologic DMARD (MTX, sulphasalazine, or leflunomide), followed by addition of a biologic DMARD (any medication inhibiting TNF-alpha, T-cell co-stimulation, IL-6, or B cells) if there is an inadequate response at the 3, 6, or 12 month assessment.
- This plan allows for an increase in dose or change in the non-biologic DMARD.
- Oral steroids can be started at the time of initiation of treatment. It is recommended that steroids be tapered off as quickly as possible. Patients can also receive intra-articular steroid injections.
- This plan is most similar to what is recommended by the 2011 American College of Rheumatology (ACR) JIA treatment guidelines for polyarticular JIA

Early Combination Treatment Plan

- A non-biologic DMARD and biologic DMARD are both started within 1 month of treatment initiation.
- The non-biologic DMARD can be increased in dose or changed at each assessment point if needed. The biologic DMARD can also be changed.
- Similar to the Step Up Plan, oral steroids and intra-articular steroids can be used.

Biologic First Treatment Plan

- The patient is started on a biologic DMARD at initiation of treatment without starting a non-biologic DMARD.
- If the patient does not achieve an adequate response, the biologic DMARD can be changed or a non-biologic DMARD can be added beginning at the 3-month assessment point.
- Oral and intra-articular steroids can be used, again with the goal of discontinuing steroids as soon as possible.
- Dosing and safety monitoring guidelines for each non-biologic and biologic DMARD were agreed upon.

Limitations

- In contrast to the 2011 ACR JIA treatment recommendations, the CTPs are based mostly on consensus opinion rather than evidence-based data and expert opinion. In addition, the CTPs only address treatment during the 1st year of disease.
- The CTPs reflect opinions of CARRA members, a North-American-based network of pediatric rheumatologists and may not be generalizable to other areas of the world.
- These CTPs do not take into account features of poor prognosis (such as positive rheumatoid factor, axial joint disease, or erosions on imaging) that traditionally alter treatment regimes. These features are addressed in the ACR JIA treatment recommendations.

Implications

- There is a great deal of variability in how patients with polyarticular JIA are being treated. The CTPs aim to reduce this variability through the creation of three consensus-based plans that rheumatologists can follow.
- The CTPs reflect the current treatment practices of North American pediatric rheumatologists, in contrast to the ACR JIA treatment recommendations which are limited in their scope by the current evidence base (or lack thereof).
- Data collected using these CTPs can be used to compare the effectiveness and safety of these different treatment strategies, as is being done in the CARRA Start Time Optimization of biologics in Poly-JIA (STOP-JIA) study currently underway as a sub-study of the CARRA Registry, and will likely help to inform evidence-based recommendations, such as the ACR JIA guidelines, over time.

Key references

Beukelman T, Patkar NM, Saag KG, *et al.* 2011 American College of Rheumatology recommendations for the treatment of Juvenile Idiopathic Arthritis: Initiation and safety monitoring of therapeutic agents for the treatment of arthritis and systemic features. *Arthritis Care & Research.* 2011; 63(4): 465–482.

Ringold S, Weiss PF, Colbert RA, *et al.* Childhood arthritis and rheumatology research alliance consensus treatment plans for new-onset polyarticular juvenile idiopathic arthritis. *Arthritis Care & Research.* 2014; 66(7): 1063–72.

The CARRA consensus treatment plans for systemic JIA

Purpose

- There is a great deal of variability in the treatment of systemic JIA.
- As new medications are made available, it is important to understand their effectiveness and safety in treating this disease.
- By creating CTPs, the Childhood Arthritis and Rheumatology Research Alliance (CARRA) aims to standardize the most commonly used treatment regimes in order to subsequently allow for comparative effectiveness studies to be carried out.

Development

- CARRA members in the JIA Research Committee were surveyed regarding their treatment choices for 4 clinical scenarios of new-onset systemic JIA patients that represented mild, moderate, moderate-high, and high-level disease activity. The members voted on first, second, and third line treatment options for each of the scenarios. As expected, the survey results showed that there was significant variability in treatment approaches, but several common preferences were identified.
- During the 2010 CARRA Annual Scientific Meeting, these responses and literature review were used by the JIA Research Committee to agree upon CTPs using a combination of discussion and modified nominal group technique, followed by continued refinement by an expert workgroup that met by conference calls. After a series of reevaluations and discussions, the plans were presented to the entire CARRA membership via an online survey and this feedback helped to finalize the systemic JIA CTPs.
- 92.6% of the entire CARRA membership was willing to follow the CTPs that were created.
- Following approval of canakinumab by the FDA for use in systemic JIA, the IL-1 inhibitor CTP was updated in 2014 to include the use of canakinumab in addition to anakinra.

Inclusion and exclusion criteria, endpoints, reasons to change approach (all CTPs)

- Inclusion criteria: age 6 months to 18yrs, fever for at least 2 weeks, arthritis in at least 1 joint, and at least one of the following: evanescent erythematous rash, generalized lymphadenopathy, hepatomegaly or splenomegaly, or serositis (pericarditis, pleuritis, or peritonitis).
- Exclusions: infection, malignancy, positive TB screening, recent live virus vaccination (within the past 4 weeks), or prior treatment for systemic JIA aside from NSAIDs or a short course of steroids.
- Treatment response is assessed at 1–2 weeks and 1, 3, 6, and 9 months after initiation of treatment.
- Reasons to change treatment approach include inadequate response, the glucocorticoid (GC) dose cannot be weaned below 50% of the starting dose by 3 months, and/or if the disease activity has worsened at any point.

- The assessment of disease activity and treatment response is measured by the physician assessment of whether the patient has improved, stayed the same or worsened at each time point.
- The CTPs suggest measuring quality of life, physical function, Physician Global Assessment Score (PGAS), active joint count, presence of systemic features (fever, rash, hepatosplenomegaly, serositis), and laboratory tests (CBC, ESR, CRP, ferritin, LDH) at each standardized time point.
- The primary endpoint is inactive disease off glucocorticoids at 12 months.

The CTPs
- Four plans were created: Glucocorticoid Only, MTX, IL-1 Inhibitor (anakinra or canakinumab), and IL-6 Inhibitor (tocilizumab) Treatment Plans. GC can be given with any of the CTPs. Medication dosing and steroid tapering guidelines were included in the plans.
- Glucocorticoid Only Treatment Plan:
  - Patients are started on prednisone 1 mg/kg (max 60 mg) daily. Patients can be treated with 3 days of pulse methyprednisolone (MP) (30 mg/kg/day) prior to initiation of oral steroids.
  - At each assessment (beginning at 1–2 weeks, then 1, 3, 6, and 9 months), if the patient is worsening, the physician can add or repeat pulse MP or increase oral prednisone to 2 mg/kg (max 100 mg) daily. If the patient is improved, the steroids can be tapered. If there is no change, the current dose of prednisone can be continued or pulse MP can be considered.
  - At the 3-month assessment point, if the patient is unchanged, doing worse and/or still on >50% of the starting steroid dose, the physician should consider adding additional therapy (changing CTPs to MTX, IL-1 inhibitor or IL-6 inhibitor). If the patient is on <50% of the starting dose, the steroid taper can be continued.
- MTX Treatment Plan:
  - Patients are started on MTX 0.5 mg/kg (max 15 mg) PO or SC weekly. Patients can also be treated with prednisone 1 mg/kg/day or pulse MP 30mg/kg/day (maximum dose 1g/day) for 3 days.
  - At each assessment (beginning at 1–2 weeks, then 1, 3, 6, and 9 months), if the disease activity is worsened, prednisone should be added or the dose increased to 2 mg/kg daily if they are already on prednisone. The physician can also consider giving pulse MP. If the patient is unchanged, the same dose of MTX and prednisone are continued and pulse MP can be considered. If the patient is improved, the same dose of MTX is continued and the steroids can be tapered.
  - Beginning at the 1-month assessment point, if the patient has worsened, the MTX dose is increased to 1 mg/kg SC weekly.
  - At the 3-month reassessment, if the patient is unchanged, doing worse, or the steroid dose is >50% of the starting dose, the physician should consider adding additional therapy (changing CTPs to IL-1 inhibitor or IL-6 inhibitor). If the patient is improved, the prednisone can be tapered while continuing MTX.

- IL-1 Inhibitor Treatment Plan:
  - Patients are started on anakinra 2 mg/kg (max 100 mg) SC daily or canakinumab 4 mg/kg (max 300 mg) SC monthly. As with the MTX plan, patients can also be treated with oral or pulse steroids.
  - At each assessment (beginning at 1–2 weeks, then 1, 3, 6, and 9 months), if the patient is worsening, the anakinra dose is increased to 4 mg/kg (max 200 mg) SC daily (canakinumab dose is maintained). Prednisone can be started, maintained at the current dose (1 mg/kg), increased to 2 mg/kg daily, or pulse MP can be given. If the status is unchanged, the current dose of anakinra/canakinumab and steroids are continued. If improved, the GC can be tapered.
  - The physician can also consider switching IL-1 inhibitors at any time point.
  - At the 3-month assessment point, if the patient is unchanged, doing worse, or the steroid dose is >50% of the starting dose, the physician should consider adding additional therapy (changing CTPs to MTX or IL-6 inhibitor).
- IL-6 Inhibitor Treatment Plan:
  - The patient is started on tocilizumab 8 mg/kg (if weight >30 kg) or 12 mg/kg (if <30 kg) IV every 2 weeks. PO or IV steroids can also be given as with the previous plans.
  - At each assessment (beginning at 1–2 weeks, then 1, 3, 6, and 9 months), if the patient has worsened, the current dose of tocilizumab is maintained and prednisone is started or increased to 2 mg/kg daily (or pulse MP can be given). If unchanged, the current regimen is continued. If improved, tocilizumab is continued and prednisone can be tapered if applicable.
  - At the 3-month reassessment, if the patient is unchanged, doing worse, or the steroid dose is >50% of the starting dose, the physician should consider adding additional therapy (changing CTPs to MTX or IL-1 inhibitor).

Limitations

- Many patients with new-onset systemic JIA do not initially fulfil the International League of Associations of Rheumatology (ILAR) criteria for the diagnosis of systemic JIA (i.e. do not have arthritis), but still need to be treated. The CTPs require at least 2 weeks of fever and at least 1 active joint.
- The CTPs only address treatment of patients during the first 9 months of disease.
- They do not address tapering of medications other than prednisone.
- The CTPs differ from the 2011 & 2013 ACR JIA recommendations in several respects. The CTPs are mostly based on consensus opinion, not strictly on evidence-based data combined with expert opinion as are the ACR recommendations. The ACR recommendations also address the treatment of macrophage activation syndrome in systemic JIA, and consider a broader array of medication options (TNF inhibitors, abatacept, calcineurin inhibitors) whereas the CTPs focus on standardizing the most commonly used treatments for moderate-severe patient with new-onset disease. The CTPs consider

treatment of systemic features and arthritis together, while the ACR recommendations consider these to be two separate issues with different treatment approaches.

• The CTPs reflect opinions of CARRA members, a North-American based network of paediatric rheumatologists and may not be generalizable to other areas of the world. The CARRA CTPs differ to European practice and are useful to compare and contrast.

Implications

• There is a great deal of variability in how patients with systemic JIA are being treated. The CTPs aim to reduce this variability through the creation of four consensus-based plans that rheumatologists can follow in treating patients with new-onset systemic forms of JIA.

• The CTPs reflect the current treatment practices of North American paediatric rheumatologists, in contrast to the ACR JIA treatment recommendations which are limited in what can be recommended by the existing evidence base (or lack thereof).

• Data collected using these CTPs can be used to compare the effectiveness and safety of different treatment strategies as is being done in the CARRA FiRst line treatment Options in Systemic JIA Treatment (FROST) study currently underway as a sub-study of the CARRA Registry. A pilot study was completed to assess the feasibility of conducting a comparative effectiveness study of the systemic JIA CTPs. The FROST study will likely help to inform evidence-based recommendations, such as the ACR JIA guidelines, over time.

Key references

Beukelman T, Patkar NM, Saag KG, et al. 2011 American College of Rheumatology recommendations for the treatment of Juvenile Idiopathic Arthritis: Initiation and safety monitoring of therapeutic agents for the treatment of arthritis and systemic features. Arthritis Care & Research. 2011; 63(4): 465–82.

DeWitt EM, Kimura Y, Beukelman T, et al. Consensus treatment plans for new-onset systemic juvenile idiopathic arthritis. Arthritis Care Res, 2012; 64: 1001–10.

Kimura, Y., DeWitt, E.M., Beukelman, T., et al. Adding canakinumab to the Childhood Arthritis and Rheumatology Research Alliance consensus treatment plans for systemic juvenile idiopathic arthritis: Comment on the article by DeWitt et al. Arthritis Care Res, 2014. 66(9): 1430–4.

Ringold, S., Weiss, P.F., Beukelman, T., et al. 2013 Update of the 2011 American College of Rheumatology recommendations for the treatment of juvenile idiopathic arthritis. Arthritis Rheum 2013; 65(10): 2499–512.

Kimura Y, Grevich S, Beukelman T, Morgan E, Mieszkalski K, et al. Pilot study results comparing the Childhood Arthritis and Rheumatology Research Alliance (CARRA) Consensus Treatment Plans for new-onset Systemic Juvenile Idiopathic Arthritis (JIA) Pediatric Rheumatology (2017) 15:23.

Clinical guidelines and protocols: SHARE guidelines: summary

From 2012-2015, Single Hub and Access point for paediatric Rheumatology in Europe (SHARE), a European Union funded initiative from the Execution Agency for Health and Consumers Authority, was executed with the aim of:

- Optimizing care and perspectives of paediatric rheumatology patients throughout Europe.
- Formulating clear recommendations to help clinicians in the care of patients with paediatric rheumatic diseases (PRD); currently there is no international consensus regarding diagnosis and treatment for most of the PRD
- Developing and disseminating diagnostic and management regimens (so called 'best practice') for children and young people with PRD.
  - This initiative included JIA, JDM, JSLE, and anti-phospholipid syndrome (APS), childhood vasculitis, and localized and systemic scleroderma
  - In addition, the monogenic periodic fever syndromes familial Mediterranean fever (FMF), the cryopyrin associated periodic fever syndromes (CAPS), mevalonate kinase deficiency (MKD) and tumour necrosis factor receptor associated periodic syndrome (TRAPS)
- SHARE also mapped the current state of care for PRD in the EU member and candidate member states (as of 2014) via questionnaires to both care providers and patients.
  - Doing this, SHARE aimed to provide EU member states and candidate member states with specific recommendations on aspects of care, research and access to therapy (DMARDS or biological drugs) in order to optimize and provide equity of access to care for PRD throughout Europe.

Methodology

- The SHARE recommendations on diagnosis and treatment are evidence based where possible (following the EULAR standard operating procedures on systematic literature reviews), and consensus based where needed.
- Evidence based recommendations, and consensus finding on non-evidence based recommendations were developed in a transparent and structured way.
  - This involved disease experts from all over Europe and further abroad (for example from Turkey and Israel for FMF).

Box 9.2 and 9.3 display the prerequisites and rules that were followed in the process of developing the guidelines.

Dissemination

- From 2015 on, the SHARE recommendations are published or soon to be submitted for publication in peer reviewed journals (See References).
- Besides the disease specific recommendations, SHARE also developed overarching recommendations, largely consensus based, by all involved

Box 9.2 Systematic literature reviews
- Inclusion criteria:
  - English literature, > 1970
  - Separate analysis of paediatric patients
- Exclusion criteria:
  - Case reports < 3 paediatric patients
  - Reviews
  - Meeting abstracts

Box 9.3 Consensus-finding process for SHARE recommendations
1. Development of recommendations by a core team of disease experts is based upon systematic literature review.
2. Pre-testing consensus-finding potential, by web based survey of recommendations.
3. Two face to face meetings, chaired by a non-voting disease expert. Discussion of the recommendations by Nominal Group Technique (2).
4. Only recommendations with > 80% consensus were accepted in the final guidelines.

disease experts (more than 50 international acknowledged experts in paediatric rheumatology).
- Importantly, for these overarching recommendations, expert advice was also obtained by inviting consultants from clinically related medical subspecialties (ophthalmology, haematology, adult rheumatology, paediatric nephrology, exercise physiology, and physiotherapy).

Overarching principles
Below, the most important overarching principles from the SHARE guidelines are listed.
- Children with rheumatic disease should be cared for by paediatric rheumatologists. This may be done by means of shared care, which must include a robust mechanism for communication between teams.
- Clear guidelines of referral to paediatric rheumatology are needed for all centres in fostering the prompt and early diagnosis and management of PRD.
  - Patients should be assessed by a paediatric rheumatologist and, depending on the clinical presentation of the PRD, members of a multidisciplinary team. This team should consist as a minimum of:
    —a nurse specialized in PRD
    —a physiotherapist
    —an occupational therapist
    —and access to a psychologist and/or psychosocial worker.

- Paediatric rheumatology patients would have timely access to all medical subspecialties with paediatric expertise, and clinically related medical and surgical specialties.
- Patients and caregivers should be helped in finding age-appropriate and accurate information about their condition and its management.
- All children and young people with PRD should have regular disease activity assessed using the disease appropriate tools.
- Disease activity monitoring should be standardized, so that treatment efficacy can be closely monitored at each visit.
- All children with PRD should have a damage assessment on a regular (at least annual) basis using disease-appropriate tools, where these exist.
- All PRD patients should have access to, and reimbursement for treatment with EMA approved DMARDS and/or biologicals when indicated.
- Paediatric rheumatologists should direct the prescription of biologics or DMARDs for registered PRD indications.
- Paediatric rheumatologists at tertiary care/ referral centres should direct the off-label use of biologics/ DMARDs.
- In children using biologics/ DMARDS, clinical outcome and pharmacovigilance data should be included in high quality registries, whenever possible. Given the rarity of certain side effects, international collaboration is key.
- A coordinated transition programme including paediatric and adult rheumatology (and clinically related) teams is crucial for ensuring continuity of care and adherence to treatments in order to optimize longterm outcome.

Further reading

Time to share. Pediatr Rheumatol Online J. 2013 Feb 15;11(1):5. Wulffraat NM, Vastert SJ; SHARE consortium.

Dougados, M., Betteridge, N., Burmester, G. R. et al. EULAR standardised operating procedures for the elaboration, evaluation, dissemination, and implementation of recommendations endorsed by the EULAR standing committees. Ann Rheum Dis. 2004;63:1172–1176.

The nominal group as a research instrument for exploratory health studies. Am J Public Health. 1972;62:337–342. Van de Ven, A. H. and Delbecq, A. L.

Evidence-based recommendations for genetic diagnosis of familial Mediterranean fever. Ann Rheum Dis. 2015 Apr;74(4):635–41. Giancane G, Ter Haar NM, Wulffraat N, Vastert SJ, Barron K, Hentgen V, Kallinich T, Ozdogan H, Anton J, Brogan P, Cantarini L, Frenkel J, Galeotti C, Gattorno M, Grateau G, Hofer M, Kone-Paut I, Kuemmerle-Deschner J, Lachmann HJ, Simon A, Demirkaya E, Feldman B, Uziel Y, Ozen S.

Recommendations for the management of autoinflammatory diseases. Ann Rheum Dis. 2015 Sep;74(9):1636–44.Ter Haar NM, Oswald M, Jeyaratnam J, Anton J, Barron KS, Brogan PA, Cantarini L, Galeotti C, Grateau G, Hentgen V, Hofer M, Kallinich T, Kone-Paut I, Lachmann HJ, Ozdogan H, Ozen S, Russo R, Simon A, Uziel Y, Wouters C, Feldman BM, Vastert SJ, Wulffraat NM, Benseler SM, Frenkel J, Gattorno M, Kuemmerle-Deschner JB.

Evidence Based Recommendations for the Management of Juvenile Dermatomyositis. Under revision, Ann Rheumatic Dis. Bellutti Enders, F, Bader-Meunier, B, Baildam, E, Constantin, T, Dolezalova, P, Feldman, BM, Lahdenne, P, Magnusson, B, Nistala, K, Pilkington, C, Ozen, S, Ravelli, A, Russo, R, Uziel, Y, Van Brussel, M, Van der Net, JJ, Vastert, SJ, Wedderburn, LR, Wulffraat, NM, McCann, LJ, and Van Royen-Kerkhof, A.

EULAR/PReS recommendations for transitional care

- Juvenile onset rheumatic and musculoskeletal diseases are not confined to childhood. At least 50% of patients will have active disease or require treatment when entering adulthood and 25–50% have morbidity and sequelae due to the disease itself or to the adverse effects of treatment. The risk of disease relapse and further damage and disability continues beyond adolescence [1].
- Most patients therefore require transition from paediatric to adult healthcare. However, many young people with rheumatic diseases do not have a successful transfer to adult rheumatology and are therefore at particular risk of unfavourable outcomes.
- The period around transfer from child-centred to adult health services coincides with development of adolescent identity, increasing awareness of healthcare and the need to balance such needs against the many other demands on a young person's development and interests.
- Understanding transition as a process needs to address the wider needs of young people and has focused attention on understanding the holistic well-being and participation of young people as they move to adulthood (Fig. 9.4). See ➔ Transition, pp. 430–2.

Paediatric rheumatology →	Adult rheumatology
1. Transition policy	1. Young Adult Transition and Care Policy
2. Transition Tracking and Monitoring	2. Young Adult Tracking and Monitoring
3. Transition Readiness Assessment	3. Transition Readiness/Orientation to Adult Practice
4. Transition Planning	4. Transition Planning/Integration into Adult Practice
5. Transfer of Care	5. Transfer of Care/Initial Visit
6. Transfer Completion	6. Transfer Completion/Ongoing Care

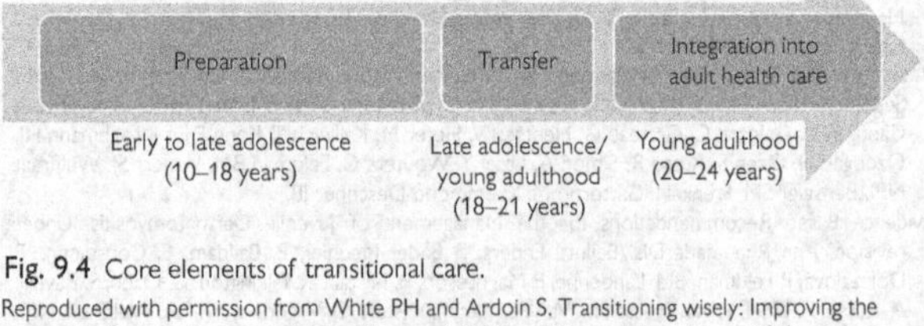

Preparation	Transfer	Integration into adult health care
Early to late adolescence (10–18 years)	Late adolescence/ young adulthood (18–21 years)	Young adulthood (20–24 years)

Fig. 9.4 Core elements of transitional care.

Reproduced with permission from White PH and Ardoin S. Transitioning wisely: Improving the connection from pediatric to adult health care. *Arthritis and Rheumatolgy*, Volume 68, Issue 4, pp. 789-94, Copyright © 2016 American College of Rheumatology.

- There is need to support young people and enable them to take control of their healthcare needs, to engage successfully with adult healthcare services, and to emerge into adulthood with maximal function and potential.
- A recent initiative funded by EULAR aims to increase the profile of transition, optimize delivery of transitional care and improve patient experience.
- Our EULAR/PReS Recommendations (Box 9.4) were derived by an international expert panel (young people and multidisciplinary representatives from adult and paediatric rheumatology), following

Box 9.4 EULAR/PReS recommendations for transitional care

- Young people (YP) should have access to high quality, coordinated transitional care, delivered through partnership with healthcare professionals, YP and their families, to address needs on an individual basis.
- The transition process should start as early as possible; in early adolescence or directly after the diagnosis in adolescent-onset disease
- There must be 'direct' communication between the key participants (and as a minimum, to include the YP, parent/carer, and a member each of the paediatric and adult rheumatologist teams) during the process of transition. Before and after the actual transfer there should be 'direct' contacts between paediatric and adult rheumatologist teams.
- Individual transition processes and progress should be carefully documented in the medical records and planned with YP and their families.
- Every rheumatology service and clinical network—paediatric and adult—must have a written, agreed, and regularly updated transition policy.
- There should be clear written description of the multidisciplinary team (MDT) involved in transitional care, locally and in the clinical network. The MDT should include a designated transition coordinator.
- Transition services must be YP focused, be developmentally appropriate and address the complexity of YP development.
- There must be a transfer document.
- Health care teams involved in transition and adolescent-young adult care must have appropriate training in generic adolescent care and childhood onset rheumatic diseases.
- There must be secure funding for dedicated resources to provide uninterrupted clinical care and transition services for YP entering adult care.
- There must be a freely accessible electronic-based platform to host the recommendations, standards, and resources for transitional care.
- Increased evidence-based knowledge and practice is needed to improve outcomes for YP with childhood onset rheumatic diseases.

a systematic literature review, process mapping to generate draft Recommendations and then achieving consensus with Delphi methodology to gauge opinion from clinicians within adult and paediatric rheumatology.

- The Recommendations target young people from early adolescence (defined as 10 to 13 years), mid adolescence (14 to 16 years), late adolescence (17 to 19 years) to young adulthood (20 to 24 years).
- The Recommendations are accompanied by standards, quality indicators and to aid implementation into clinical practice in different healthcare settings they have been stratified into 'essential' (the minimum to be acceptable) and 'ideal' (optimal) components (see Further Reading).

Further reading

Clemente D, Leon L, Foster HE, et al. Systematic review and critical appraisal of transitional care programmes in rheumatology. Sem Arthritis Rheum 2016;46: 372–9.

Foster HE, Minden K, Clemente D, et al. EULAR/PReS standards and recommendations for the transitional care of young people with juvenile onset rheumatic diseases. Ann Rheumatic Dis 2017;76:639–646.

References

1. Hersh A, von Scheven E, Yelin E. Adult outcomes of childhood-onset rheumatic diseases. Nat Rev Rheumatol 2011; 7(5):290–95.
2. White PH, Ardoin S. transitioning wisely: improving the connection from pediatric to adult health care. Arthritis Rheumatol. 2016;68(4):789–94.

Rashes in paediatric rheumatology

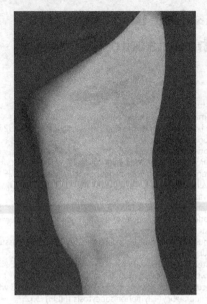

Fig. 10.1 Systemic JIA. Note the rash occurring in linear streaks and exhibiting Koebner phenomenon (also see color plate).

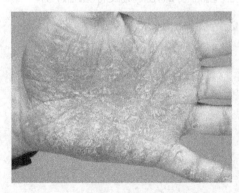

Fig. 10.2 Palmar psoriasis in a patient with psoriatic JIA (also see color plate).

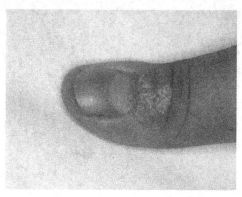

Fig. 10.3 Nail pits and psoriasis in a patient with psoriatic JIA (also see color plate).

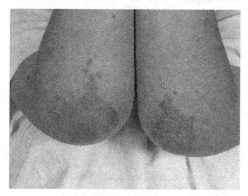

Fig. 10.4 Psoriatic JIA (elbows) (also see color plate).

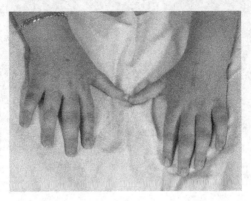

Fig. 10.5 Psoriatic JIA (hands) (also see color plate).

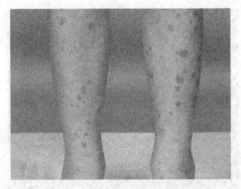

Fig. 10.6 HSP with bilateral ankle swelling (also see color plate).

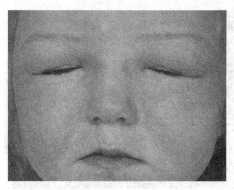

Fig. 10.7 Juvenile dermatomyositis with periorbital oedema (also see color plate).

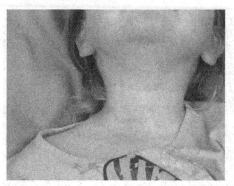

Fig. 10.8 Severe juvenile dermatomyositis with anterior chest wall vasculitis—'shawl sign' (also see color plate).

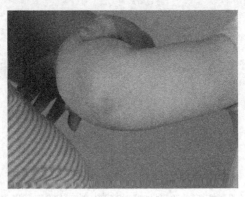

Fig. 10.9 Extensor surface vasculitis in juvenile dermatomyositis (also see color plate).

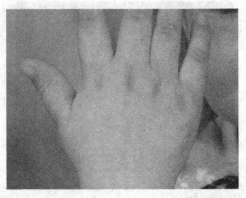

Fig. 10.10 Subtle Gottron's papules in a patient with severe juvenile dermatomyositis (also see color plate).

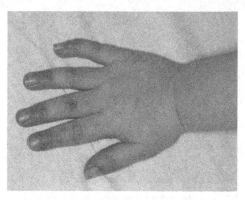

Fig. 10.11 Periungual erythema in undifferentiated connective tissue disease (also see color plate).

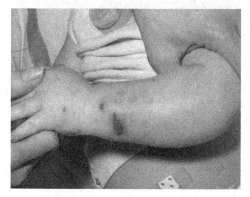

Fig. 10.12 Systemic vasculitis with pyrexia, livido reticularis, vasculitic rash with skin necrosis (also see color plate).

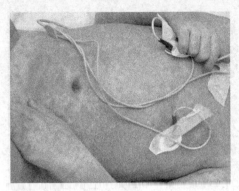

Fig. 10.13 Maculo-papular rash of Epstein–Barr virus associated with haemophagocytic lymphohistiocytosis (HLH) (also see color plate).

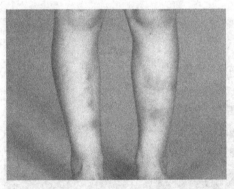

Fig. 10.14 Erythema nodosum (also see color plate).

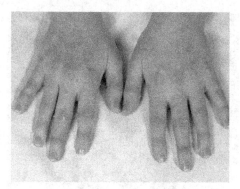

Fig. 10.15 Generalized peeling in Kawasaki disease (also see color plate).

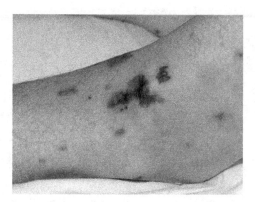

Fig. 10.16 Purpura in granulomatosis with polyangiitis (GPA; formerly known as Wegener's granulomatosis) (also see color plate).

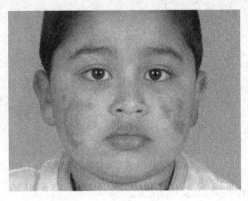

Fig. 10.17 SLE associated with congenital C1q deficiency (also see color plate).

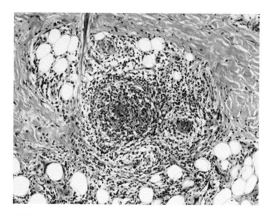

Fig. 4.6 PAN—skin biopsy.

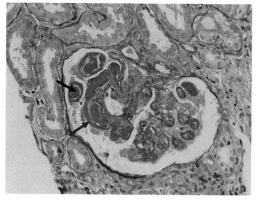

Fig. 4.12 ISN/RPS Class IV LN (PAS stain, original magnification ×250). Wire loop lesion (denoted by lower arrow) and hyaline droplet (upper arrow) change representing massive subendothelial deposits when seen on light microscopy.

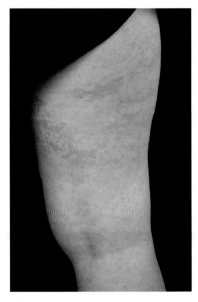

Fig 10.1 Systemic JIA. Note the rash occurring in linear streaks and exhibiting Koebner phenomenon.

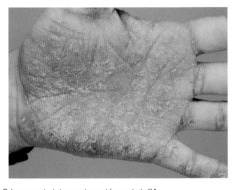

Fig 10.2 Palmar psoriasis in a patient with psoriatic JIA.

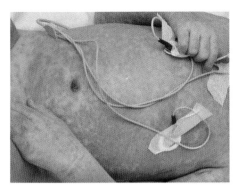

Fig. 10.13 Maculo-papular rash of Epstein–Barr virus associated with haemophagocytic lymphohistiocytosis (HLH).

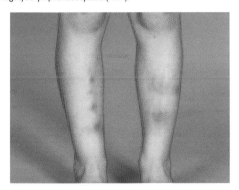

Fig. 10.14 Erythema nodosum.

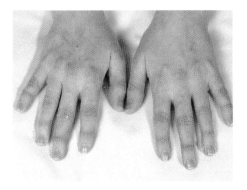

Fig. 10.15 Generalized peeling in Kawasaki disease.

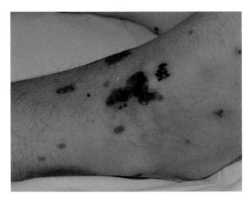

Fig. 10.16 Purpura in granulomatosis with polyangiitis (GPA; formerly known as Wegener's granulomatosis).

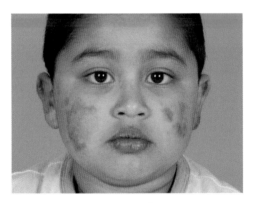

Fig. 10.17 SLE associated with congenital C1q deficiency.

Index